Practical Evidence-Based Physiotherapy

SECOND EDITION

Rob Herbert BAppSc MAppSc PhD
Professor, The George Institute for Global Health and
Sydney Medical School, The University of Sydney, Sydney, Australia

Gro Jamtvedt PT MPH PhD
Executive Director, Norwegian Knowledge Centre for the Health Services, Oslo, Norway

Kåre Birger Hagen PT PhD
Professor, National Resource Centre for Rehabilitation in Rheumatology,
Diakonhjemmet Hospital, Oslo, Norway

Judy Mead MCSP
Formerly Head of Research and Clinical Effectiveness, Chartered Society of
Physiotherapy, London, UK

Foreword by

Sir Iain Chalmers
Editor, James Lind Library, Oxford, UK

Edinburgh   London   New York   Oxford   Philadelphia   St Louis   Sydney   Toronto   2011

ELSEVIER
CHURCHILL
LIVINGSTONE

First edition 2005
Second edition 2012
  Reprinted 2013, 2014, 2015

ISBN 9780702054501

British Library Cataloguing in Publication Data
A catalogue record for this book is available from the British Library

Library of Congress Cataloging in Publication Data
A catalog record for this book is available from the Library of Congress

ELSEVIER your source for books,
journals and multimedia
in the health sciences
www.elsevierhealth.com

Working together to grow
libraries in developing countries
www.elsevier.com | www.bookaid.org | www.sabre.org
ELSEVIER   BOOK AID International   Sabre Foundation

The
Publisher's
policy is to use
**paper manufactured
from sustainable forests**

Printed in China

Contents

Foreword by Sir Iain Chalmers vii

Preface to the first edition ix

Preface to the second edition xi

1 Evidence-based physiotherapy: what, why and how? 1
   What is 'evidence-based physiotherapy'? 1
   Why is evidence-based physiotherapy important? 4
   History of evidence-based health care 5
   How will this book help you to practise evidence-based physiotherapy? 5

2 What do I need to know? 9
   Relevant clinical questions 9
   Refining your question 11

3 What constitutes evidence? 15
   What constitutes evidence about effects of interventions? 15
   What constitutes evidence about experiences? 26
   What constitutes evidence about prognosis? 30
   What constitutes evidence about the accuracy of diagnostic and screening tests? 32

4 Finding the evidence 39
   Search strategies 39
   Finding evidence of effects of interventions 43
   Finding evidence of prognosis and diagnostic tests 51
   Finding evidence of experiences 55
   Getting full text 58
   Finding evidence of advances in clinical practice (browsing) 60

5 Can I trust this evidence? 61
   A process for critical appraisal of evidence 62
   Critical appraisal of evidence about the effects of intervention 64
   Critical appraisal of evidence about experiences 81
   Critical appraisal of evidence about prognosis 84
   Critical appraisal of evidence about diagnostic tests 87

6 What does this evidence mean for my practice? 93
   What does this randomized trial mean for my practice? 93
   What does this systematic review of effects of intervention mean for my practice? 114
   What does this study of experiences mean for my practice? 122
   What does this study of prognosis mean for my practice? 124
   What does this study of the accuracy of a diagnostic test mean for my practice? 127

7 Clinical guidelines as a resource for evidence-based physiotherapy 135
   What are clinical guidelines? 135
   History of clinical guidelines and why they are important 136
   Where can I find clinical guidelines? 137
   How do I know if I can trust the recommendations in a clinical guideline? 138

8 When and how should new therapies be introduced into clinical practice? 143
The life cycle of a medical innovation 143
A case study 145
Proposal for a protocol for introduction of new therapies 145
Anticipation of some objections 146

9 Making it happen 149
What do we mean by 'making it happen'? 149
Changing is hard 150
Evidence-based implementation 154
Evidence-based physiotherapy in the context of continuous quality improvement 159

10 Am I on the right track? 161
Assessing patient outcomes: clinical measurement 161
Assessing the process of care: audit 164
Concluding comment 168

Index 169

A few years ago, I wrote an article about what I want from health research when I am a patient (Chalmers 1995). I tried to make clear that I want decisions about my care to be based on reliable evidence about the effects of treatments. I can't imagine that many patients or health professionals would suggest that this is an unreasonable wish, but they might well vary quite a lot in what they regard as 'reliable evidence'.

I illustrated the issue by noting that, after about five treatments from a chiropractor to whom she had been referred by her general practitioner, my wife believed that she had reliable evidence that chiropractic could help relieve her chronic shoulder and back pain. By contrast, although I was delighted that her longstanding symptoms had subsided, I noted that I would begin to believe in the benefits of chiropractic when a systematic review of the relevant controlled trials suggested that it could be helpful.

Sometimes the effects of treatments are dramatic, as they had been for my wife. For example, after my general practitioner referred me for physiotherapy for a very painful right shoulder injury, the experienced physiotherapist tried a number of technological approaches using some impressive-looking kit; nothing seemed to be helping. Then she decided to treat my right supraspinatus tendon with what I understand are called Cyriax's frictions. The relief was instantaneous and dramatic, and I needed no persuasion that it was as the result of the treatment.

If treatments never did any harm and were universally available in unlimited variety and supply, basing decisions in health care on the individual experiences of patients and professionals would not present any problems. But treatments do have the capacity for doing harm. Chest physiotherapy in very low birthweight infants, for example, came under suspicion of causing brain damage (Harding et al 1998). Even though doubt remains as to whether the associations observed at the time reflected an adverse effect of neonatal physiotherapy (Knight et al 2001), it would have been reassuring if it had been possible to point to a strong evidence base justifying the use of physiotherapy in these fragile infants. Even if treatments don't harm the people for whom they are prescribed,

if they don't do any good they use limited resources that could be deployed more profitably elsewhere.

I don't know how frequently physiotherapy has dramatic effects. But if it is anything like medical care, dramatic effects of treatment are very rare. In these circumstances, it is important to assess whether particular forms of care are likely to do more good than harm, and this entails doing carefully designed research.

A decade ago, I sustained a fractured fibula while on holiday in the USA. The orthopaedic surgeon there advised me that, when the swelling had subsided after my impending return to the UK, I would have a plaster cast applied for 6 weeks. Two days later a British orthopaedic surgeon said that the advice that I had received was rubbish, and that I was to have a supportive bandage and to walk on the ankle until it hurt, and then some more! When I asked whether I might be entered into a randomized trial to find out whether he or his 'colleague' across the Atlantic was correct, he told me dismissively that randomized trials were for people who were uncertain whether or not they were right, and he was certain that he was right!

Several questions were posed in the account of this experience published in the *Journal of Bone and Joint Surgery* (Chalmers et al 1992). Which of these orthopaedic surgeons was right? Were they both right, but interested in different outcomes of treatment? What were the consequences, in terms of short- and long-term pain and function (and the costs of treatment), of acquiescing in the advice of the second rather than the first? And what was known about the effects of the various forms of physiotherapy that were subsequently prescribed (Chalmers et al 1992)? In the decade since that experience there has been a welcome increase in the likelihood of patients and professionals obtaining answers to questions like these, and this impressive new book constitutes an important milestone in these developments.

Reliable identification of the modest but worthwhile effects of physiotherapy poses a substantially greater challenge than reliable evaluation of the effects of most drugs and some other forms of health care. Not only is it often difficult to characterize physiotherapy interventions in words that allow readers to understand what was done, but taking account of the social and psychologically mediated effects of physiotherapists themselves may also pose interpretive conundrums. I remember being impressed by the results of a randomized comparison of routine instruction for post-natal pelvic floor exercises with personal encouragement from a physiotherapist, done by colleagues in a unit where I worked at the time (Sleep & Grant 1987). No differences were detected in the frequency of urinary or faecal incontinence between the two groups of women 3 months after delivery, but those who had received personal advice

and encouragement from the physiotherapist were less likely to report perineal pain and feelings of depression.

Physiotherapists who recognize that they have a professional responsibility to do their best to ensure that their treatments are likely to do more good than harm, and that they are a sensible use of limited resources for health care, will find that *Practical Evidence-Based Physiotherapy* is a veritable goldmine of useful information. I am confident that next time I am referred for physiotherapy this book will have helped to ensure that I will be offered treatment that is likely to be good value for both my time and my taxes.

Sir Iain Chalmers

References

Chalmers, I., 1995. What do I want from health research and researchers when I am a patient? BMJ 310, 1315–1318.

Chalmers, I., Collins, R., Dickersin, K., 1992. Controlled trials and meta-analyses can help to resolve disagreements among orthopaedic surgeons. J. Bone Joint Surg. Br. 74-B, 641–643.

Harding, J.E., Miles, F.K., Becroft, D. M., et al., 1998. Chest physiotherapy may be associated with brain damage in extremely premature infants. J. Pediatr. 132, 440–444.

Knight, D.B., Bevan, C.J., Harding, J.E., et al., 2001. Chest physiotherapy and porencephalic brain lesions in very preterm infants. J. Paediatr. Child Health 37, 554–558.

Sleep, J., Grant, A., 1987. Pelvic floor exercises in postnatal care. Midwifery 3, 158–164.

How does it come to happen that four physiotherapists from three countries write a book together? We first met at the World Confederation of Physical Therapy's (WCPT) Expert Meeting on Evidence-Based Practice in London in 2001. By then we knew of each other's work, but at that meeting we discovered kindred spirits who had been thinking about similar issues, albeit from quite different perspectives.

We had all been thinking and writing about evidence-based practice. Judy Mead had co-edited and co-authored the first textbook on evidence-based health care in 1998 (Bury & Mead 1998). Kåre Birger Hagen and Gro Jamtvedt were working on a Norwegian textbook on evidence-based physiotherapy (subsequently published as Jamtvedt et al 2003). And Rob Herbert and his colleagues at the Centre for Evidence-Based Physiotherapy had launched the PEDro database on the internet late in 1999. Together we had been teaching skills of evidence-based practice, carrying out clinical research and advising health policy makers. The ground had been laid for collaboration on a text with a broader perspective than any of us could write on our own.

The catalyst for the book was Heidi Harrison, commissioning editor at Elsevier. During the WCPT Congress at Barcelona in 2003, Heidi twisted eight arms and extracted four commitments to the writing of this book. We are grateful to Heidi for getting us started, and for providing ongoing support over the year that it took to write the book.

Is there a need for another textbook on evidence-based practice? We think so. Few textbooks on evidence-based practice have been written with physiotherapists in mind. This book considers how physiotherapists can use clinical research to answer questions about physiotherapy practice. In that respect at least we think this book is unique.

We hope this book can meet the needs of a diverse readership. We want it to provide an introduction to the skills of evidence-based practice for undergraduate students and practising physiotherapists who have not previously been exposed to the ideas of evidence-based practice. Throughout the book we have highlighted critical points in the hope that those who are new to these ideas will not 'lose the forest for the trees'. We also hope to provide a useful resource for those who already practise physiotherapy in an evidence-based way. We do that by providing a more detailed presentation of strategies for searching for evidence, critical appraisal of evidence, and using clinical practice guidelines than is available in other texts. We have gone beyond the boundaries that usually encompass texts on evidence-based practice by considering how evidence about feelings and experiences can be used in clinical decision-making. There is an extensive use of footnotes that we hope will stimulate the interest of advanced readers.

Some books are great labours. This one was exciting, challenging and fun. It has been a shared process in which all contributed their different perspectives. We have discussed, struggled with difficult ideas, resolved disagreements, and learned a lot. We also learned about each other and became good friends. For two wonderful weeks we met and worked together intensively: first in the snowy mountains of Norway in mid-winter, and later in a quiet village near Oxford in spring.

We would like to thank the people who reviewed part or all of the manuscript and gave useful feedback. They are, in alphabetical order, Trudy Bekkering, Mark Elkins, Claire Glenton, Mark Hancock, Hans Lund, Sue Madden, Chris Maher, Anne Moore, Anne Moseley and Cathie Sherrington. All remaining shortcomings are our own.

Rob Herbert, Gro Jamtvedt,
Judy Mead and Kåre Birger Hagen, 2005

References

Bury, T.J., Mead, J.M. (Eds.), 1998. Evidence based healthcare: a practical guide for therapists. Butterworth-Heinemann, Oxford.

Jamtvedt, G., Hagen, K.B., Bjørndal, A., 2003. Kunnskapsbasert Fysioterapi. Metoder og Arbeidsmåter. Gyldendal Akademisk.

Preface to the second edition

Since the first edition of *Practical Evidence-Based Physiotherapy* was published 5 years ago there have been many changes in the profession of physiotherapy. Remarkably, the number of published reports of randomized trials has more than tripled (from 4100 in July 2004 to 13 700 in August 2010), as has the number of systematic reviews of randomized trials (from 780 to 2500 over the same period). Commensurate increases have occurred in the volume of reports of qualitative research studies, cohort studies and cross-sectional studies of diagnostic test accuracy relevant to the practice of physiotherapy. This has been accompanied by an increase in the quality of research, demonstrably so in the case of randomized trials (Moseley et al, in press). The huge increase in volume and relatively modest increase in quality of clinical research means that now, more than ever before, it is possible to inform the practice of physiotherapy with high-quality clinical research.

There have also been other changes relevant to the practice of evidence physiotherapy. Our impression is that there is now a healthier, less antagonistic and more co-operative relationship between those interested in quantitative and qualitative research. Electronic access to full-text journals has improved, particularly in developing countries, although it is still less than satisfactory for many physiotherapists. There has been a growing interest in using 'clinical prediction rules' to identify those patients most likely to benefit from intervention. (Unfortunately much of the discussion around this issue ignores the extensive earlier literature on subgroup analyses in medical trials.) Another area of growing interest has been the development of methods for determining how big the effects of interventions must be for recipients of care (patients) to perceive that intervention is worthwhile. We anticipate that, in the long run, this will have a big impact on which interventions physiotherapists choose to offer to their patients. Important contributions have been made to discussions about the nature, extent and significance of placebo effects, the role of blinding in randomized trials, and methods of appraising quality of trials of complex interventions. There has been a growth in 'implementation research' that investigates the effectiveness of strategies for translating findings of high-quality research into clinical practice. And there have been substantial methodological advances, notably into methods for dealing with missing data, repeated measurements in clinical trials, and meta-regression techniques.

The second edition of *Practical Evidence-Based Physiotherapy* incorporates discussion of most of these emerging issues. References and examples that had become anachronistic have been replaced with more contemporary references and examples. A new chapter (Chapter 8) discusses when and how new interventions should become routine clinical practice.

Writing books can be hard work, but it's not all hard. In a tradition established with the first edition, the authors spent an idyllic week working together in a rustic cottage in an olive grove in rural Tuscany. Once again we were able to discuss intricacies of evidence-based practice and enjoy the pleasure of each other's company.

We thank Rita Demetriou-Swanwick and Ailsa Laing from Elsevier for their support and assistance. Ingvild Kirkehei, a librarian at the Norwegian Knowledge Centre for the Health Services in Oslo, Norway, updated the chapter on searching for evidence (Chapter 4). We are grateful for the great care with which she checked and updated content, and for her thoughtful and substantial contributions to that chapter.

Rob Herbert, Gro Jamtvedt,
Kåre Birger Hagen and Judy Mead
September 2010

Reference

Moseley, A.M., Herbert, R.D.,
Maher, C.G., et al., 2010. Reported
quality of randomised controlled trials
of physiotherapy interventions has
improved over time. J. of Clin.
Epidemiol. Epub ahead of print.
doi: 10.1016/j.jclinepi.2010.08.009.

Evidence-based physiotherapy: what, why and how?

1

CHAPTER CONTENTS

Overview 1
What is 'evidence-based physiotherapy'? 1
   What do we mean by 'high-quality
   clinical research'? 2
   What do we mean by 'patient
   preferences'? 2
   What do we mean by 'practice
   knowledge'? 3
   Additional factors influencing
   clinical decisions 3
   The process of clinical decision-making 3
Why is evidence-based physiotherapy
important? 4
   For patients 4
   For physiotherapists and the
   profession 4
   For funders of physiotherapy services 4
History of evidence-based health care 5
How will this book help you to practise
evidence-based physiotherapy? 5
   Steps for practising evidence-based
   physiotherapy 6
   Chapter 2: What do I need to know? 6
   Chapter 3: What constitutes evidence? 6
   Chapter 4: Finding the evidence? 6
   Chapter 5: Can I trust this evidence? 6
   Chapter 6: What does this evidence
   mean for my practice? 6
   Chapter 7: Clinical practice guidelines 6
   Chapter 8: When and how should new
   therapies be introduced into clinical
   practice? 6
   Chapter 9: Making it happen 6
   Chapter 10: Am I on the right track? 6
References 7

OVERVIEW

Evidence-based physiotherapy is physiotherapy informed by relevant, high-quality clinical research. The *practice* of evidence-based physiotherapy should involve integration of evidence (high-quality clinical research) with patient preferences and practice knowledge. This chapter provides a brief outline of the history of evidence-based health care and argues that clinical practice should be evidence-based wherever high-quality clinical research is available. A five-step process for practising evidence-based physiotherapy is described. This process provides a framework for the rest of the book.

What is 'evidence-based physiotherapy'?

The aim of this book is to provide physiotherapists with a practical guide to evidence-based physiotherapy. What is 'evidence-based physiotherapy'?

> Evidence-based physiotherapy is physiotherapy informed by relevant, high-quality clinical research.

This implies that when we refer to 'evidence' we mean high-quality clinical research.

Our definition of evidence-based physiotherapy differs from earlier definitions of evidence-based physiotherapy and evidence-based health care. Previous authors considered that practice was evidence based when it involved the use of the *best available* evidence (Bury & Mead 1998, Sackett et al 2000). The best available evidence might be high-quality clinical research, but where high-quality clinical research is not available the best available evidence could consist of poor-quality clinical research, consensus views or clinical experience. That is, according to earlier definitions, evidence-based practice could be practice based on poor-quality clinical research, consensus views or clinical experience. We recognize that there is often insufficient relevant, high-quality research to inform clinical decisions and that, when this is the case, decisions still need to be made. Sometimes best practice can be informed only by poor-quality clinical research, consensus views or clinical experience. However, in our view, such practices cannot be considered to be evidence based. The term 'evidence-based physiotherapy' should be reserved for physiotherapy that is based on high-quality clinical research.

A premise of this book is that, wherever possible, clinical decisions should be informed by high-quality clinical research. This does not mean that clinical decisions should be informed *only* by high-quality clinical research. Good decisions must take into account patients' expectations, desires and values (patient 'preferences'; Haynes et al 2002). In addition, experienced health professionals can use past experiences and procedural knowledge ('practice knowledge'; Higgs et al 2004) to inform clinical decision-making.

> Wherever possible, clinical decisions should be informed by high-quality clinical research, but never just by clinical research. Good clinical decisions, whether evidence based or not, should involve consideration of patient preferences and therapists' practice knowledge.

What do we mean by 'high-quality clinical research'?

The term clinical research is usually used to mean research conducted on patients in clinical settings.[1] Clinical research is empirical in nature, which means that it uses experiment or observation rather than theory to generate knowledge.

An enormous amount of clinical research has been conducted, but not all clinical research is of high quality. High-quality clinical research distinguishes itself from low-quality research by being designed, conducted and reported in a way that allows us to trust the results. That is, high-quality research is that which can be expected to have a low risk of bias.[2] In reality, much clinical research is of neither a very high nor a very low quality; most research is of high quality in some respects and of low quality in others. A degree of judgement is needed to determine whether a particular piece of research is of sufficiently high quality to inform clinical decision-making.

What do we mean by 'patient preferences'?

The traditional model of clinical decision-making has been one in which physiotherapists make decisions about therapy for their patients. In recent years there has been greater consumer involvement in decision-making and now many patients expect to be given an opportunity to contribute to, and share, decisions involving their health (Edwards & Elwyn 2001). In contemporary models of clinical decision-making, patients are encouraged to contribute information about their experiences and values – what it is that matters most to them. In this way patient 'preferences' can inform decision-making. There has been a move away from the situation in which the physiotherapist or doctor alone makes decisions for the patient, towards a situation in which the patient and the physiotherapist or doctor make shared decisions. Some patients do not like intervention and would consider intervention to be worthwhile only if it conferred very large beneficial effects, whereas other patients would like to have intervention even if the effects were very small. Therefore decisions about the acceptability of an intervention need to be negotiated with each individual patient. Each patient needs to be told of the expected effect of intervention and asked whether they feel that effect is large enough that they would choose to have the intervention This is an important cultural change. It requires that physiotherapists exercise communication skills, empathy and flexibility needed to communicate to patients the risks and benefits of alternative actions.

---

[1]Clinical research may not always be carried out on patients. It could include in-depth interviews with carers, for example. Similarly, the setting may not always be clinical – the research may be conducted in patients' homes or other community environments, or it may involve public health activities such as community-based health promotion programmes.

[2]One definition of bias is a systematic deviation from the truth.

What do we mean by 'practice knowledge'?

Practice knowledge is knowledge arising from professional practice and experience (Higgs & Titchen 2001). Consciously or subconsciously, physiotherapists add to their personal knowledge base during each patient encounter. This knowledge is used on a day-to-day basis, along with other sources of information such as high-quality clinical research, to inform practice. Practice knowledge 'underpins the practitioner's rapid and fluent response to a situation' (Titchen & Ersser 2001). It is what differentiates well-educated new graduates and experienced physiotherapists.

Practice knowledge is not 'evidence' as we have defined it. Nonetheless, practice knowledge should always be brought to the decision-making process, and sometimes practice knowledge should dominate evidence. For example, there is some evidence that upper extremity casting can increase the quality and range of upper extremity movement for children with cerebral palsy (Law et al 1991). However, an experienced physiotherapist might suggest alternative interventions for a particular child if his or her practice knowledge suggested that casting would cause that child distress, or if the child or the child's parents were unlikely to tolerate the intervention well.

Additional factors influencing clinical decisions

We have discussed how good clinical decision-making involves integration of high-quality clinical research, patient preferences and practice knowledge. But other factors can also influence decisions. Good practice is responsive to a range of contextual factors.

The availability of resources often influences clinical decisions. For example, the most effective intervention for a particular problem could require large amounts of staff time or an expensive piece of equipment that is not available, in which case a less effective intervention might have to be used. Another resource to be considered may be the skills of the physiotherapist. In making shared decisions about an appropriate intervention, physiotherapists need to judge whether they have the skills and competence needed to provide treatment safely and effectively. If not, it might be appropriate to refer the patient to another physiotherapist who does have the necessary skills and expertise. Consideration might also need to be given to whether services are available in other settings (for example, in the community instead of a hospital) and, if there is a choice, which setting would provide the greater benefit for the patient.

If we look at physiotherapy from a global perspective we can see huge variations in the spectrum of conditions that are treated and in the resources provided for health care. Global comparisons of mortality and disability (Murray & Lopez 1997, World Health Organization 2004), perceptions of disability (Üstün et al 1999) and the level of physiotherapy services, clearly show how important these factors are. These regional factors have huge implications for what kinds of patient and problem physiotherapists should be concerned with, and how clinical decisions are made.

In addition, there are important cultural influences that shape how physiotherapy should be practised. Culture affects patient and physiotherapist expectations, attitudes to illness, the provision of health care, communication and patient–physiotherapist interaction, and the ways in which interventions are administered. This means that it might be quite appropriate for physiotherapy to be practised very differently in different countries. We acknowledge that some cultures, particularly those with strong social hierarchies, provide contexts that are less conducive to evidence-based practice or shared decision-making. In multicultural societies physiotherapists may need to be able to accommodate the range of cultural backgrounds of their patients.

The process of clinical decision-making

At the heart of the practice of evidence-based physiotherapy is the process of clinical decision-making. Clinical decision-making brings together information from high-quality clinical research, information from patients about their preferences, and information from physiotherapists within a particular cultural, economic and political context.

Clinical decision-making is complex. Clinical reasoning must be used to analyse, synthesize and interpret relevant information. Evidence, information from patients and practice knowledge must be integrated using professional judgement. 'Clinical reasoning needs to be seen as a pivotal point of knowledge management in practice, utilizing the principles of evidence-based practice and the findings of research, but also using professional judgement to interpret and make research relevant to the specific patient and the current clinical situation' (Higgs et al 2004: 193). Only when physiotherapy is practised in this way can we 'claim to be adopting credible practice that is not only evidence-based, but also client-centred and context-relevant' (Higgs et al 2004: 194).

While acknowledging the importance of clinical reasoning and the development of practice knowledge, the focus of this book is narrower – we aim to help physiotherapists inform their practice with relevant, high-quality clinical research. Readers who are specifically interested in clinical reasoning and development of practice knowledge could consult Higgs & Jones (2000) and Higgs et al (2004).

Why is evidence-based physiotherapy important?

For patients

A premise of evidence-based practice, though one that is hard to demonstrate empirically, is that practice that is informed by high-quality research is likely to be safer and more effective than practice that is not based on high-quality research. The expectation is that physiotherapy will produce the best possible clinical outcomes when it is evidence based.

Patients are increasingly demanding information about their disease or clinical problem and the options available for treatment. Many patients have access to a wide range of information sources, but not all of these sources provide reliable information. The most widely used source of information is the internet, but the internet provides the full spectrum of information quality. If patients are to make informed contributions to decisions about the management of their conditions, they will need assistance to identify high-quality clinical research.

In some countries, such as the UK, patients' demands for information have been nurtured and encouraged. A number of high-priority government programmes have promoted shared decision-making and choice by providing consumers of health care services access to reliable evidence (Coulter et al 1999, National Institute for Health and Clinical Excellence), and by supporting patients to help each other understand about disease processes (NHS Executive 2001).

For physiotherapists and the profession

Physiotherapists assert that they are 'professionals'. Koehn (1994) argues that a particularly unique characteristic of being a professional is trustworthiness, by which is meant that professionals can be expected to strive to do good, have the patient's best interests at heart and have high ethical standards. A tangible demonstration of a profession's interests in the welfare of its patients is its preparedness to act on the basis of objective evidence about good practice, regardless of how unpalatable the evidence might be. A prerequisite is that the profession must be aware of what the evidence says. Practitioners who don't know whether the evidence indicates that the interventions they offer are effective may have a questionable claim to being 'professionals'. Physiotherapy qualifies as a profession in so far as practice is informed by evidence. And in so far as it is not, there is a risk that physiotherapists will lose the respect and trust of patients and the public at large.

The profession of physiotherapy has changed enormously in the last 60 years. There has been a transition from a role in which physiotherapists did what doctors told them to do to the current role in which, in many countries, physiotherapists act as autonomous or semi-autonomous health professionals. This new-found professional autonomy should be exercised responsibly. With autonomy comes responsibility for ensuring that patients are given accurate diagnoses and prognoses, and are well informed about benefits, harms and risks of intervention.

For funders of physiotherapy services

Physiotherapy should do more good than harm. This is true whether physiotherapy services are funded by the public, through taxes, or by individuals in a fee-for-service or insurance payment. Policy-makers, managers and purchasers of health services have an interest in ensuring value for money and health benefits in situations where health resources are always scarce. Decisions have to be made about where and how to invest to benefit the health of the population as a whole. Where possible, decisions on investment of health services should be based on evidence (Gray 1997).

History of evidence-based health care

The term 'evidence-based medicine' was first introduced in 1992 by a team at McMaster University, Canada, led by Gordon Guyatt (Evidence-Based Medicine Working Group 1992). They produced a series of highly influential guides to help those teaching medicine to introduce the notion of finding, appraising and using high-quality evidence to improve the effectiveness of the care given to patients (Guyatt et al 1994, Jaeschke et al 1994, Oxman et al 1993).

Why did the term evolve? What were the drivers? There had been growing concern in some countries that the gap between research and practice was too great. In 1991, the Director of Research and Development for the Department of Health in England noted that 'strongly held views based on belief rather than sound information still exert too much influence in health care' (Department of Health 1991). High-quality medical research was not being used in practice even though evidence showed the potential to save many lives and prevent disability. For example, by 1980 there were sufficient studies to demonstrate that prescription of clot-busting drugs (thrombolytic therapy) for people who had suffered heart attacks would produce a significant reduction in mortality. But in the 1990s thrombolytic therapy was still not recommended as a routine treatment except in a minority of medical textbooks (Antman 1992). Similarly, despite high-quality evidence that showed bed rest to be ineffective in the treatment of acute back pain, physicians were still advising patients to take to their beds (Cherkin et al 1995).

Another driver was the rapidly increasing volume of literature. New research was being produced too quickly for doctors to cope with it. At the same time, there was a recognition that much of the published research was of poor quality. Doctors had a daily need for reliable information about diagnosis, prognosis, therapy and prevention (Sackett et al 2000).

One way of dealing with the growing volume of literature has been the development of systematic reviews, or systematically developed summaries of high-quality evidence. Systematic reviews will be discussed in several chapters in this book. In 1992, the Cochrane Collaboration[3] was established. The Cochrane Collaboration's purpose is the development of high-quality systematic reviews, which are now conducted by 52 Cochrane Review Groups, supported by 26 Cochrane Centres around the world. The Collaboration has had a huge impact on making high-quality evidence more accessible to large numbers of people.

One of the early drivers of evidence-based physiotherapy was the Department of Epidemiology at the University of Maastricht in the Netherlands. Since the early 1990s this department has trained several 'generations' of excellent researchers who have produced an enormous volume of high-quality clinical research relevant to physiotherapy. In 1998, the precursor to this book, *Evidence-Based Healthcare: A Practical Guide for Therapists* (Bury & Mead 1998), was published, providing a basic text to help therapists understand what evidence-based practice was and what it meant in relation to their clinical practice. And from 1999 PEDro, a database of randomized trials, has given physiotherapists easy access to high-quality evidence about effects of intervention.

Today, most physiotherapists have heard of evidence-based practice, and evidence-based practice has initiated much discussion and also some skepticism. Some feel the concept threatens the importance of skills, experience and practice knowledge and the pre-eminence of interaction with individual patients. We will discuss these issues further in this book.

How will this book help you to practise evidence-based physiotherapy?

This book provides a step-by-step guide to the practice of evidence-based physiotherapy. The focus is on using evidence to support decision-making that pertains to individual patients or small groups of patients, but much of what is presented applies equally to decision-making about physiotherapy policy and public health issues.

---

[3]The Cochrane Collaboration was named after Archie Cochrane, a distinguished British epidemiologist who assessed the effectiveness of medical treatments and procedures. More information about Archie Cochrane and the Cochrane Collaboration can be found at http://www.cochrane.org/index0.htm

Steps for practising evidence-based physiotherapy

Evidence-based practice involves the following steps (Sackett et al 2000):

Step 1 Converting information needs into answerable questions.

Step 2 Tracking down the best evidence with which to answer those questions.

Step 3 Critically appraising the evidence for its validity impact and applicability.

Step 4 Integrating the evidence with clinical expertise and with patients' unique biologies, values and circumstances.

Step 5 Evaluating the effectiveness and efficiency in executing steps 1–4 and seeking ways to improve them both for next time.

These steps form the basis for the outline of this book, which is structured as follows.

Chapter 2: What do I need to know?

Evidence-based physiotherapy will occur only when two conditions are met: there has to be a sense of uncertainty about the best course of action, and there has to be recognition that high-quality clinical research could resolve some of the uncertainty. Once these conditions are met, the first step in delivering evidence-based physiotherapy is to identify, possibly with the patient, what the clinical problem is. Framing the problem or question in a structured way makes it easier to identify information needs. Chapter 2 is designed to help you to frame answerable questions. We focus on four types of clinical question: those about the effects of intervention, attitudes and experiences, prognosis, and the accuracy of diagnostic tests.

Chapter 3: What constitutes evidence?

Each type of clinical question is best answered with a particular type of research. Chapter 3 considers the types of research that best answer each of the four types of clinical question raised in Chapter 2.

Chapter 4: Finding the evidence

You will need to do a search of relevant databases to find evidence to answer your clinical questions. Chapter 4 makes recommendations about which databases to search, and how to search in a way that will be most likely to give you the information you need in an efficient way.

Chapter 5: Can I trust this evidence?

Not all research is of sufficient quality to be used for clinical decision-making. Once you have accessed the research evidence, you need to be able to assess whether or not it can be believed. Chapter 5 describes a process for appraising the trustworthiness or validity of clinical research.

Chapter 6: What does this evidence mean for my practice?

If the research is of high quality, you will need to decide whether it is relevant to the particular clinical circumstances of your patient or patients, and, if so, what the evidence means for clinical practice. Chapter 6 considers how to assess the relevance of clinical research and how to interpret research findings.

Chapter 7: Clinical practice guidelines

Properly developed clinical guidelines provide recommendations for practice that are informed, wherever possible, by high-quality research evidence. Chapter 7 describes how to decide whether clinical practice guidelines are sufficiently trustworthy to apply in practice.

Chapter 8: When and how should new therapies be introduced into clinical practice?

This chapter describes a protocol that should be followed before new therapies are introduced into clinical practice.

Chapter 9: Making it happen

It can be hard to get high-quality clinical research into practice. Chapter 9 discusses barriers to changing practice and ways of improving professional practice.

Chapter 10: Am I on the right track?

Lifelong learning requires self-reflection and self-evaluation. In Chapter 10 we discuss self-evaluation, both of how well evidence is used to inform practice and of how well evidence-based practices are implemented. In addition, we consider clinical evaluation of the effects of intervention on individual patients.

References

Antman, D., 1992. A comparison of results of meta-analyses of randomized control trials and recommendations of clinical experts. Treatments for myocardial infarction. JAMA 268 (2), 240–248.

Bury, T., Mead, J., 1998. Evidence-based healthcare: a practical guide for therapists. Butterworth-Heinemann, Oxford.

Cherkin, D.C., Deyo, R.A., Wheeler, K., Ciol, M.A., 1995. Physicians' views about treating low back pain: the results of a national survey. Spine 20, 1–10.

Coulter, A., Entwistle, V., Gilbert, D., 1999. Sharing decisions with patients: is the information good enough? BMJ 318, 318–322.

Department of Health, 1991. Research for health: a research and development strategy for the NHS. Department of Health, London.

Edwards, A., Elwyn, G., 2001. Evidence-based patient choice. Oxford University Press, Oxford.

Evidence-Based Medicine Working Group, 1992. A new approach to teaching the practice of medicine. JAMA 268 (17), 2420–2425.

Gray, J.A.M., 1997. Evidence-based healthcare: how to make policy and management decisions. Churchill Livingstone, Edinburgh.

Guyatt, G.H., Sackett, D.L., Cook, D.J., 1994. Users' guides to the medical literature. II. How to use an article about therapy or prevention. B. What are the results and will they help me in caring for my patients?

Evidence-Based Medicine Working Group. JAMA 271 (1), 59–63.

Haynes, B., Devereaux, P.J., Guyatt, G.H., 2002. Physicians' and patients' choices in evidence based practice: evidence does not make decisions, people do. Editorial. BMJ 324, 1350.

Higgs, J., Jones, M., 2000. Clinical reasoning. In: Higgs, J., Jones, M. (Eds.), Clinical reasoning in health professions. Butterworth-Heinemann, Oxford, pp. 3–23.

Higgs, J., Titchen, A., 2001. Rethinking the practice–knowledge interface in an uncertain world: a model for practice development. Br. J. Occup. Ther. 64 (11), 26–533.

Higgs, J., Jones, M., Edwards, I., et al., 2004. Clinical reasoning and practice knowledge. In: Higgs, J., Richardson, B., Dahlgren, M.A. (Eds.), Developing practice knowledge for health professionals. Elsevier, Oxford, pp. 181–200.

Jaeschke, R., Guyatt, G.H., Sackett, D.L., 1994. Users' guides to the medical literature. III. How to use an article about a diagnostic test. B. What are the results and will they help me in caring for my patients? Evidence-Based Medicine Working Group. JAMA 271 (9), 703–707.

Koehn, D., 1994. The ground of professional ethics. Routledge, London.

Law, M., Cadman, D., Rosenbaum, P., et al., 1991. Neurodevelopmental therapy and upper extremity inhibitive casting for children with cerebral palsy. Dev. Med. Child. Neurol. 33 (5), 379–387.

Murray, C.J., Lopez, A.D., 1997. Alternative projections of mortality and disability by cause 1990–2020: Global Burden of Disease Study. Lancet 349, 1498–1504.

National Institute for Health and Clinical Excellence, NHS evidence. Online. Available:http://www.nice.org.uk.

NHS Executive, 2001. The expert patient: a new approach to chronic disease management for the 21st century. Department of Health, London.

Oxman, A.D., Sackett, D.L., Guyatt, G.H., 1993. Users' guides to the medical literature. I. How to get started. The Evidence-Based Medicine Working Group. JAMA 270 (17), 2093–2095.

Sackett, D.L., Straus, S.E., Richardson, W.S., et al., 2000. Evidence-based medicine: how to practice and teach EBM. Churchill Livingstone, Edinburgh.

Titchen, A., Ersser, S., 2001. The nature of professional craft knowledge. In: Higgs, J., Titchen, A. (Eds.), Practice knowledge and expertise in the health professions. Butterworth-Heinemann, Oxford, pp. 35–41.

Üstün, T.B., Rehm, J., Chatterji, S., et al., 1999. Multiple-informant ranking of the disabling effects of different health conditions in 14 countries. WHO/NIH Joint Project CAR Study Group. Lancet 354, 111–115.

World Health Organization, 2004. The global burden of disease: 2004 Update. WHO, Geneva.

References

What do I need to know?

2

CHAPTER CONTENTS

Overview 9
Relevant clinical questions 9
Refining your question 11
  Effects of intervention 11
  Experiences 12
  Prognosis 12
  Diagnosis 12
References 13

OVERVIEW

The first step in evidence-based practice is to ask relevant clinical questions. In this chapter we consider how to structure questions about the effects of intervention, experiences, prognosis and the accuracy of diagnostic tests. By structuring questions well, relevant evidence can be found more efficiently and easily.

Let us imagine that you are a full-time practitioner in an outpatient clinic. One day you are faced with the following patient:

> Mr Y is 43 years old. He presents with low back pain of relatively acute onset (about 2 weeks) with pain radiating down his left leg. He has no apparent neurological deficits. The problem has arisen during a period of heavy lifting at work and has become progressively worse over subsequent days. Mr Y's general practitioner prescribed analgesics, anti-inflammatory drugs and bed rest for 5 days, but this brought little improvement. Mr Y was then referred to you for treatment to relieve his pain and restore physical functioning.

This scenario will probably make many physiotherapists think how they would manage this patient. Most of us will admit that there is quite a lot we do not know about what the evidence says is the best treatment for patients with back pain. That is a good thing: uncertainty prompts clinical questions, so it is a precondition for evidence-based physiotherapy.

Relevant clinical questions

A well-known saying is that 'the beginning of all wisdom lies not in the answer, but in the question'. The first step in evidence-based practice is to formulate a specific question. The question you have concerning your practice should be formulated so it is possible to find a scientific answer to the question. Posing specific questions relevant to a patient's problem provides a focus to thinking, and it helps in the formulation of search strategies and in the process of critical appraisal of evidence.

Typically physiotherapists confront a wide variety of questions during patient encounters. Some answers, such as those about how the patient's problem affects his or her day-to-day life, are best obtained by asking the patient. Other information needs are met by practice knowledge that is at our fingertips. But some information needs are best provided by high-quality clinical research. This information may be hard to find, and tracking it down is always difficult in the pressurized atmosphere of a busy practice. The intention of this book is to help physiotherapists find important evidence quickly.

In the scenario we have before us, you are faced with the problem of a man with low back pain of relatively acute onset. What questions does this scenario stimulate you to ask? You may have thought of some or all of the following:

- Is heavy lifting the cause of this man's problem?
- Could this problem have been prevented?
- How can I decide whether he has nerve root involvement?
- Which tests would be useful to rule out more serious conditions, such as malignancy?
- What is his principal underlying concern about the condition?
- If my aim is to improve his functional capacity, should I advise him to stay active or to rest in bed?
- What does he feel about staying in bed or returning to work?
- What is the probability that the problem will resolve by itself within a month?
- What can I do to relieve his pain during this period?
- Is there anything I can do to speed up his recovery?

All of these questions are important. Each is answered with a different kind of evidence. The questions can be categorized as shown in Table 2.1.

Often the most important clinical questions concern:

- **effects of intervention**
- **patients' experiences**
- **the course of a condition (prognosis)**
- **the accuracy of diagnostic tests.**

Clinical research that answers these sorts of question is therefore the most important research for clinical practice. In this book we consider how to answer such questions with high-quality clinical research.

We have chosen to start by considering questions about the effects of intervention. One justification is that questions about effects of intervention arguably have the most important implications for practice. Most of the thinking and concepts in evidence-based physiotherapy have been developed from research on the effects of intervention. After considering questions about effects of intervention we will consider questions about patients' experiences, because these questions are often complementary to and closely linked with questions about effectiveness. Finally we consider questions regarding prognosis and diagnosis.

The separation of clinical questions into those about intervention, experiences, prognosis and accuracy of diagnostic tests is a little contrived. In practice, many clinical questions are complex and require the synthesis of findings of several types of research. A clinical question about whether or not to apply a particular intervention may require information about the effects of that intervention, but it may also need to be informed by studies about prognosis and about patients' experiences. For example, consider a middle-aged man who presents to a physiotherapy department with acute neck pain. He has been told by his general practitioner that a course of cervical mobilization and manipulation will relieve his pain. When deciding how to proceed, his physiotherapist could consider evidence from studies of the effectiveness of mobilization and manipulation,

Table 2.1 Categorization of questions

Question	Requires evidence about
• Could this problem have been prevented? • If my aim is to improve his functional capacity, should I advise him to stay active or to rest in bed? • What can I do to relieve his pain during this period? • Is there anything I can do to speed up his recovery?	Effects of intervention
• What does he feel about staying in bed or returning to work? • What is his principal underlying concern about the condition?	Experiences
• What is the probability that the problem will resolve by itself within a month?	Prognosis
• How can I decide whether he has nerve root involvement? • Which tests would be useful to rule out more serious conditions, such as malignancy?	Diagnosis
• Is heavy lifting the cause of his problem?	Harm or aetiology

which show a moderate effect on pain and disability (Gross et al 2004), as well as research on the natural course of this condition, which indicates a fairly favourable prognosis (Borghouts et al 1998). The physiotherapist might also be interested in what the evidence has to say about patients' expectations of manual therapy, and what it is that most patients hope to be able to achieve with physiotherapy. For the patient, these issues are closely entwined. However, if the physiotherapist is to think clearly about these issues and find relevant research, he or she will do better to take the global question about how to treat and break it up into its components concerning effects of intervention, prognosis and experiences.

Our impression is that physiotherapists frequently ask another class of question, about harm or aetiology. (One of the questions in our example was a question about aetiology: we asked about whether heavy lifting was the most likely cause of the patient's problem.) These questions are of great theoretical importance, but they are usually not immediately relevant to practice. To see why, consider the following example. A substantial body of evidence suggests that being overweight exacerbates symptoms of osteoarthritis of the knee (for example, Coggon et al 2001, Felson et al 1992). Although that is useful information for researchers, it does not, on its own, indicate that interventions aimed at weight loss are indicated. This is because the causes of most diseases are multifactorial, so intervention that modifies one aetiological factor may have little effect on the course of the disease. In addition, interventions aimed at producing weight loss may not have sufficient long-term effects to be worthwhile. In general, studies of aetiology suggest interventions but do not confirm their effectiveness. Questions about aetiology could be considered *preclinical* questions. Consequently, we shall not consider questions about aetiology further in this book.

However, there is one type of aetiological research that is of immediate clinical importance: research into unintended harmful effects of intervention. Physiotherapists seldom believe that their treatment could cause harm, but it might be possible for some modalities to do so. Cervical manipulation is one intervention that is known to produce occasional harm (Di Fabio 1999). It causes harm so infrequently that studies of effects of cervical manipulation do not provide a useful estimate of the harm that is caused. The research on harm caused by cervical manipulation is, therefore, most often of the same type as the traditional aetiological research. In general,

evidence of the harmful effects of intervention often comes from aetiological research.

Refining your question

Before we begin the hunt for evidence that relates to our clinical questions, we need to spend some time making the questions specific. Structuring and refining the question makes it easier to find an answer. One way to do this is to break the problem into parts. Below we provide some suggestions for breaking questions about effects of intervention, experiences, prognosis and diagnosis into parts. We will use some simple tables to help us formulate well-structured questions.

Effects of intervention

We usually break questions about the effects of intervention into four parts (Sackett et al 2000):

- Patient or problem
- Intervention or management strategy
- Comparative intervention
- Outcome.

A useful mnemonic is PICO (Glasziou et al 2003).

The first part (**P**) identifies the patient or the problem.[1] This involves identifying those characteristics of the patient or problem that are most likely to influence the effects of the intervention. If you specify the patient or problem in a very detailed way, you will probably not get an answer, because the evidence is usually not capable of providing very specific answers (more on this in Chapter 6). So a compromise has to be reached between specifying enough detail to get a relevant answer, but not too much detail to preclude getting any answer at all.

The second (**I**) and third (**C**) parts concern interventions. Here we specify the intervention that we are interested in and what we want to compare the effect of that intervention with. We may want to compare the effect of an intervention with no intervention, or with a sham intervention (more on sham interventions in Chapter 5) or with another active intervention.

---

[1] The example we use is one of an individual patient. However, health care interventions do not always concern patients. For example, questions related to organizing and funding health services may also be of interest to physiotherapists. This book will, however, focus on problems of individual patients.

The fourth part of the question (**O**) specifies what outcomes we are interested in. In some circumstances it may be worth spending some time with the patient to identify precisely what outcomes they are interested in. For example, when considering whether to refer an injured worker to a work-hardening programme, it may be important to determine whether the patient is interested primarily in reductions in pain, or reductions in disability, or returning to work, or some other outcome. Traditionally there has been little involvement of patients when it comes to defining the desired outcomes of intervention. There is now an increasing recognition that the patient is the main stakeholder when it comes to choosing outcome measures, and involvement of patients in setting the goals of intervention is an important element in a shared decision-making process.

Let us return to the scenario of the man who presents with acute back pain and ask a question about the effects of intervention. You are considering whether to advise this man to stay in bed or to continue his daily routine as actively as possible. He has been explicit that he wants you to do something to relieve his pain and restore his physical functioning. Consequently, your four-part question is: 'In patients with acute low back pain, does bed rest or advice to stay active produce greater reductions in pain and disability?'

Patient	Intervention	Comparison intervention	Outcome
Adult with acute low back pain	Bed rest	Advice to stay active	Pain and disability

Experiences

Questions about experiences can relate to any aspect of clinical practice. Because such questions are potentially very diverse, they must be relatively open. We recommend that, when formulating questions about experiences, you specify the patient or problem and the phenomena of interest.

Returning to our example, you may be interested in your patient's attitudes to his condition. In a similar scenario in your own practice you recently heard a patient expressing concern about whether his complaint might become chronic, or whether he might have a serious illness. You become interested in knowing more about the concerns of patients with acute low back pain. Consequently your two-part question is: 'What are the principal concerns of adults with acute low back pain?'

Patient	Phenomena
Adult with acute low back pain	Principal concerns

Prognosis

When asking questions about prognosis you should specify (again) the patient or problem, and the outcome you are interested in. The question may be about the expected *amount* of the outcome or about the *probability* of the outcome. (We will consider this distinction in more depth in Chapter 6.) Often it is worthwhile specifying the timeframe of the outcome as well. In general we can ask questions about the prognosis of people who do not receive treatment (the natural history of the condition) or about the prognosis of people receiving intervention (the clinical course of the condition).

When you discuss different management strategies with your patient, he asks you whether he is likely to recover within the next 6 weeks, because he has some important things planned at that time. So your first question about prognosis is a broad question about the prognosis in the heterogeneous population of people with acute low back pain. The question is: 'In patients with acute low back pain, what is the probability of being pain-free within 6 weeks?'

Patient	Outcome and timeframe
Adult with acute low back pain	Probability of being pain-free within 6 weeks

It is important to understand that questions about prognosis are questions about what will happen in the future, not questions about the causes of what will happen in the future. When we ask questions about the clinical course of a person's condition we want to know what that person's outcome will be, not why it will be what it will be.

Diagnosis

Even the best diagnostic tests occasionally misclassify patients. Misclassification and misdiagnosis are an unavoidable part of professional practice. It is useful to know the probability of misclassification so that we can know how much certainty to attach to diagnoses based on a test's findings. The research literature can help us to obtain relatively unbiased estimates of the accuracy of diagnostic tests. When asking questions about diagnostic test accuracy it is useful to specify the patient or problem, the diagnostic test and the diagnosis for which you are testing.

Our patient's general practitioner has told him that he does not have sciatica. You first interpret this to mean there were no neurological deficits, but after the patient describes radiating pain corresponding with the L5 dermatome you are not sure. You are aware that general practitioners often do not examine patients with low back pain very thoroughly, so you start thinking about doing further clinical

examinations, perhaps using Lasègue's test, amongst others, to find out whether there is nerve root compromise. So you ask: 'In adults with acute low back pain, how accurate is Lasègue's test as a test for nerve root compromise?'

Patient	Test	Diagnosis
Adult with acute low back pain	Lasègue's test	Nerve root compromise

These four clinical questions are best answered with different types of research. Chapter 3 will describe the sorts of research that best answer each type of question.

References

Borghouts, J.A., Koes, B.W., Bouter, L.M., 1998. The clinical course and prognostic factors of non-specific neck pain: a systematic review. Pain 77 (1), 1–13.

Coggon, D., Reading, I., Croft, P., et al., 2001. Knee osteoarthritis and obesity. Int. J. Obes. Relat. Metab. Disord. 25 (5), 622–627.

Di Fabio, R.P., 1999. Manipulation of the cervical spine: risks and benefits. Phys. Ther. 79 (1), 50–65.

Felson, D.T., Zhang, Y., Anthony, J.M., et al., 1992. Weight loss reduces the risk for symptomatic knee osteoarthritis in women. The Framingham Study. Ann. Intern. Med. 116 (7), 535–539.

Glasziou, P., Del Mar, C., Salisbury, J., 2003. Evidence-based medicine workbook. BMJ Publishing, London.

Gross, A.R., Hoving, J.L., Haines, T.A., et al., 2004. Cervical overview group.

Manipulation and mobilisation for mechanical neck disorders (Cochrane review). In: The Cochrane Library, Issue 2. Wiley, Chichester.

Sackett, D.L., Straus, S.E., Richardson, W.S., et al., 2000. Evidence-based medicine: how to practice and teach EBM. Churchill Livingstone, Edinburgh.

What constitutes evidence?

3

CHAPTER CONTENTS

Overview 15

What constitutes evidence about effects
of interventions? 15

Clinical observation 16
Theories about mechanisms 18
Clinical research 19
Case series and controlled trials 19
Randomized trials 21
N-of-1 randomized trials 22
Systematic reviews 23
Systematic reviews, meta-analysis,
meta-analysis of individual patient data, and
prospective systematic reviews 25
Section conclusion 26

What constitutes evidence about
experiences? 26

Clinical observation 26
Clinical research 27
Systematic reviews 29

What constitutes evidence about
prognosis? 30

Clinical observation 30
Clinical research 30
Prospective and retrospective
cohort studies 31
Clinical trials 31
Systematic reviews 32

What constitutes evidence about the
accuracy of diagnostic and screening
tests? 32

Clinical observation 32
Clinical research 33
Cross-sectional studies 33

Randomized trials 34
Screening 34
Systematic reviews 34
References 35

OVERVIEW

Readers looking for evidence of the effects of intervention, experiences, prognosis or accuracy of diagnostic tests should look first for relevant systematic reviews. If relevant systematic reviews cannot be found, the reader can consult reports of individual studies. The best (least biased) individual studies of effects of intervention are randomized clinical trials. Evidence of experiences can be obtained from qualitative research that typically involves in-depth interviews, observation of behaviours, or focus groups. Evidence of prognosis can be obtained from longitudinal studies. The preferred study type is the prospective cohort study, but sometimes good prognostic information can be obtained from retrospective cohort studies or clinical trials. Evidence of the accuracy of diagnostic tests comes from cross-sectional studies that compare the findings of the test of interest with a reference standard.

What constitutes evidence about effects of interventions?

The preceding chapter described four important types of clinical question: questions about the effects of intervention, experiences, prognosis and diagnostic tests. In this chapter we consider the types of clinical research that can be used to answer these questions.

Clinical observation

The practice of physiotherapy has always been based, at least in part, on clinical observation. Day-to-day clinical practice provides physiotherapists with many observations of their patients' conditions. Some physiotherapists supplement their clinical observations with careful measures of outcomes using validated measurement tools. Over time, experienced practitioners accumulate large numbers of such observations. Distillation of clinical observations generates 'practice knowledge' or 'professional craft knowledge' (Higgs et al 2001). The practice knowledge of veteran physiotherapists may be shared with less experienced colleagues in practice or at conferences or workshops.

The simplest way to interpret observations of clinical outcomes is as the effect of intervention. If the condition of most patients improves with intervention then, according to this simple interpretation, the intervention must be effective. Alternatively, if the intervention is designed to prevent adverse outcomes, the observation that most people who receive the intervention do not experience an adverse outcome might be interpreted as indicating that the intervention is effective. The confusion of outcomes and effects of interventions is reinforced by patients. Patients often interpret an improvement in their condition as evidence that intervention was effective, and patients whose condition does not improve may feel dissatisfied with the intervention.

This way of reasoning is attractive but potentially seriously misleading. Many factors determine clinical outcomes.

> It may be incorrect to interpret clinical observations of successful outcomes as evidence of a beneficial effect of intervention because sometimes factors other than the intervention are the primary determinants of outcome.

In epidemiology-speak, the effects of intervention are 'confounded' by 'extraneous factors'. What extraneous factors confound simple cause–effect interpretations of interventions and outcomes?

One important source of confounding is natural recovery. Natural recovery occurs when conditions resolve without intervention. Examples of conditions that can resolve without intervention are acute low back pain and post-surgical respiratory complications. People with these conditions can experience satisfactory outcomes even if they are not given any intervention, or if they are given ineffective interventions. Clinical observations are not always helpful

in determining the effects of intervention because it can be difficult, in the course of normal clinical practice, to determine what part of the improvement was due to intervention and what would have occurred without intervention.

Natural recovery may occur because the underlying course of the condition is one of gradual improvement, but it will also tend to occur in chronic conditions that are episodic or that tend to fluctuate in severity. Two common examples of episodic conditions are arthritic pain and respiratory infections. By their very nature, episodic conditions tend to resolve even without intervention, and then they relapse again.

Statisticians consider the spontaneous resolution of episodic disease as an example of a more general phenomenon called statistical regression. The statistical way of thinking about episodic disease is that the disease has a random component to its severity. Sometimes, when the symptoms become particularly bothersome or serious (when random fluctuations are in the direction of worsening of symptoms), patients are driven to seek care. At this stage, when the patient's condition is more severe than usual, still more severe symptoms are relatively unlikely – it is more likely that subsequent random fluctuations will be towards more average symptom levels (Figure 3.1) (Bland & Altman 1994). Consequently conditions of fluctuating intensity, once they become severe, are most likely to resolve, even without intervention.[1]

A third confounder of clinical observations applies when information about outcomes is supplied by the patient rather than directly observed by the physiotherapist. In practice, most useful information about clinical outcomes is obtained in this way.[2] (Two important examples are information about pain severity and function, both of which are almost always supplied by the patient.) The only practical way to find out about these types of outcome is to ask patients to tell us whether or not their condition has improved. But self-reports of outcomes are potentially misleading because patients' responses

---

[1]Of course, the opposite is also true. When a patient with episodic disease is in remission (when their symptoms are particularly mild) subsequent random fluctuations are likely to be in the direction of increasing severity. Patients rarely seek care when in remission, so statistical regression rarely acts to make disease severity worse in the period soon after seeking care.

[2]The real test of most physiotherapy interventions is how they make recipients of the intervention feel (more on this in Chapter 6). Consequently the constructs that we most need to know about are intrinsically subjective. The subjectiveness of many clinical outcome measures is a strength, not a weakness, of the measures.

Figure 3.1 • Statistical regression. Patients with episodic disease seek intervention when the severity of the condition exceeds some threshold value. Subsequent fluctuations are more likely to be in the direction of a reduction in disease severity, even if the intervention does not have any effect on the course of the condition.

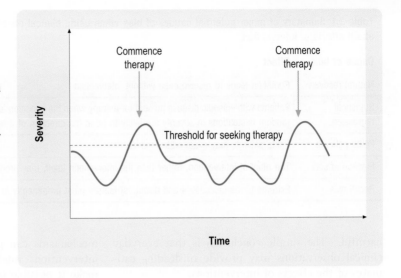

to questioning about outcomes can be distorted by the social mores that guide interactions between therapists and patients (Kienle & Kiene 1997). Patients understand that most therapists try hard to do their best for their patients, and some patients may find it difficult to report that their condition has not substantially improved. Politeness or a sense of obligation may cause some patients to report improvements that did not occur, or to report exaggerated improvements. In this way, sensitive and polite patients can make intervention look more effective than it truly is. The confounding effect of polite patients is an example of a more general phenomenon, sometimes called the 'Hawthorne effect', which refers to the fact that participants in research may change their behaviours as a result of knowing that their behaviours are under study (Wickstrom & Bendix 2000).

A closely related confounder is the placebo effect (Beecher 1955, Hrobjartsson & Gotzsche 2003, Kienle & Kiene 1997). Placebo effects are improvements in the patient's condition that result from the 'treatment ritual' (Hrobjartsson 2002), as evidenced by effects of inert (sham) interventions. It is widely believed that placebo effects contribute substantially to the benefits of most interventions. For example, a survey showed that many Australian physiotherapists believe that the apparent effects of ultrasound are due largely to placebo effects (Chipchase & Trinkle 2003). Insofar as ultrasound exerts placebo effects, there must be powerful mechanisms that convert the psychological phenomenon of an expectation of effective therapy into the biopsychosocial phenomenon of recovery. But there is considerable

controversy surrounding the placebo effect. One point of disagreement is whether placebo effects should be considered confounders or effects of therapy in their own right (Vickers & de Craen 2000). A more radical point of view holds that much of what has been ascribed to the placebo effect is an artefact of poorly designed research. We will examine the placebo effect in more detail in Chapter 5.

Interpretations of clinical observations of outcomes may also be confounded by recall bias. Recall bias occurs because the task of keeping track of clinical observations is difficult: experienced physiotherapists who have applied an intervention many times need to maintain an accurate mental ledger of typical outcomes with that therapy. In practice, patients who fared particularly well or particularly badly may feature most prominently in memory. We tend to remember our most successful and most disastrous cases, so our memories of clinical outcomes may be unduly optimistic or unduly pessimistic. Thus accumulation of large numbers of observations of clinical outcomes does not guarantee a reduction in bias.

The preceding paragraphs suggest that simple cause–effect interpretations of clinical observations can be biased (Table 3.1). Most of the biases we have considered act to inflate estimates of effects of interventions; that is, simple cause–effect interpretations of clinical observations tend to overestimate effects of interventions. History points to the same conclusion. There are many examples from the history of medicine where clinical observations have suggested that a therapy was effective yet subsequent investigations have shown the therapy to be ineffective or

Table 3.1 Summary of major potential causes of bias when using clinical observations to make inferences about effects of intervention

Cause of bias	Effect
Natural recovery	Condition tends to resolve even without intervention
Statistical regression	Patients with episodic disease present for therapy when the condition is severe, but when the condition is severe random fluctuations in severity are likely to be in the direction of a reduction of severity
Polite patients	Polite patients may exaggerate recovery
Placebo effects	The ritual of intervention, rather than the intervention itself, may produce beneficial effects
Recall bias	Extreme cases (successes and disasters) feature most prominently in memory

harmful.[3] The simple conclusion is that everyday clinical observations may provide misleading estimates of the effects of interventions.

Theories about mechanisms

In some areas of physiotherapy practice the primary justification for intervention is provided not by clinical observations but by theory. The justification is not that the intervention has been observed to be effective but that what we know about the mechanisms of the intervention leads us to believe that intervention should be effective.

There are many examples: physiotherapists began to use ultrasound to treat musculoskeletal lesions back in the 1950s because they believed that ultrasound increased the permeability of cell membranes, which was thought to facilitate healing (Wedlick 1954). The techniques of proprioceptive neuromuscular facilitation (Voss et al 1985), and their successors such as the muscle energy techniques (Chaitow 2001), are based on neurophysiological concepts such as reciprocal inhibition. And many people stretch after sport because they have been told that stretching reduces muscle spasm which causes delayed onset muscle soreness (de Vries 1961).

We need to have theories about the mechanisms of interventions. Properly used, theories about

mechanisms can provide hypotheses about which interventions might be effective. Good theories make it possible for us to administer interventions that have the greatest chance of being effective. But theories about mechanisms, on their own, provide very inferior evidence of the effects of intervention. Why?

Physiotherapy involves the application of complex interventions to complex problems, so it should not be surprising that our theories are almost always incomplete. Theories about mechanisms usually have the status of working hypotheses rather than comprehensive and accurate representations of the truth. Theories should be, and usually are, subject to frequent revision. We can rarely know, with any certainty, that theories about intervention are true.

There is another problem with using theory to justify intervention. Theories might tell us about the *direction* of effects of interventions, but they can never tell us about the *size* of effects of interventions. Laboratory studies of the effects of ultrasound might show that insonation of fibroblasts increases their secretion of collagen, or that ultrasound hastens ligament healing, and these findings might suggest that ultrasound will bring about clinically useful effects such as returning subjects to sport faster than would otherwise occur. But how much faster? The theory, even if true, cannot tell us whether the application of ultrasound therapy will have a patient fit to return to sport one week sooner, or one day sooner, or one minute sooner. We might consider a therapy that gets patients fit to return to sport one week sooner is effective, but a therapy that gets patients fit to return to sport just one minute sooner is ineffective. Theory cannot distinguish between the two. Making rational treatment decisions involves considering the size of

---

[3]For an extreme example of misleading clinical observations, see Whitehead's description, in 1901, of the use of a tape seton for treatment of migraine. Whitehead treated migraine by passing a dressmaker's tape through an incision in the skin on the back of the neck. He wrote of his experiences with this therapy (Whitehead 1901: 335): 'During the last five and twenty years I have never failed to treat successfully the most inveterate and severe cases of migraine.'

treatment effects, and theory cannot tell us about the size of treatment effects.

> Theories of mechanisms can help us develop and refine interventions, but they provide a very poor source of information about the effects of intervention.

We need more than theory.

Clinical research

Clinical research potentially provides us with a better source of information about the effects of intervention than clinical observation or theories about mechanisms. High-quality clinical research is able to prevent ('control for') much of the bias associated with simplistic interpretations of clinical observations and, unlike theories about mechanisms, can provide us with estimates of the size of treatment effects.

> High-quality clinical research can provide us with *unbiased* estimates of the *size* of the effects of intervention, so it potentially provides us with the best way of assessing effectiveness of interventions.

The systematic and critical use of high-quality clinical research in clinical decision-making is what differentiates evidence-based physiotherapy from other models of physiotherapy practice. That is why, in this book, we use the word 'evidence' to mean high-quality clinical research.

Unfortunately most clinical research is not of high quality. Surveys of the methodological quality of clinical research have invariably found that most published research does not satisfy basic requirements of good research design (see Chapter 5). One of the consequences is that the findings of many studies cannot be relied upon. It is possible to find studies that purport to demonstrate clinically important effects of particular interventions alongside other studies that draw exactly the opposite conclusions. Undiscriminating readers may find this disconcerting! Readers who have the ability to discriminate between high-quality and low-quality studies will be more able to make sense of the literature, and should be more able to discern the true effects of interventions. A prerequisite of evidence-based physiotherapy is the ability to discriminate between low-quality and high-quality clinical research. One of the aims of this book is to provide readers with that skill.

What sorts of clinical research give us the best answers about effects of intervention? There are many ways to design clinical studies of the effectiveness of interventions, but some research designs are more suitable than others.

Case series and controlled trials

The simplest studies of the effects of intervention simply involve assessing patients presenting with the condition of interest, applying the intervention, and determining whether, on average, the patients' condition improves. Such studies are sometimes called 'case series'. The simplistic interpretation often applied by authors of such studies is that if, on average, patients get better, the intervention is, on average, effective.

These very simple studies just involve systematic recording of normal clinical practice. Like clinical practice, they involve the accumulation of observations. And, like any clinical observations of the effects of intervention, they are prone to bias because extraneous factors, other than treatment, can masquerade as effective treatment. These sorts of study are prone to serious bias from natural recovery, statistical regression, placebo effects and polite patients. Therefore they provide very weak evidence of the effects of intervention.

More sophisticated studies compare outcomes in people who do and do not receive the intervention of interest. In such studies the focus is on whether people who receive the intervention of interest have better outcomes than patients who do not receive the intervention. Comparison of outcomes in people who do and do not receive the intervention of interest is thought to provide better 'control' of bias than case series, so these studies are called controlled trials.

Controlled trials potentially provide control of bias because both groups (the group that receives the intervention of interest and the group that does not) experience natural recovery and both groups experience statistical regression (and, depending on other features of the design, both groups' outcomes may be influenced by placebo effects or patients' politeness). Therefore, it is reasoned, the *differences* in outcomes of the two groups cannot be due to natural recovery or statistical regression or, in some studies, to placebo effects or polite patients. As these sources of bias have been controlled for, it is more reasonable to attribute differences between the groups' outcomes to the intervention.

A common misunderstanding is the belief that the control group in a controlled trial must receive 'no intervention'. This is not the case. In fact we can distinguish three sorts of controlled study that differ in the nature of intervention and control:

1. One group receives intervention and the other group receives no intervention.
2. One group receives standard intervention and the other group receives standard intervention plus a new intervention.
3. One group receives a particular intervention and the other group receives a different intervention.[4]

In the rest of this book we will refer, when discussing controlled trials, to the 'intervention group' and 'control group', although we acknowledge that, in the third type of study at least, it may not be clear which group is which.

A common feature of all three designs is that differences in outcomes of the two groups are attributed to differences in the interventions the groups receive. Thus the first sort of study tells us about the effects of intervention over and above no intervention. The second tells about whether there is any benefit in adding the new intervention to standard intervention. The third tells us which of the two interventions is most effective. All three designs potentially tell us something useful, but each tells us something different.

An important assumption of controlled studies is that the two groups are comparable. That is, it is assumed that had the two groups received the same intervention they would experience the same outcomes. When this condition is not met (when the groups consist of subjects that are different in some important way so that they would experience different outcomes even if they received the same intervention) then differences between the groups' outcomes could be attributable, at least in part, to subject characteristics. That is, when the groups are not comparable, differences between outcomes of the two groups cannot be assumed to reflect solely the effects of intervention. (This is called 'allocation bias' or sometimes, less accurately, 'selection bias'. Another way of saying the same thing is to say that the effects of the intervention are confounded by subject characteristics.)

> Controlled studies can only be assumed to provide unbiased estimates of the effects of intervention if the two groups are comparable.

In many studies, groups are self-selected. That is, the grouping occurs naturally, without the intervention of the researcher. For example, in a study of the effects of a movement and swimming programme on respiratory outcomes in children with cerebral palsy, Hutzler and colleagues (1998) compared outcomes of children attending two kindergartens that offered a movement and swimming programme with outcomes of children attending two kindergartens that offered a standard land-based exercise programme. The study found greater improvements in respiratory outcomes among the children receiving the movement and swimming programme. However, this study is unconvincing because it is quite plausible that the differences in outcomes might be due to different characteristics of the children at the different kindergartens, rather than to the greater effectiveness of the movement and swimming programme. In general, when groups self-select, the groups will not have identical characteristics; some characteristics of the subjects or their experiences causes them to be allocated to one group rather than the other. If those characteristics are related to outcome, the groups will not be comparable. Consequently, controlled trials in which subjects self-select groups are particularly prone to allocation bias.

How is it possible to assemble two groups of comparable patients? Some researchers try to 'match' subjects in treatment and control groups on characteristics that are thought to be important. For example, in their study of the effects of exercise on lipid profiles in children, Tolfrey and colleagues (1998) matched children undergoing exercise with maturity-matched children not undergoing exercise. Matching on its own is generally unsatisfactory for two reasons. First, there are limitations to the number of variables that can be matched – it is practically impossible to match subjects on more than two or three variables – so the groups may not have equal distributions of other variables that were not matched. Some statistical techniques allow the researchers to match the two groups statistically on many more variables, although these techniques are also limited in the number of variables that can be matched. And, anyhow, it is still necessary to measure all of those variables on all subjects in the study, which may not be practical.[5]

---

[4]In Chapter 5 we shall examine variants of all three designs that involve the provision of sham interventions.

[5]There is another, more technical, limitation of these statistical techniques. They can properly adjust for imbalances in prognostic variables only when the prognostic variable is measured without error. In practice most prognostic variables, and almost all prognostic variables measured on a continuous scale, are measured with error. As a consequence, the statistical techniques tend to underadjust. This is called regression dilution bias.

Moreover, we usually do not know what all the important prognostic variables are. And if we don't know what is important, we can't match the groups with respect to those variables. In general, the approach of attempting to match groups of patients is generally unsatisfactory because we can never be satisfied that this will produce groups that are comparable in all important respects.

Randomized trials

> There is only one way we can assemble intervention and control groups that will give us the expectation of comparable groups, and that is to randomize subjects to groups.

In a randomized trial, subjects agree to be allocated to either the intervention or the control group. Then, when they enter the trial, a random process (sometimes just coin-tossing, but usually a computer-generated random process) allocates each subject to one group or the other.

Random allocation is a marvellous thing. Paradoxically, even though each subject's allocation is indeterminate, the effect of randomizing many subjects is predictable. When many subjects are randomized to groups we can expect that the groups will be comparable. That is, we can expect that randomized groups would have similar outcomes if they were treated in a similar way. This means that randomization protects against allocation bias; it prevents confounding of the effects of the intervention by differences between groups.

While randomization ensures groups will be comparable, it does not ensure that they will be identical. There will always be small random differences between groups, which means that randomized trials may underestimate or overestimate the true effects of intervention. Herein lies another important benefit of randomization: random processes can be modelled mathematically. This means that it is possible to determine how much uncertainty is associated with estimates of the size of the effects of intervention. We will look at how to ascertain the degree of uncertainty associated with estimates of effects of intervention in Chapter 6.

There are many examples in which randomized and non-randomized trials have examined the effectiveness of the same intervention and have come up with different conclusions. A particularly clear example comes in studies of extracorporeal shock therapy

for treatment of plantar fasciitis. Several early but non-randomized studies had shown impressive effects for extracorporeal shock therapy (for example, Chen et al 2001) but subsequent randomized trials found that this therapy had little or no effect (Buchbinder et al 2002, Haake et al 2003). Indeed, some data suggest that this is usually the case: there is a general tendency for randomized trials to be less biased than non-randomized trials. Kunz & Oxman (1998) systematically reviewed studies that had compared estimates from randomized and non-randomized trials of effects of particular interventions and found that non-randomized controlled trials tended to show larger treatment effects than randomized trials. In contrast, systematic reviews of individual trials by Concato et al (2000) and Benson & Hartz (2000) found that studies with non-randomized but contemporaneous controls produced similar estimates of effects to those of randomized trials.

The existing data are, therefore, ambivalent. While there is a substantial body of evidence that suggests non-randomized trials tend to be biased, this has not been demonstrated unequivocally, and there are some examples where non-randomized trials give similar answers to randomized trials. Nonetheless, there is a strong justification for relying on randomized trials for evidence of the effects of intervention.[6] Randomization produces the *expectation* of comparable groups. Therefore randomized trials provide the only way of obtaining estimates of effects of interventions that can be expected to be unbiased. For this reason we should look to randomized trials for evidence of the effects of intervention. There are of course ethical and practical considerations that preclude the conduct of randomized trials in some situations (Box 3.1); in those situations we may have to rely on less rigorous evidence.

Randomized trials come in different flavours and colours. In the simplest designs, subjects are allocated randomly to either a treatment or a control group and outcomes are measured only at the end of the trial. In other trials, measurements may be taken before and after the intervention period, or at several time points during and after the intervention period. Some trials allocate subjects randomly to

---

[6]Taken to its extreme, the view that only randomized trials can provide unbiased estimates of the effects of therapy is clearly untenable. Some interventions are obviously effective. Smith & Pell (2003) make this case in their systematic review of 'Parachute use to prevent death and major trauma related to gravitational challenge.'

Box 3.1

Ethical and practical impediments to the conduct of randomized trials

It is often said that some randomized trials cannot be carried out because it is not ethical to conduct them. When is it not ethical to conduct randomized trials of the effects of interventions?

The ethics of randomized trials has been discussed intensely for many decades. One point of view is that it is unethical to randomize subjects to intervention and control conditions unless the clinician is completely ambivalent about which intervention is the better of the two. (This is sometimes called 'equipoise'.) A problem with the requirement of equipoise is that it permits randomization to be vetoed by the clinician, rather than the patient. Arguably, decisions about the acceptability of randomization should be made by properly informed patients, not by clinicians (Lilford 2003). In addition, it has been argued that the requirement of equipoise is impractical (clinicians rarely express complete ambivalence), inconsistent with many other apparently ethical behaviours, and not necessarily in the individual patient's best interests (Piantadosi 1997). A more practical and arguably more consistent position is that randomization of properly informed, consenting patients could be considered provided there is no clear evidence that one alternative is superior to the other. In our opinion it becomes unethical to randomize subjects to groups only when it is not plausible that, from an informed patient's perspective, either alternative could be the best available therapy.[7]

There are some situations in which randomized trials cannot be conducted practically (Black 1996). Some interventions, such as the introduction of management strategies, are conducted at the level of organizations. In theory it may be possible to randomize parts of an organization to receive reforms and others not, but in most circumstances this would be logistically impossible. Other circumstances in which randomized trials cannot be conducted are when the intervention involves significant lifestyle modifications, particularly those that must be implemented over long periods of time, or when the outcome of interest is very rare. For example, it may be impossible to use randomized trials to determine whether decades of regular exercise increase longevity because few people would be prepared to exercise regularly or not for decades on the basis of random allocation. Also, it could be prohibitively expensive to monitor large numbers of subjects over decades. When the outcome of interest is a rare event it is necessary to study large numbers of subjects, so it is often difficult to use randomized trials to determine the effects of interventions designed to prevent rare events. At the other extreme, it may be wasteful to perform a randomized trial to investigate the effects of a simple, inexpensive and harmless intervention that supplements other therapies, because there may be little to be gained from knowing of the intervention's effects.

---

more than two groups,[8] perhaps a control and two intervention groups. Other trials (called *factorial trials*) examine the effects of more than one intervention by randomly allocating all subjects to receive either one intervention or its control and then randomizing the same subjects also to receive another intervention or its control. (For example, van der Heijden et al (1999) randomized subjects with painful shoulders to receive either interferential or sham interferential therapy *and* ultrasound or sham ultrasound therapy. This made it possible to assess the effects of both interferential therapy and ultrasound, and the combination of both in one trial.)

In randomized *crossover trials*, all subjects receive both the treatment and control conditions in random order. (For example, Moseley (1997) randomly allocated head-injured patients with plantar flexor contractures to receive either a period of serial casting followed by a period of no casting, or to a period of no casting followed by a period of casting.) In some types of trial *(cluster randomized trials)*, small groups (clusters) of subjects, rather than individual subjects, are allocated randomly to intervention and control conditions. (For example, in their study of over 6000 people with low back pain, Scheel and colleagues (2002) randomized 65 municipalities of subjects to one of two groups.) Although the designs of these studies differ, they all have a common characteristic. All are protected from allocation bias by randomization.

N-of-1 randomized trials

Randomized trials give us probabilistic answers about average effects of interventions: they tell us about the

---

[7]There should be systems in place to safeguard the rights, dignity and welfare of people participating in research. The most common mechanism is a Research Ethics Committee (REC) within a hospital or other health care facility. Members of a REC usually include patients and members of the public as well as health professionals, academics and people with specific ethical expertise.

[8]The groups in a clinical trial are sometimes referred to as 'arms'. Thus a clinical trial that compares three groups might be called a three-armed trial.

expectation of the effects of intervention.[9] But most patients are uninterested in this technical point. They want to know: 'Will the treatment benefit me?' Unfortunately, randomized trials cannot usually tell us what the effect of intervention will be on any individual patient.

There is one way to determine rigorously whether a particular treatment is beneficial for an individual patient. This involves conducting a trial on that patient. If the patient receives both the treatment and control condition in random order it is possible to determine whether the intervention is more effective than a control condition *for that patient*. To distinguish random effects from real effects, both the treatment and control conditions are administered to the subject several times, or even many times, and a comparison is made between the average outcomes during treated and control conditions. This approach, called the n-of-1 randomized design,[10] has been described in detail (Sackett et al 1991; see also Barlow & Herson 1984).

As with conventional trials, it is necessary to control for potential sources of bias in single-subject trials. If the order of the experimental and control treatment is randomized and the treatment assignment is concealed from the patient and outcome assessor (and perhaps also the therapist), the most important sources of bias are eliminated. We will discuss these features of clinical trials in more detail, in the context of conventional randomized trials, in Chapter 5.

As with cross-over trials, n-of-1 trials are suitable only for certain sorts of conditions and interventions. First, the condition should be chronic, because there is little point in conducting a trial if the condition resolves during the trial. In addition, the intervention should be one that produces only transient effects so that when the intervention is withdrawn the condition returns to its baseline level. The beneficial effect should appear relatively quickly when the treatment starts and disappear quickly when the treatment is withdrawn, otherwise the relationship between intervention and outcome will be obscured. As a consequence, n-of-1 trials are most useful for palliative interventions for chronic conditions.

The physiotherapy literature contains many n-of-1 trials, but very few are n-of-1 *randomized* designs. Some examples are trials of orthoses for growing pains in children (Evans 2003) and a trial contrasting effects of graded exposure and graded activity approaches to management of chronic low back pain (Vlaeyen et al 2001).

The strength of n-of-1 trials is also their limitation. N-of-1 trials permit inferences to be made about the effects of intervention on a particular patient, but they provide no logical basis upon which the findings on a single patient can be extrapolated to other patients. Thus n-of-1 trials are of most use for making decisions about that patient, but may be less use for making broader inferences about the effects of an intervention. Some investigators replicate n-of-1 trials on a number of patients, in the belief that this may enable broader inference about the effects of therapy. Replication of n-of-1 trials may enable some degree of generalization.

Systematic reviews

A well-designed randomized trial can provide strong evidence for the effects of an intervention. However, readers are entitled to be unconvinced by a single randomized trial. With any single trial there is always the concern that there was some feature of the trial, perhaps a feature that is not apparent in the trial report, that provided aberrant results. For example, there may have been some characteristic of the subjects in the trial that made them unusually responsive or unresponsive to therapy. Alternatively, the intervention may have been administered by an outstanding therapist or, for that matter, a very unskilled therapist. We will consider these issues at greater length in Chapter 6. For now, it is sufficient to say that factors that are not easily discerned on reading a trial report may cause an individual trial to represent unfairly the true effects of intervention.

It is reassuring, then, when several trials have investigated the effects of the same intervention and provide data that support the same conclusion. In that case the findings are said to be 'robust'. Conversely, when several trials produce data supporting different conclusions the findings of any one of those trials must be considered less convincing.

---

[9]We will consider what is meant by 'probabilistic answers about average effects of interventions' in Chapter 6.

[10]There is a long history of n-of-1 trials that precedes their recent discovery in medicine. The methodology was extensively developed by psychologists, notably Herson & Barlow (1984). Psychologists call these studies 'single-case experimental designs'. But the terminology is used inconsistently: the term 'n-of-1 design' is sometimes used inappropriately to describe case series or case studies that do not involve experimental alternation of treatment conditions, and the term 'single-case experimental design' is often used to described studies that are not true experiments because they do not involve random assignment of conditions.

The combined evidence provided by many clinical trials may provide a truer picture of the effects of intervention than any individual trial. This is one reason why it is best, wherever possible, to use reviews of several trials, rather than individual trials, to answer questions about the effects of interventions.

There is another reason why reviews may provide a better source of information about the effects of intervention than an individual clinical trial. Literature reviews have at their disposal all of the data from all of the trials they review. One of the consequences of having more data is an increase in precision – literature reviews potentially provide more precise estimates of the size of the effects of therapy. This will be considered in more detail in Chapter 6.

We can distinguish two types of review. In the traditional type of review, now called a 'narrative review', an expert in the field locates relevant studies and writes a synthesis of what those studies have to say. Narrative reviews are attractive to readers because they often summarize a vast literature. However, narrative reviews have fallen out of favour because of concerns about bias.

Serious problems with narrative reviews were becoming apparent to psychologists in the late 1970s. By that time the psychological literature had grown to an enormous size and it had become impossible for practising psychologists to read all of the relevant studies pertaining to a particular clinical question; they were forced, instead, to rely on reviews of the literature. But unfortunately there were examples where reviewers had gone to the same literature and come to very different conclusions. For example, Glass and colleagues describe three reviews, completed within about 5 years of one another, that compared effects of drug therapy plus psychotherapy to drug therapy alone. The reviews variously concluded that 'the advantage for combined treatment is striking' and 'there is little difference between psychotherapy plus drug and drug therapy alone' and 'the existing studies by no means permit firm conclusions as to the nature of the interaction between combined psychotherapy and medication' (Glass et al 1981: 18–20).

It is worthwhile contemplating why the different reviewers came up with different conclusions. One explanation is that reviewers had different philosophical orientations that made them see the problems, interventions and outcomes in different ways. Perhaps they were attracted to different parts of the literature and they made different judgements about which studies were and were not important.

Unfortunately, the way in which reviewers selected studies and made judgements about study quality was usually not transparent. This is a characteristic of narrative reviews: the process of narrative reviews is usually inscrutable.

The inscrutability of the review process and the inconsistency of review conclusions led to a crisis of confidence. Methodologists began to look for alternatives to narrative reviews. In a short space of time in the late 1970s and early 1980s there was a rapid development of new methods of conducting reviews (Glass et al 1981, Hedges & Olkin 1985, Hunter et al 1982). Soon afterwards, these methods were discovered by medical researchers, and they have since become widely adopted in all areas of health care, including physiotherapy. The new approach to the conduct of reviews is called the 'systematic review' (Egger et al 2001). In systematic reviews the aim is to make the review methodology transparent to the reader and to minimize potential sources of bias.

As their name implies, systematic reviews are conducted using a systematic and explicit methodology. They are usually easily recognizable because, unlike narrative reviews, there is a section of the systematic review that describes the methods used to conduct the review. Typically the Methods section outlines the precise review question and describes criteria used to select studies for inclusion in the review and methods used to assess the quality of those studies, extract data from the studies, and synthesize findings of the studies. As the best studies of effects of intervention are randomized trials, most (but not all) systematic reviews of the effects of interventions review only randomized trials.[11]

High-quality systematic reviews provide comprehensive, transparent and minimally biased overviews of the research literature. Systematic reviews of randomized trials often constitute the best single source of information about the effects of particular interventions.

A particularly important source of systematic reviews of the effects of health interventions is the Cochrane Collaboration, an international network of researchers dedicated to producing systematic reviews of effects of interventions in all areas of health care. Between its inception in 1993 and August 2010 the Collaboration produced 6264 reviews. Cochrane reviews tend to be of high quality

---

[11]In other areas, such as social policy research, most systematic reviews include non-randomized trials.

(Jadad et al 1998, Moseley et al 2009), so they are a very useful source of information about the effects of intervention. Where available, relevant Cochrane systematic reviews often provide the best single source of information about effects of particular health interventions.

Systematic reviews, meta-analysis, meta-analysis of individual patient data, and prospective systematic reviews

There is some inconsistency in the terminology used to describe systematic reviews. The first systematic reviews were called 'meta-analyses'. But, over time, the term meta-analysis came to mean a class of statistical methods used in systematic reviews (Hedges & Olkin 1985). Now the term meta-analysis is usually reserved to describe certain statistical methods, and the term is no longer used as a synonym for systematic reviews. In contemporary parlance, a meta-analysis is *part of* a review. Meta-analysis can be part of a systematic review or part of a non-systematic (narrative) review. The relationship between systematic reviews, non-systematic reviews and meta-analysis is shown in Figure 3.2. In the conventional systematic review, published data from randomized trials are used to make inferences about the effects of therapies. Unfortunately, many trial reports provide incomplete data, present data in an ambiguous way, or present data in a way that is not easily combined with or compared with other studies. To circumvent these problems some reviewers ask the authors of individual trial reports to provide the reviewers with raw data from the original trial. This

enables the reviewers to re-analyse the data in an optimal and consistent way. The resulting *systematic reviews of individual patient data* are generally considered more rigorous than conventional systematic reviews. There are, however, very few systematic reviews of individual patient data relevant to physiotherapy. (For an example, see Kelley & Kelley 2004.)

One concern with systematic reviews is that they are usually conducted retrospectively. That is, the review is usually designed and conducted after most of the relevant trials have been conducted. When this is the case it is possible that the reviewers' knowledge of the trials, prior to designing the review, could influence the criteria used to select studies for inclusion in the review, assess the quality of those studies, and extract data. A new kind of systematic review, the *prospective* systematic review, has been designed to control for these kinds of bias (for example, Sacks et al 2000). As the name suggests, prospective reviews are designed before the completion of the trials that they review. This ensures that the design of the review cannot be influenced by knowledge of trial results. Prospective reviews of individual patient data from high-quality trials potentially provide the strongest possible evidence of effects of an intervention. Unfortunately, prospective systematic reviews tend to be very difficult to perform and take many years to complete, so they are very rare. An example relevant to physiotherapy, and possibly the first ever prospective systematic review, is the prospective meta-analysis of the FICSIT (Frailty and Injuries Cooperative Studies of Intervention Techniques) trials of measures to reduce the risk of falls (Province et al 1995).

Figure 3.2 • The relationship between systematic reviews and meta-analyses. In contemporary terminology a meta-analysis is a statistical technique used in some reviews. Some, but not all, systematic reviews contain meta-analyses. Meta-analyses can also be found in non-systematic reviews.

Section conclusion

In the preceding section we considered a number of sources of information about effects of intervention. It was argued that high-quality clinical research usually provides better information about effects of intervention than clinical observations and theory. In general, case series and non-randomized controlled studies do not provide trustworthy sources of information about the effects of therapy so they do not, in our opinion, constitute substantial evidence. The best evidence of effects of interventions is provided by randomized trials or systematic reviews of randomized trials.

There are differing points of view about whether the best evidence of effects of a therapy is provided by a systematic review of relevant trials or by the best individual trial. The answer must be that it depends on how well the review and the best trial were conducted. We encourage physiotherapists seeking answers to clinical questions first to seek systematic reviews relevant to their questions. If the review indicates that there is one trial that is clearly superior to other relevant trials, it may be worthwhile consulting that trial as well.

We conclude this section on evidence of effects of intervention with a comment about a limitation of randomized trials and systematic reviews. The experimental control and lack of bias provided by randomized trials and systematic reviews comes at a cost (Herbert & Higgs 2004). Freedom from bias is achieved by quantifying differences in outcomes of subjects in intervention and control groups. But the act of quantification precludes a deep exploration of subjects' experiences of the intervention (and, for that matter, their experiences of the control condition). Even in trials that examine quality of life or perceptions of the effects of therapy, trials can provide only low-dimensional descriptions of outcomes. A deep understanding of patients' experiences of therapy, and of a number of other clinical phenomena, requires different research approaches. This is the subject of the next section.

What constitutes evidence about experiences?

Questions about effects of physiotherapy are crucial in everyday practice. Physiotherapists and patients alike seek information about whether a particular intervention is effective or whether one kind of intervention is better than another. They might also want to know whether an intervention causes harmful side-effects. Heads of departments might seek information about cost-effectiveness to help prioritize activities among staff. Where available, evidence of effectiveness and cost-effectiveness from high-quality randomized trials should be used to inform decisions about intervention.

But you might have other information needs as well. You might be concerned about how to set up an interdisciplinary team to run an asthma school, how the team should be organized, what opposition you might meet from staff in setting up an interdisciplinary team, or how to handle conflicting views. You may also have questions about which elements of the interventions are the most important and what should be core content. At the same time you might like to know about the experiences of children attending asthma schools, and the experiences of the parents of those children, or how you could motivate families from deprived areas to attend. Most of these questions cannot be answered by clinical trials. Randomized trials and systematic reviews of randomized trials can tell us whether particular interventions are effective, but they cannot provide deep insights into patients' experiences of those interventions.

Questions such as these, about experiences, attitudes and processes, constitute a separate class of clinical question. How can we answer these questions? We could start by asking our professional colleagues, or the patients and users of health services, or we could draw on our own observations in practice. Or we could use high-quality clinical research designed to answer these questions in a systematic way.

Clinical observation

You can learn a great deal by asking your patients about their experiences. Skilled physiotherapists develop strategies and skills to ascertain patients' thoughts and values because this information is important for everyday practice. With practice, most physiotherapists become better at understanding how patients regard therapy and how experiences differ between patients. By talking and listening to patients and observing and reflecting on their responses, skilled physiotherapists learn to better interact and communicate with their patients, and they develop a better understanding of their patients' feelings and perceptions.

However, if you really need to explore a social phenomenon, or dig deep into a question that involves feelings or experiences, there are limitations to what you can find out from clinical observations. Two important limitations are time and resources. Deep exploration of experiences is difficult in the course of everyday clinical practice. An alternative to relying on clinical observations is to look for relevant high-quality clinical research.

Clinical research

> Questions about experiences are best answered by qualitative methods.

Qualitative research methods, also called methods of naturalistic inquiry, were developed in the social and human sciences and refer to theories on interpretation (hermeneutics) and human experience (phenomenology) (Malterud 2001). Qualitative methods are useful for the study of human and social experience, communication, thoughts, expectations, meanings, attitudes and processes, especially those related to interaction, relations, development, interpretation, movement and activity (Malterud 2001). Often an aim is to understand the meaning that underpins behaviours.

Qualitative methods can be used to address a diverse spectrum of clinical questions. In this book we refer to those questions as questions about 'experiences'. This term is used as a shorthand for referring to many sorts of questions, including questions about communication, thoughts, expectations, meanings, attitudes and behaviours.

Qualitative research paradigms are rooted in a different philosophical tradition to that of quantitative research. Consequently, qualitative and quantitative research methods provide complementary ways of understanding the world (Herbert & Higgs 2004). Qualitative research focuses on 'understanding the complex world of lived experience from the point of view of those who live it' (Jones 1995: 2). It is concerned with understanding the views of those being researched. Typically these studies answer questions about 'what it is like' for patients when they experience health care. Answering these sorts of questions requires moving beyond an objective view of the world. Unlike quantitative research, which may aim to find out about 'the' truth, qualitative research aspires to understand a variety of truths. Thus, qualitative and quantitative research methods are based on different ways of knowing, and they produce different types of knowledge (Seers 2004).

> The term 'qualitative methods' is an umbrella term for a broad range of approaches and strategies for collecting, analysing and interpreting data. Each has its own philosophical perspective and its own methodologies.

Gibson and Martin's useful overview of research questions and qualitative approaches is shown in Table 3.2 (Gibson & Martin 2003). The reader who is interested in reading further about qualitative research methods could consult Pope & Mays (2000).

The data that are analysed in qualitative research may be collected using in-depth interviews of individuals or groups (focus groups), through observation with or without the participation of the observer, by keeping field notes, by means of open-ended survey

Table 3.2 Research questions and qualitative approaches (Gibson & Martin 2003)

Research question	Qualitative approach	Common methods
What is the meaning attached to this phenomenon?	Phenomenology (philosophy)	In-depth interviews Analysis of personal writings
What is life like for this group?	Ethnography (anthropology)	Participant observation Formal and informal interviews Video or photographic analysis
What is happening? Why is it happening?	Grounded theory (sociology)	In-depth interviews Focus groups
What are they communicating? How are they communicating?	Discourse analysis (sociology, linguistics)	Document analysis

questions, or from action research, where data sources are multiple and complex (Malterud 2001).

> Qualitative research can contribute to evidence-based practice in a number of ways. It can challenge taken-for-granted practices, illuminate factors that shape client and clinical behaviour, suggest new interventions based on clients' experiences, identify and evaluate optimal measures of care, enhance understanding of organizational culture and the management of change, and evaluate service delivery (Popay et al 1998).

Common areas of research relevant to clinical practice include the motives, assumptions and perceptions of individuals and groups, and interactions between individuals or between groups. A topic of particular importance is the influence of patient–physiotherapist relationships on health care outcomes. Many studies of patient–physiotherapist relationships have demonstrated the importance of effective communication skills within physiotherapy (Klaber Moffett & Richardson 1997, Potter et al 2003). Such studies can suggest ways of improving therapeutic relationships.

Another area in which qualitative research methods have been used widely in physiotherapy is in the development of theory. An important part of this research has used qualitative research to inform theories of occupation, particularly about the processes of generating practice knowledge and professional knowledge. We regard this kind of research as important for developing professional practice and clinical expertise but, in the main, this research does not address questions that arise in everyday clinical practice. Physiotherapists in clinical practice will probably find the most immediately useful qualitative research is that which explores patients' health-related perceptions and feelings, particularly those that are a consequence of physiotherapy interventions.

By combining qualitative and quantitative research methods, the shortcomings of both approaches can be offset. Consequently it is not surprising that many research projects combine qualitative and quantitative methods. Morgan (1998) classifies combinations of qualitative and quantitative research into four categories: preliminary qualitative methods in a quantitative study, preliminary quantitative methods in a qualitative study, follow-up qualitative methods in a quantitative study, and follow-up quantitative methods in a qualitative study. Qualitative research may be conducted prior to quantitative research to set the direction for exploration with quantitative methods, or as follow-up to quantitative studies,

where it can aid in interpretation. Researchers frequently use qualitative methods to develop projects, interventions and outcome measures. Before carrying out a survey, qualitative methods are often used to develop a questionnaire, and in-depth interviews can be used to identify attitudes and barriers to phenomena (such as regular exercise) before the development of an intervention that aims to influence it.

Some qualitative research that accompanies quantitative research is not of immediate clinical importance; its primary importance is that it provides insights for researchers into requirements for design and analysis. But other qualitative research is directly relevant to clinical decision-making because it provides insights into the way in which an intervention is experienced by those involved in developing, delivering or receiving the intervention. Qualitative research can also help identify which aspects of the intervention are valued, or not, and why (Cochrane Qualitative Research Methods Group & Campbell Process Implementation Methods Group 2003). So it can be useful to read both a study evaluating the effects of an intervention and a complementary study exploring participants' experiences of the intervention.

Such studies can also help by explaining why some patients do not 'comply' with intervention. This information can be used to tailor interventions to individual needs. For example, researchers evaluating the effectiveness and cost-effectiveness of a progressive exercise programme for patients with low back pain carried out a study that explored associations between factors that influence changes in physical activity and the way individuals perceive and behave with their low back pain, and the impact of those perceptions and behaviours on physical activity (Keen et al 1999). The study found that an aversion to physical activity and fear of pain were the two main factors that hindered increases in physical activity, even though the majority of informants believed strongly that being physically active was beneficial. The study suggests (but does not prove) that it may be helpful to identify an aversion to physical activity or fear of pain at the earliest stage in order to tailor advice accordingly.

Another example of how qualitative research can complement quantitative research comes from a study of a sports injury prevention programme. The study sought to describe lessons learned from the implementation of a rugby injury prevention programme carried out as a cohort study (Chalmers et al 2004). Qualitative research methods, including informant interviews, participant observation and the scrutiny of written, visual and archival material, were used to describe the process of implementation of the programme. Among the lessons learned were the difficulties in implementing complex interventions, the advantages of a formal agreement between partners in the implementation of a programme, the central role played by coaches in promoting injury prevention strategies, and the value of describing the process of implementation and monitoring injury outcomes and changes in knowledge, attitudes and behaviour. The authors suggested that professionals wishing to develop injury prevention programmes in other sports could learn from these experiences.

Qualitative research can influence how outcomes are measured and interpreted, as in a trial that tested the effect of a package of physiotherapy interventions for patellofemoral osteoarthritis. This study identified discrepancies in outcomes assessed with qualitative in-depth interviews and a quantitative questionnaire (Campbell et al 2003). The lack of agreement between the two measures provided some insights into how interventions benefit patients, how clinicians could measure outcomes of therapy, and the need for patient-centred outcome measures. It is obvious that this knowledge is of importance for researchers and teachers, and for promoting new high-quality studies, but it might also be helpful to clinicians by suggesting relevant dimensions of health outcome measures.

There are other areas of qualitative research that are highly relevant to practice. Studies that have as their objective to understand clients' health-related perceptions and explore patients' experiences with therapy can be very useful. For example, a study describing how parents experienced living with a child with asthma uncovered four main themes related to management of asthma (Trollvik & Severinsson 2004). One important finding was that parents felt they were not respected by health professionals and that their competence was questioned. The findings emphasize the importance of a mutual dialogue between health care professionals and parents to enable parents to develop the competence necessary for the care of their children. Another study explored how the process of discharge from physiotherapy following stroke was managed and experienced by patients and physiotherapists (Wiles et al 2004). The study found that patients' expectations and optimism about recovery were not confronted at discharge. The notion of natural recovery that was raised with patients by physiotherapists

at discharge, and the information physiotherapists gave about exercise post-discharge, had the effect of maintaining patients' high expectations and hopes for recovery. This might suggest that physiotherapists can make a positive contribution to the process of adaptation and adjustment that stroke survivors experience following discharge.

Qualitative research can also form a basis for developing patient information based on patients' information needs. Much information has been developed over the years based on health professionals' perceptions of patients' needs without asking patients themselves what they perceive their needs to be. By integrating valid and relevant results from research carried out with qualitative methods into clinical practice, physiotherapists may be more able to understand their patients, develop empathy and understanding with them, and convey relevant information to them. Two examples of studies that can inform provision of health information are projects designed to develop patient information for people with low back pain (Glenton 2002, Skelton et al 1995). These studies concluded that patient information should be presented in the user's own language, at several levels of understanding, and should include both evidence-based and experience-based knowledge.

Importantly, although qualitative research gives insights into attitudes to and experiences of therapy and prevention, this evidence cannot provide definitive answers to questions about effects of interventions. There is a particular danger in using research that is designed to describe patients' experiences as justification for a particular intervention. For example, evidence that patients with low back pain enjoy massage should not necessarily be interpreted as indicating that massage should be used to treat back pain. It is often easy to 'jump' directly from information about experiences and attitudes to making inferences about practical interventions. Such interpretations should be made carefully.

Systematic reviews

If clinicians are going to use qualitative research in decision-making, the findings of qualitative research need to be accessible and aggregated in a meaningful way. Summaries of existing studies facilitate the dissemination of findings of qualitative research. Gibson & Martin (2003) have called for international collaboration among qualitative researchers to develop methods for meta-synthesis and the translation of evidence into practice. This is difficult because there are many challenges in combining different philosophical approaches in qualitative research syntheses.

There have been attempts to integrate studies with qualitative methods into systematic reviews of interventions. The Cochrane Collaboration has established a methods group, the Cochrane Qualitative Methods Group, focusing on the inclusion of evidence from qualitative studies into systematic reviews (Cochrane Qualitative Research Methods Group & Campbell Process Implementation Methods Group 2003). The group argues that studies of qualitative methods can provide insight into 'internal' factors, including aspects of professional, managerial or consumer behaviour, and 'external' factors such as policy developments, which facilitate or hinder successful implementation of a programme or service and how it might need to be adapted for large scale roll-out. Such studies can also generate qualitative data on the outcomes of interventions.

> The findings from qualitative research studies can therefore help to answer questions about the impact, appropriateness and acceptability of interventions and thus enhance the scope, relevance and utility of effectiveness reviews (Cochrane Qualitative Research Methods Group & Campbell Process Implementation Methods Group 2003).

The Cochrane Collaboration's 'sister' organization, the Campbell Collaboration, which aims to prepare systematic reviews of social and educational policies and practices, is currently investigating how to review studies of qualitative methods that have evaluated health programmes and health service delivery. Some organizations have published reports that integrate qualitative research with trials in systematic reviews (Thomas et al 2004). An example is a review of the effects of interventions to promote physical activity among children and young people. The review includes an overview of the barriers and motivators extracted from qualitative research (Evidence for Policy and Practice Information and Co-ordinating Centre 2003).

What constitutes evidence about prognosis?

Often our patients ask us when or whether or how much their condition will improve. These are questions about prognosis. How can we learn to make accurate prognoses?

In general we can obtain information about prognosis from clinical observation and from clinical research. We consider these in turn.

Clinical observation

One source of information about prognosis is clinical observation. Experienced clinicians accumulate many observations of patients with a particular condition over the course of their careers. Some therapists may be able to distil their experiences into an accurate statement about typical outcomes. That is, some physiotherapists gain accurate impressions of the prognosis of conditions they see. Astute physiotherapists may go one step further. They may be able to see patterns in the characteristics of patients who subsequently have good outcomes and those who do not. In other words, some physiotherapists may develop the ability to recognize prognostic factors.

Several factors make it difficult for physiotherapists to generate accurate estimates of prognosis or the importance of prognostic factors from clinical observations alone. First, we are often particularly interested in long-term prognoses, and many physiotherapists do not routinely see patients for long-term follow-up. Second, follow-up is usually conducted on a subset of patients, rather than on all patients, and the subset on whom follow-ups are conducted may not be representative, in terms of their prognoses, of all patients initially seen by the physiotherapist. Lastly, in order to obtain reasonably accurate estimates of the prognoses of some conditions, it may be necessary to see several hundred patients with the condition of interest, and, if the condition is not very common, few physiotherapists may ever see enough of the condition to gain accurate impressions of the prognosis (de Bie 2001). For these reasons, deriving prognoses for particular patients or conditions often necessitates supplementing clinical experience with clinical research.

Clinical research

The requirements of a good study of prognosis are less stringent than the requirements of a good study of the effects of intervention. To generate good information about prognosis, researchers must identify a group of people with the condition of interest and see how those people's condition changes over time. Such studies are called longitudinal studies – the term 'longitudinal' implies that observations on any one subject are made at more than one point in time.

The particular type of longitudinal study that involves observing representative samples of people with specific characteristics is called a 'cohort' study. Here the term 'cohort' simply refers to a group of people with some shared characteristics, such as a shared diagnosis. Cohort studies can provide us with information about prognosis, and may also provide us with information about how we can refine the prognosis based on certain prognostic factors.

Prospective and retrospective cohort studies

If the cohorts are identified before the follow-up data are obtained (that is, if subjects are followed forwards in time) then the study is a 'prospective cohort study'.[12]

> Prospective cohort studies are a particularly useful source of information about prognosis.[13]

In other sorts of cohort study, follow-up data are obtained before the cohort has been identified. For example, outcome data may have been collected in the course of routine clinical care and archived in medical records before the researcher initiated the study. In that case the researcher can extract follow-up data that pre-existed identification of the cohort. Such studies are called 'retrospective cohort studies'. Sometimes retrospective cohort studies can also provide us with useful prognostic data.

An example of a prospective cohort study was reported by Albert et al (2001). These authors monitored the presence or absence of pelvic pain in 405 women who had pelvic pain at 33 weeks of pregnancy. In this study each subject was identified as eligible for participation in the study before her outcome measures had been obtained, so this was a prospective cohort study. In contrast, Shelbourne & Heinrich (2004) performed a retrospective cohort study to determine the prognosis of patients with meniscal tears that were not treated at the time of knee reconstruction for anterior cruciate ligament injury. Outcome data were obtained from a database of clinical outcomes measured over a 13-year period prior to the study. As the data were obtained before identification of the cohort, this study was retrospective.

Clinical trials

We can obtain information about prognosis from other sorts of longitudinal study too. Another sort of longitudinal study design that can provide information about prognosis is the clinical trial. Clinical trials are designed to determine the effects of intervention, but they almost always involve longitudinal observation of specific cohorts. Even though the aim of clinical trials is to determine the effects of intervention, they can sometimes generate useful information about prognosis along the way.

The fact that prognostic information exists incidentally in some studies that are designed with a different purpose means that the authors of a clinical trial may not even appreciate that the study contains prognostic information. So prognostic information may be buried, unrecognized and hidden, in reports of clinical trials.[14] This makes finding prognostic information more difficult than finding information about effects of intervention.

Importantly, clinical trials do not have to be *randomized* trials to provide prognostic information. They do not even have to be *controlled* trials. Studies of the effects of intervention must have control groups to distinguish the effects of intervention from the effects of other variables that affect outcomes, but studies of prognosis do not require control groups

---

[12]Some authorities make a slightly different distinction between prospective and retrospective studies. According to Rothman & Greenland (1998), prospective studies are those in which exposure status is measured prior to the onset of disease. We prefer to define prospective studies as those in which the cohort is identified prior to the measurement of outcome because this definition is more broadly applicable: it applies just as well to studies of prognosis (where exposure might be of no interest, and where we may be interested in the evolution of the severity of disease) as it does to studies of aetiology.

[13]Prospective cohort studies are often also the best design for answering another sort of question: questions about aetiology (or 'harm'). Questions about aetiology concern what *causes* disease (that is, they identify factors that are the last-satisfied component in a series of components necessary for the disease; Rothman & Greenland 1998). Establishing causation is more difficult than describing or predicting outcomes. And, although understanding aetiology is important for the development of interventions, it is of less immediate importance to clinical practice than obtaining accurate prognoses. This is because even if we know about risk factors it is not always obvious how to change those risk factors, nor is it necessarily true that changing the risk factors will substantively reduce risk. We will not consider questions about aetiology any further in this book.

[14]Another reason that prognostic information may be hard to find is that many researchers are more interested in prognostic factors (factors that are related to prognosis) than in the prognosis itself. Consequently many research reports contain detailed presentations of information about prognostic factors but little or no information about the prognosis.

because the aim of studies of prognosis is not to determine what caused the outcome, just to describe what the outcome is.

An example of a clinical trial that contains useful information about prognosis is a randomized trial of the effects of specific stabilizing exercises for people with first-episode low back pain (Hides et al 2001). The primary aim of this study was to determine the effectiveness of a particular type of exercise, so subjects were allocated randomly to a group that exercised or a group that did not. But, because this study followed subjects for 3 years, it incidentally provided information about the 3-year prognosis for people with first-episode low back pain.

Although randomized trials provide the best (least biased) estimates of effects of interventions, they often provide less satisfactory estimates of prognosis. This, as we shall see in Chapter 6, is because good estimates of prognosis rely heavily on obtaining representative samples. Randomized trials, and clinical trials in general, often require considerable commitment from participants, and consequently often involve highly selected groups of participants that are not representative of any easily identifiable population. When that is the case, clinical trials provide less useful estimates of prognosis.

Systematic reviews

Some authors have reviewed the literature on prognosis for particular conditions. Narrative reviews of prognosis are prone to the same sorts of bias as narrative reviews of the effects of intervention. Consequently over the last decade, methodologists have begun to develop methods for conducting systematic reviews of prognosis (see, for example, Altman 2001).[15]

> High-quality systematic reviews potentially provide us with a transparent and minimally biased overview of all the best data on the prognosis of a particular condition, so, when they are available, they may constitute the best single source of information about the prognosis for that condition.

Some examples of systematic reviews of prognosis are those by Scholten-Peeters et al (2003), on

the prognosis of whiplash-associated disorders, and Pengel et al (2003), on the prognosis of acute low back pain.

In summary, we can obtain information about prognosis from prospective and retrospective cohort studies and clinical trials, or from systematic reviews of these studies. Of course, not all such studies provide good information about prognosis. In Chapter 5 we shall examine how to differentiate high-quality and low-quality information about prognosis.

What constitutes evidence about the accuracy of diagnostic and screening tests?

How can we get good information about the accuracy of diagnostic tests? Again, we could rely on clinical observations or we could consult the research literature.

Clinical observation

To find out about the accuracy of a diagnostic test we need to apply the test to many people and then see how well the test's findings correspond with what subsequently proves to be the correct diagnosis. It may be possible to do this in routine clinical practice, but more often than not circumstances conspire to make it difficult to obtain unbiased estimates of the accuracy of diagnostic tests in the course of routine clinical practice. Why is that so?

In routine clinical practice, the true diagnosis may be obtained from subsequent investigations. For example, a clinician's impressions about the presence of a rotator cuff tear, based on tests such as O'Brien's test, may subsequently be confirmed or refuted by arthroscopy Usually, however, information about the correct diagnosis is not *routinely* available, because usually not *all* patients are subjected to subsequent investigation. Consequently, clinical observations of the concordance of clinical tests and the true diagnosis are almost always based on a (sometimes small) subset of patients that are tested. Insofar as it is possible that the accuracy of the diagnostic test may be higher or lower in that subgroup, clinical observations of the accuracy of the diagnostic test may underestimate or overestimate the accuracy of the test. This makes it difficult to generate accurate estimates of diagnostic accuracy on the basis of unstructured clinical observations alone.

[15]The chapter by Altman (2001) is concerned primarily with studies of prognostic factors, rather than prognosis itself. Nonetheless much of it is relevant to systematic reviews of prognosis.

Better estimates of the accuracy of diagnostic tests may be obtained from high-quality clinical research.

Clinical research

Cross-sectional studies

Like clinical observations, clinical studies of the accuracy of diagnostic tests involve applying the test to many people and then determining how well the test's findings correspond with the correct diagnosis. Such study designs are usually called cross-sectional studies, to distinguish them from longitudinal studies. Studies of the accuracy of diagnostic tests are cross-sectional studies because they are concerned with how accurately a test can determine whether a disease or condition is present at the time the test is conducted (Knottnerus 2002).

In cross-sectional studies of diagnostic tests, a group of subjects is subjected to the test of interest. We will call this the clinical test. The same subjects are also tested with some other test that is thought to establish the true diagnosis. The test used to establish the correct diagnosis is often called the 'gold standard' or 'reference standard' test. Reference standards are often tests that are more invasive or more expensive than the clinical test that is the subject of the research. For example, a recent study compared the findings of a range of simple clinical tests for lumbosacral nerve root compression in people with sciatica (the clinical tests included questions such as whether pain was worse in the leg than in the back, straight leg raise test, weakness, absence of tendon reflexes, and so on) with the findings of magnetic resonance imaging (MRI) (Vroomen et al 2002). In this study, MRI was the reference standard.

Sometimes the reference standard is hindsight, because the true diagnosis becomes apparent only with time. An example is provided by studies of 'red flags' used in the assessment of low back pain (Deyo & Diehl 1988, Henschke et al 2009). Red flags such as recent unexplained weight loss may be suggestive of cancer. But there is no satisfactory reference standard for immediate diagnosis of cancer in people presenting with low back pain. It is possible that some sorts of cancer might not be detected easily, even with invasive or expensive diagnostic tools. The diagnosis might be established only some time later when the disease has advanced. In that case the reference standard may involve extended monitoring of patients. The correct diagnosis at the time of the initial test may be considered to be cancer if

extended follow-up subsequently detects cancer, and the diagnosis is considered to be something other than cancer if extended follow-up does not detect cancer.[16,17]

Two sorts of cross-sectional study can be distinguished, based on how the researchers go about recruiting ('sampling') subjects for the study. The most useful sorts of study seek to sample from the population of subjects suspected of the diagnosis. For example, the study of clinical tests for lumbosacral nerve root compression cited above (Vroomen et al 2002) recruited subjects with back pain radiating into the leg because this is the population in which the diagnosis of lumbosacral nerve root compression is suspected. As expected, MRI subsequently confirmed nerve root compression in some but not all subjects. The true diagnosis for each subject was not known until after the subject had entered the study. Such studies are sometimes called, somewhat confusingly, 'cohort studies'.[18]

In an alternative approach, the researchers recruit two groups of subjects: one group consists of subjects who are thought to have the diagnosis, and the other group consists of subjects thought not to have the diagnosis. For example, Bruske et al (2002) investigated the accuracy of Phalen's test for diagnosis of carpal tunnel syndrome by recruiting two groups of subjects: one group had clinically and electromyographically confirmed carpal tunnel syndrome and the other was a group of volunteers who did not complain of any hand symptoms. The researchers sought

---

[16]Technically, such studies are cross-sectional studies and not, as it first appears, longitudinal studies, even though they involve following patients over time (Knottnerus 2002). This is because the focus of the study is the test findings and diagnosis at the time that the initial test was conducted. In studies of diagnostic tests, extended follow-up is intended to provide information about the *diagnosis* at the time of the initial test, not the subsequent *prognosis*.

[17]One problem with diagnostic test studies in which the reference standard involves extended follow-up is that the disease may develop between the time of the initial testing and the follow-up. This would cause the study to be biased in the direction of making the test appear less accurate than it really is.

[18]The application of the terms 'cohort study' and 'case–control study' to cross-sectional studies is confusing because many people think of cohort studies and case–control studies as types of longitudinal study. Epidemiologists who apply the terms 'cohort study' and 'case–control study' to cross-sectional studies of diagnostic tests argue that the essential characteristic of cohort studies and case–control studies is the method of sampling. In cohort studies the researcher seeks to sample in a representative way from the population about which inferences are to be made. In case–control studies of diagnostic tests the researcher intentionally samples separately from two populations: a population with the diagnosis and a population without the diagnosis.

to determine whether Phalen's test could discriminate accurately between the two groups of subjects. Studies such as these are sometimes called 'case–control' studies, although again the terminology is a little confusing. In Chapter 5 we shall see that cohort studies provide a much better source of information about the accuracy of diagnostic tests than case–control studies.

Randomized trials

Theoretically we could use randomized trials to tell us about the usefulness of diagnostic tests. Trials do not necessarily tell us about the accuracy of diagnostic tests, but they can tell us about the effects of using a diagnostic test on patients' outcomes.

The principle of using randomized trials to investigate the effects of diagnostic tests is simple. Subjects are allocated randomly to groups that either receive or do not receive the diagnostic test of interest[19] and the outcomes of the two groups are compared. If the test provides accurate diagnostic information that supports better decisions about management, this will be reflected in better health outcomes in the group that is tested. On the other hand, if the diagnostic test does not provide accurate information, or if it does provide accurate information but that information does not contribute to better management, the tested group will not have better outcomes.

Several randomized trials have been conducted to determine the value of routine X-rays in primary care of people with low back pain. In the trials by Kerry et al (2000) and P Miller et al (2002), patients presenting to general medical practitioners with low back pain were either routinely referred for X-rays or not, and the outcomes of the two groups (such as disability, subsequent medical consultations and health care costs) were compared.

Screening

We can differentiate two sorts of diagnostic testing. The first is the sort of diagnostic testing we considered in the preceding section: the test is applied when people present with a particular problem and we use the test to determine a diagnosis to explain that problem. A second sort of test is a screening test. Screening tests are tests that we apply to people who we have no particular reason to

suspect of having the diagnosis. The screening may be practice-based (for example, all patients presenting with low back pain may be screened for depression; Levy et al 2002) or it may be part of a community-based programme (for example, in some countries adolescent girls are screened for scoliosis in school-based screening programmes; Yawn et al 1999). The potential value of screening is that it makes it possible incidentally to detect disease early. And for some diseases early detection may enable more effective management.

Screening programmes are best evaluated with randomized trials because randomized trials provide information about the end-benefit of screening. The screening test will produce demonstrable beneficial effects only if it is capable of accurately detecting the condition of interest *and* detection occurs significantly earlier than it otherwise would *and* early detection means that intervention can be more effective *and* these beneficial effects are not outweighed by the harm produced by false-positive and false-negative screening test results.

Most of the randomized trials of diagnostic procedures have been trials of medical screening tests. Some important examples are randomized trials of the effects of mammogram screening for breast cancer and PAP smears for cervical cancer (Batal et al 2000, Miller et al 2002). Clinical trials of screening tests usually have to study very large numbers of patients, so they are often very expensive. Consequently there are very few randomized trials of diagnostic or screening tests conducted by physiotherapists – possibly none! Until randomized trials are conducted, many physiotherapists will continue to screen for a range of conditions in the absence of evidence of a beneficial effect. (An example is the practice, in some countries, of screening first-grade school pupils for clumsiness or minimal cerebral dysfunction.)

As there are very few randomized trials of screening tests in physiotherapy, this book will concentrate on evaluating studies of diagnostic test accuracy, and we will not consider randomized trials of screening tests further. In the next few years we hope to see the publication of randomized trials of screening tests used by physiotherapists.

Systematic reviews

In recent years the first systematic reviews of studies of the accuracy of diagnostic tests have been published. Examples are systematic reviews of tests

---

[19]Alternatively, both groups could be tested but the results of the tests made available for only one group.

for anterior cruciate ligament injury (Scholten et al 2003), the Ottawa ankle rules (Bachmann et al 2003), and tests for carpal tunnel syndrome (d'Arcy & McGee 2000). Like systematic reviews of studies of the effects of intervention or of prognosis, systematic reviews of studies of the accuracy of diagnostic tests potentially provide transparent and unbiased assessments of studies of diagnostic test accuracy, and some provide precise estimates of test accuracy, so they potentially provide the best single source of information about the accuracy of diagnostic tests. The Cochrane Collaboration recently began to publish systematic reviews of the accuracy of diagnostic tests in the Cochrane Library. Examples include reviews on clinical tests for radiculopathy (van der Windt et al 2010) and red flags for vertebral fracture (Henschke et al 2010) in people with low back pain.

Enough talk. It's time for some action. Let's find some studies with which to answer our clinical questions.

References

Albert, H., Godskesen, M., Westergaard, J., 2001. Prognosis in four syndromes of pregnancy-related pelvic pain. Acta Obstet. Gynecol. Scand. 80, 505–510.

Altman, D.G., 2001. Systematic reviews of evaluations of prognostic variables. In: Egger, M., Davey Smith, G., Altman, D.G. (Eds.), Systematic reviews in health care. Meta-analysis in context. BMJ Books, London, pp. 228–247.

Bachmann, L.M., Kolb, E., Koller, M.T., et al., 2003. Accuracy of Ottawa ankle rules to exclude fractures of the ankle and mid-foot: systematic review. BMJ 326, 417.

Barlow, D.H., Herson, M., 1984. Single case experimental designs: strategies for studying behavior change. Allyn and Bacon, Boston.

Batal, H., Biggerstaff, S., Dunn, T., et al., 2000. Cervical cancer screening in the urgent care setting. J. Gen. Intern. Med. 15, 389–394.

Beecher, K.H., 1955. The powerful placebo. JAMA 159, 1602–1606.

Benson, K., Hartz, A.J., 2000. A comparison of observational studies and randomized, controlled trials. N. Engl. J. Med. 342, 1878–1886.

Black, N., 1996. Why we need observational studies to evaluate the effectiveness of health care. BMJ 312, 1215–1218.

Bland, J.M., Altman, D.G., 1994. Statistics notes: some examples of regression towards the mean. BMJ 309, 780.

Bruske, J., Bednarski, M., Grzelec, H., et al., 2002. The usefulness of the Phalen test and the Hoffmann–Tinel sign in the diagnosis of carpal tunnel syndrome. Acta Orthop. Belg. 68, 141–145.

Buchbinder, R., Ptasznik, R., Gordon, J., et al., 2002. Ultrasound-guided extracorporeal shock wave therapy for plantar fasciitis: a randomized controlled trial. JAMA 288, 1364–1372.

Campbell, R., Quilt, B., Dieppe, P., 2003. Discrepancies between patients' assessments of outcome: qualitative study nested within a randomised controlled trial. BMJ 326, 252–253.

Chaitow, L., 2001. Muscle energy techniques. Churchill Livingstone, Edinburgh.

Chalmers, D.J., Simpson, J.C., Depree, R., 2004. Tackling rugby injury: lessons learned from the implementation of a five-year sports injury prevention program. J. Sci. Med. Sport 7, 74–84.

Chen, H.S., Chen, L.M., Huang, T.W., 2001. Treatment of painful heel syndrome with shock waves. Clin. Orthop. Relat. Res. 387, 41–46.

Chipchase, L.S., Trinkle, D., 2003. Therapeutic ultrasound: clinician usage and perception of efficacy. Hong Kong Physiother. J. 21, 5–14.

Cochrane Qualitative Research Methods Group & Campbell Process Implementation Methods Group, 2003. http://www.joannabriggs.edu.au/cqrmg/role.html 6 Nov 2010.

Concato, J., Shah, N., Horwitz, R.I., 2000. Randomized controlled trials, observational studies, and the hierarchy of research designs. N. Engl. J. Med. 342, 1887–1892.

d'Arcy, C.A., McGee, S., 2000. Does this patient have carpal tunnel syndrome? JAMA 283, 3110–3117.

de Bie, R., 2001. Critical appraisal of prognostic studies: an introduction. Physiother. Theory Pract. 17, 161–171.

de Vries, H.A., 1961. Prevention of muscular distress after exercise. Res. Q. 32, 177–185.

Deyo, R., Diehl, A., 1988. Cancer as a cause of back pain. Frequency, clinical presentation and diagnostic strategies. J. Gen. Intern. Med. 3, 230–238.

Egger, M., Davey Smith, G., Altman, D.G. (Eds.), 2001. Systematic reviews in health care. Meta-analysis in context. BMJ Books, London, pp. 228–247.

Evans, A.M., 2003. Relationship between 'growing pains' and foot posture in children. J. Am. Podiatr. Med. Assoc. 93, 111–117.

Evidence for Policy and Practice Information and Co-ordinating Centre (EPPI-Centre), 2003. Children and physical activity: a systematic review of research on barriers and facilitators. The Evidence for Policy and Practice Information and Co-ordinating Centre Social Science Research Unit (SSRU), Institute of Education, University of London. Online. Available: http://eppi.ioe.ac.uk/EPPIWeb/home.aspx 6 Nov 2010.

Gibson, B., Martin, D., 2003. Qualitative research and evidence-based physiotherapy practice. Physiotherapy 89, 350–358.

Glass, G.V., McGaw, B., Smith, M.L., 1981. Meta-analysis in social research. Sage, Beverly Hills.

Glenton, C., 2002. Developing patient-centred information for back pain sufferers. Health Expect. 5, 19–29.

Haake, M., Buch, M., Schoellner, C., et al., 2003. Extracorporeal shock wave therapy for plantar fasciitis:

randomised controlled multicentre trial. BMJ 327, 75.

Hedges, L.V., Olkin, I., 1985. Statistical methods for meta-analysis. Academic Press, Orlando.

Henschke, N., Maher, C.G., Refshauge, K.M., et al., 2009. Prevalence of and screening for serious spinal pathology in patients presenting to primary care with acute low back pain. Arthritis Rheum. 60, 3072–3080.

Henschke, N., Williams, C.M., Maher, C.G., et al., 2010. Red flags to screen for vertebral fracture in patients presenting with low-back pain. Cochrane Database Syst. Rev. (8), CD008643.

Herbert, R.D., Higgs, J., 2004. Complementary research paradigms. Aust. J. Physiother. 50, 63–64.

Herson, D.H., Barlow, M., 1984. Single case experimental designs. Strategies for studying behavior change, second ed. Pergamon, New York.

Hides, J., Jull, G.A., Richardson, C.A., 2001. Long-term effects of specific stabilizing exercises for first-episode low back pain. Spine 26, E243–E248.

Higgs, J., Titchen, A., Neville, V., 2001. Professional practice and knowledge. In: Higgs, J., Titchen, A. (Eds.), Practice knowledge and expertise in the health professions. Butterworth-Heinemann, Oxford, pp. 3–9.

Hrobjartsson, A., 2002. What are the main methodological problems in the estimation of placebo effects? J. Clin. Epidemiol. 55, 430–435.

Hrobjartsson, A., Gotzsche, P.C., 2003. Placebo treatment versus no treatment (Cochrane review). In: The Cochrane Library, Issue 2. Wiley, Chichester.

Hunter, J.E., Schmidt, F.L., Jackson, G.B., 1982. Meta-analysis: cumulating research findings across studies. Sage, Beverly Hills.

Hutzler, Y., Chacham, A., Bergman, U., et al., 1998. Effects of a movement and swimming program on vital capacity and water orientation skills of children with cerebral palsy. Dev. Med. Child Neurol. 40, 176–181.

Jadad, A.R., Cook, D.J., Jones, A., et al., 1998. Methodology and reports of systematic reviews and meta-analyses: a comparison of Cochrane reviews with articles published in paper-based journals. JAMA 280, 278–280.

Jones, R., 1995. Why do qualitative research? BMJ 311, 2.

Keen, S., Dowell, A.C., Hurst, K., et al., 1999. Individuals with low back pain: how do they view physical activity? Fam. Pract. 16, 39–45.

Kelley, G.A., Kelley, K.S., 2004. Efficacy of resistance exercise on lumbar spine and femoral neck bone mineral density in premenopausal women: a meta-analysis of individual patient data. J. Womens Health 13, 293–300.

Kerry, S., Hilton, S., Patel, S., et al., 2000. Routine referral for radiography of patients presenting with low back pain: is patients' outcome influenced by GPs' referral for plain radiography? Health Technol. Assess. 4, 1–119.

Kienle, G.S., Kiene, H., 1997. The powerful placebo effect: fact or fiction? J. Clin. Epidemiol. 50, 1311–1318.

Klaber Moffett, J.A., Richardson, P.H., 1997. The influence of the physiotherapist–patient relationship on pain and disability. Physiother. Theory Pract. 13, 89–96.

Knottnerus, J.A., 2002. The evidence base of clinical diagnosis. BMJ Books, London.

Kunz, R., Oxman, A.D., 1998. The unpredictability paradox: review of empirical comparisons of randomised and nonrandomised clinical trials. BMJ 317, 1185–1190.

Levy, H.I., Hanscom, B., Boden, S.D., 2002. Three-question depression screener used for lumbar disc herniations and spinal stenosis. Spine 27, 1232–1237.

Lilford, R.J., 2003. Ethics of clinical trials from a Bayesian and decision analytic perspective: whose equipoise is it anyway? BMJ 326, 980–981.

Malterud, K., 2001. The art and science of clinical knowledge: evidence beyond measures and numbers. Lancet 358, 397–399.

Miller, A.B., To, T., Baines, C.J., et al., 2002. The Canadian National Breast Screening Study – 1: breast cancer mortality after 11 to 16 years of follow-up. A randomized screening trial of mammography in women age 40 to 49 years. Ann. Intern. Med. 137, 305–312.

Miller, P., Kendrick, D., Bentley, E., et al., 2002. Cost-effectiveness of lumbar spine radiography in primary care patients with low back pain. Spine 15, 2291–2297.

Morgan, D., 1998. Practical strategies for combining qualitative and quantitative methods: applications for health research. Qual. Health Res. 8, 362–376.

Moseley, A.M., 1997. The effect of casting combined with stretching on passive ankle dorsiflexion in adults with traumatic head injuries. Phys. Ther. 77, 240–247.

Moseley, A.M., Elkins, M.R., Herbert, R.D., et al., 2009. Cochrane reviews use more rigorous methods than non-Cochrane reviews: survey of systematic reviews in physiotherapy. J. Clin. Epidemiol. 62, 1021–1030.

Pengel, H.L.M., Herbert, R.D., Maher, C.G., et al., 2003. A systematic review of prognosis of acute low back pain. BMJ 327, 323–327.

Piantadosi, S., 1997. Clinical trials: a methodologic perspective. Wiley, New York.

Popay, J., Rogers, A., Williams, G., 1998. Rationale and standards for the systematic review of qualitative literature in health services research. Qual. Health Res. 3, 341–351.

Pope, C., Mays, N. (Eds.), 2000. Qualitative research in health care, second ed. BMJ Books, London.

Potter, M., Gordon, S., Hamer, P., 2003. The difficult patient in private practice physiotherapy: a qualitative study. Aust. J. Physiother. 49, 53–61.

Province, M.A., Hadley, E.C., Hornbrook, M.C., et al., 1995. The effects of exercise on falls in elderly patients. A preplanned meta-analysis of the FICSIT Trials. Frailty and injuries: cooperative studies of intervention techniques. JAMA 273, 1381–1383.

Rothman, K.J., Greenland, S., 1998. Modern epidemiology. Williams and Wilkins, Philadelphia.

Sackett, D.L., Haynes, R.B., Guyatt, G.H., et al., 1991. Clinical epidemiology. A basic science for clinical medicine. Little, Brown, Boston.

Sacks, F.M., Tonkin, A.M., Shepherd, J., et al., 2000. Effect of pravastatin on coronary disease events in subgroups defined by coronary risk factors: the Prospective Pravastatin Pooling Project. Circulation 102, 1893–1900.

Scheel, I.B., Hagen, K.B., Herrin, J., et al., 2002. A call for action: a randomized controlled trial of two strategies to implement active sick leave for patients with low back pain. Spine 27, 561–566.

Scholten, R.J., Opstelten, W., van der Plas, C.G., et al., 2003. Accuracy of physical diagnostic tests for assessing ruptures of the anterior cruciate ligament: a meta-analysis. J. Fam. Pract. 52, 689–694.

Scholten-Peeters, G.G.M., Verhagen, A.P., Bekkering, G.E., et al., 2003. Prognostic factors of whiplash-associated disorders: a systematic review of prospective cohort studies. Pain 104, 303–322.

Seers, K., 2004. Qualitative research. In: Dawes, M., Davies, P., Gray, A. et al., (Eds.), Evidence-based practice. A primer for health care professionals, second ed. Churchill Livingstone, London, pp. 133–145.

Shelbourne, K.D., Heinrich, J., 2004. The long-term evaluation of lateral meniscus tears left in situ at the time of anterior cruciate ligament reconstruction. Arthroscopy 20, 346–351.

Skelton, A.M., Murphy, E.A., Murphy, R.J., et al., 1995. Patient education for low back pain in general practice. Patient Educ. Couns. 25, 329–334.

Smith, G.C.S., Pell, J.P., 2003. Parachute use to prevent death and major trauma related to gravitational challenge: systematic review of randomised controlled trials. BMJ 327, 1459–1461.

Thomas, J., Harden, A., Oakley, A., et al., 2004. Integrating qualitative research with trials in systematic reviews. BMJ 328, 1010–1012.

Tolfrey, K., Campbell, I.G., Batterham, A.M., 1998. Exercise training induced alterations in prepubertal children's lipid–lipoprotein profile. Med. Sci. Sports Exerc. 30, 1684–1692.

Trollvik, A., Severinsson, E., 2004. Parents' experiences of asthma: process from chaos to coping. Nurs. Health Sci. 6 (2), 93–99.

van der Heijden, G.J., Leffers, P., Wolters, P.J., et al., 1999. No effect of bipolar interferential electrotherapy and pulsed ultrasound for soft tissue shoulder disorders: a randomised controlled trial. Ann. Rheum. Dis. 58, 530–540.

van der Windt, D.A., Simons, E., Riphagen, I.I., et al., 2010. Physical examination for lumbar radiculopathy due to disc herniation in patients with low-back pain. Cochrane Database Syst. Rev. (2), CD007431.

Vickers, A.J., de Craen, A.J.M., 2000. Why use placebos in clinical trials? A narrative review of the methodological literature. J. Clin. Epidemiol. 53, 157–161.

Vlaeyen, J.W.S., de Jong, J., Geilen, M., et al., 2001. Graded exposure in vivo in the treatment of pain-related fear: a

replicated single-case experimental design in four patients with chronic low back pain. Behav. Res. Ther. 39, 151–166.

Voss, D.E., Ionta, M.K., Myers, B.J., 1985. Proprioceptive neuromuscular facilitation: patterns and techniques, third ed. Harper & Row, Philadelphia.

Vroomen, P.C., de Krom, M.C., Wilmink, J.T., et al., 2002. Diagnostic value of history and physical examination in patients suspected of lumbosacral nerve root compression. J. Neurol. Neurosurg. Psychiatry 72, 630–634.

Wedlick, L.T., 1954. Ultrasonics. Aust. J. Physiother. 1, 28–29.

Whitehead, W., 1901. The surgical treatment of migraine. BMJ i, 335–336.

Wickstrom, G., Bendix, T., 2000. The 'Hawthorne effect' – what did the original Hawthorne studies actually show? Scand. J. Work Environ. Health 26, 363–367.

Wiles, R., Ashburn, A., Payne, S., et al., 2004. Discharge from physiotherapy following stroke: the management of disappointment. Soc. Sci. Med. (6), 1263–1273.

Yawn, B.P., Yawn, R.A., Hodge, D., et al., 1999. A population-based study of school scoliosis screening. JAMA 282, 1427–1432.

Finding the evidence

4

CHAPTER CONTENTS

Overview 39
Search strategies 39
  The world wide web 40
  Decision support tools 40
  Selecting search terms 41
  Wild cards 42
  Combining search terms with
  AND and OR 42
Finding evidence of effects of interventions . . 43
  PEDro 44
  Simple Search 44
  Advanced Search 46
  The Cochrane Library 48
Finding evidence of prognosis
and diagnostic tests 51
Finding evidence of experiences 55
  CINAHL 55
  PubMed 56
Getting full text 58
Finding evidence of advances in
clinical practice (browsing) 60
References 60

OVERVIEW

Having formulated a clinical question it is possible to start looking for relevant evidence. This involves searching electronic databases. Evidence of effects of physiotherapy interventions is best found in PEDro or the Cochrane Library. Evidence of experiences is best found using CINAHL or PubMed. And evidence of prognosis or the accuracy of diagnostic tests is best found using the Clinical Queries function in PubMed.

Regardless of what database is searched, it is important to select search terms carefully, and to combine search terms in a way that ensures the search is optimally sensitive, specific and efficient.

Search strategies

In this chapter we explore how to find evidence that can be used to answer questions about the effects of therapy, experiences, prognosis and diagnosis.

Finding evidence involves searching computer databases of the health care literature. The chapter suggests databases to search and search strategies for each database. At the end of the chapter we consider how you can obtain the full text of the studies you have identified.

Databases come and go, and some databases are more accessible than others. We are mindful that suggestions about which database to search can quickly become obsolete, and that some readers will have access to more databases than others. For this reason we have chosen to recommend a small number of widely available databases. Wherever possible we recommend databases that can be accessed without subscription. We also recognize that the ability to access libraries and the internet varies enormously between therapists and across countries. Therefore we suggest a number of mechanisms for obtaining full text. Unfortunately, access will remain difficult for some.

The purpose of this chapter is to help busy clinicians find answers to their clinical questions. It is not intended as a guide for researchers or systematic reviewers. Clinicians need to treat patients, so, unlike systematic reviewers, they do not have the time needed to perform exhaustive searches of the literature. They should perform searches that are efficient, but not comprehensive. Consequently our goal in this chapter will be to identify strategies for finding good evidence that pertains to a clinical question (ideally, the best evidence) in as short a time as possible. We will not try to find *all* relevant evidence.

Efficient searching means performing sensitive and specific searches. By sensitive, we mean that the search finds most of the relevant studies. By specific, we mean the search does not return too many irrelevant studies. A sensitive and specific search finds most of the relevant records and leaves out most of the irrelevant records – it does not find lots of 'junk'.

You may want to read this chapter with an internet-connected computer at hand. That way you can use databases and search strategies as they are presented. Try using each database and search strategy to search for questions relevant to your clinical practice.

Keep in mind that the aim is to do quick and efficient searches. Sometimes your search will quickly yield what you are looking for. Sometimes you will have to follow a few false leads before finding a gem. And sometimes your search will yield nothing. A temptation, especially for those with more obsessive traits, is to search through screen after screen of many hundreds of studies in the hope of finding something worthwhile. Try to resist the temptation! If your search returns hundreds of hits, refine your search so that you need sift through a smaller number of hits. If you don't find evidence that relates to your question reasonably quickly, give up and resign yourself to the fact that the evidence either does not exist or you were unable to find it without difficulty. It is unproductive and discouraging to search fruitlessly. You can spend a long time looking for something that does not exist.

Like all skills, literature searching improves with practice. If you are inexperienced at searching the literature you may find your initial attempts time consuming and frustrating. (Your searches may be insensitive or non-specific.) Don't be discouraged. With practice you will become quicker and more able to find the best evidence. A reasonable goal to aspire to, at least with a fast internet connection, is to be able routinely to find the best available evidence in 3 minutes.

Some readers will be able to enlist the help of a librarian when searching. If you have this opportunity, take advantage of it. The best way to learn how to conduct efficient searches is to observe a skilled librarian conduct searches and then have the librarian give you feedback on your own search strategies. Help pages, search tips and tutorials on the homepages of the databases you are searching might also be very useful.

The world wide web

The world wide web has become an invaluable source of information. It contains information on everything from election results in Paraguay to how to build an atomic bomb. Internet-savvy people, when confronted with almost any question, will open up a web browser and search the world wide web with a search engine such as Google or Yahoo.

Google and Yahoo provide a very convenient way to find film reviews and phone numbers, but they may not be the best way of finding high-quality clinical research. Some of the sites containing high-quality clinical research cannot be searched by these search engines. And even if they can, you will often be presented with thousands of search results. Generic search engines such as Google and Yahoo do not provide a useful way of searching for high-quality clinical research because they fail to detect most relevant research.

Google Scholar is a subset of Google and an example of a freely accessible web search engine that focuses on scientific literature. It searches through different scientific publications such as peer-reviewed journals, books and reports published by scientific publishing houses as well as governmental agencies, universities and other academic institutions. Google Scholar might be useful when you want to learn more about a subject or do initial searches to get a glimpse of existing research literature. However, even though search engines like Google, Yahoo and Google Scholar are useful in many ways, they are not designed to answer clinical questions. They lack transparency regarding their content and coverage and they tend to return an overwhelming number of search results.

Decision support tools

If you want to find high-quality clinical research you will need, instead, to search databases designed to meet your specific information needs. To find a quick answer to a question about the effects of therapy, prognosis or diagnosis you could try searching BMJ

BestPractice or UpToDate. These are web-based decision support tools aimed at providing high-quality point-of-care information to busy health care professionals, including physiotherapists. They are designed for quick navigation and do not require advanced search or appraisal skills. The content is based on a combination of the best available research evidence, guidelines and expert opinions. Both BMJ BestPractice and UpToDate are available by paid subscription only. So, if you wish to access these resources, you will need to subscribe. Alternatively, if you have an affiliation with a hospital or a university library you may be able to access these resources through your library.

BMJ BestPractice is available at http://bestpractice.bmj.com/. It contains information about over 10 000 diagnoses and helps you find evidence-based recommendations about prevention, step-by-step diagnosis, treatment and follow-up. You can also learn about aetiology and epidemiology. You can quickly browse through the content or do simple searches. Clinical Evidence is a subset of BMJ BestPractice and provides evidence based systematic overviews of treatment effects (both benefits and harms). UpToDate (http://www.uptodate.com/) is another example of a clinical point-of-care tool. The structure is quite different from that of BMJ BestPractice. Through simple searching and link navigation you can read through articles covering many different topics within more than 14 medical specialties. Even though physiotherapy is not the main focus of either BMJ BestPractice or UpToDate, both databases have a broad and deep coverage of diagnoses and treatments and you might find answers to your question here. You will also find patient information and references to relevant publications.

However, these resources may not always be of help to you. Perhaps you cannot find anything relevant to your question or perhaps the topic you are looking for is not fully updated with the latest research. Also note that BMJ BestPractice and UpToDate are not designed to answer questions about experiences, and the search options are limited. Often you will need to search specialist databases of the health science literature, either with a general medical focus or with a special focus on physiotherapy. A range of these databases exists, and each is particularly suited to finding evidence pertaining to particular sorts of question. Later in this chapter we will consider which database should be searched to answer each of our four types of clinical question, and we will look at database-specific search strategies. But first it is useful to explore some generic issues that apply to searching of all databases.

Selecting search terms

Regardless of what sort of question you are seeking answers to and what sort of database you search, you will need to select search terms. That is, you will need to specify words that tell the database what you are searching for.

Herein lies the art to efficient searching. Carefully selected search terms will usually find a manageable number of relevant studies. A poorly constructed search may return thousands of studies or none at all, or it may return studies that are irrelevant to your question. Search terms should be selected carefully.

Think through the following steps before typing search terms:

1. First, identify the key elements of your question (see Chapter 2). If the question was 'Does weight-supported training improve walking performance more than unsupported walking training following stroke?', the key elements might be *weight-supported training*, *walking performance* and *stroke*.

2. Now think about which of those key elements are likely to be uniquely answered by the studies you are interested in. There are likely to be many studies on stroke, and many studies on walking, but few on weight-supported training. Consequently a search looking for studies about weight-supported training is likely to be more specific than a search for studies about stroke or walking.

3. Lastly, think about alternative terms that could be used to describe each of the key elements.

   Weight-supported training could be described as 'weight supported training' or 'weight-supported training' (note the hyphen) or 'training with weight support' or 'weight-supported walking' or 'walking with weight support', and so on – these synonyms, and most other alternative terms for weight-supported training, contain the word 'weight', suggesting that 'weight' may be a good search term.

   Alternative search terms for walking include 'walking', 'gait', and perhaps 'ambulate', 'ambulation' and 'ambulating'. As at least three distinctly different terms are used to describe walking it is a little more difficult to search for studies using the key element of walking. The same difficulty is found in searches for studies on stroke, because a stroke can also be called a cerebrovascular accident, or cerebro-vascular accident (again, note the hyphen) or CVA. The best search terms are those that have few, quite similar, synonyms.

Sometimes a particular search term is uniquely associated with the search question and has few synonyms. Then the search strategy is obvious. For example, if you wanted to know 'Does the Butenko technique reduce the incidence of asthma attacks in children?', you could use the term 'Butenko', because it is likely to be more or less uniquely associated with your question; there are few, if any, synonyms for 'Butenko'.

There are many ways of finding relevant synonyms for search terms. You can use traditional medical dictionaries (printed or online). Sometimes you might find useful information about alternative terms in the online encyclopedia Wikipedia at http://en.wikipedia.org/. A very useful tool is the MeSH function in PubMed. MeSH (Medical Subject Headings) is produced by the United States National Library of Medicine. It is a controlled index of medical terms (often called subject headings) arranged by an alphabetical and a hierarchical structure. Each term has a definition and a list of synonyms and spelling variations. The MeSH system is freely available via PubMed at http://www.ncbi.nlm.nih.gov/mesh.[1]

Wild cards

Most databases have the facility to use wild cards to identify word variants. Wild cards are characters that act as a proxy (or substitute) for a string of characters. For example, databases such as PEDro, the Cochrane Library and PubMed all use the asterisk symbol to indicate a wild card. Thus, in these databases, 'lumb*' searches for the words 'lumbar', 'lumbosacral' and 'lumbo-sacral'. Wild cards are particularly useful when it is necessary to find a number of variants of the same word stem.[2]

Combining search terms with AND and OR

All major databases can be searched by explicitly specifying more than one search term. For example, if you were interested in the recurrence of dislocation after primary shoulder dislocation you could search using two terms: 'shoulder' and 'dislocation'. This could yield a more efficient search than using either search term on its own.

When more than one search term is used, it is necessary to specify how the search terms are to be combined. For two search terms we need to specify whether we want to find studies that contain *either* of the search terms or (as in the preceding example) *both* of the search terms. For three or more search terms we can specify whether we are interested in studies that contain *any* of the search terms or *all* of the search terms.

To specify that we want to find studies that contain *any* of the search terms, we combine the search terms with OR. For example, if we were interested in studies of lateral epicondylitis we could specify 'epicondylitis OR tennis elbow'.[3,4] Alternatively, to specify that we want to find studies that contain *all* of the search terms, we combine the search terms with AND. For example, if we were interested in studies of effects of the use of ultrasound for ankle sprain we could specify 'ultrasound AND ankle'.[5]

---

[1]MeSH can also be used to search the contents of PubMed. This is described in more detail later in this chapter.

[2]Whenever a wild card facility is available you should avoid searching for the plural form of words unless you are interested only in the plural. For example, it is generally better to search for 'knee*' than 'knees', and it is better to search for 'laser*' than 'lasers'.

[3]In some databases, such as PubMed, we actually type in the word OR, just as shown. In other databases, such as PEDro, we indicate that we want to combine search terms with OR by clicking on the OR button at the bottom of the screen. (If, in PEDro, you typed 'epicondylitis or tennis elbow' and the AND button was checked (as is the default) then PEDro would go looking for studies that contain all four words, including the word 'or'!) We consider how to specify ANDs and ORs for specific databases later in this chapter.

[4]Wild cards and OR have a similar function: both enable you to search for word variants. Wild cards are efficient in the sense that they don't require as much typing, and they don't even require that you think of the possible variants of a particular word stem. But wild cards are not as flexible as OR. OR makes it possible to find variants of a word with different stems (such as 'neck' and 'cervical').

[5]Note that the search specified 'ultrasound AND ankle', not 'ultrasound AND ankle sprain'. The term 'ankle' is likely to be more sensitive than ankle sprain, because some studies will talk about 'sprains of the ankle' or 'sprained ankles' rather than 'ankle sprains'. The search term 'ankle' will capture either, but the search term 'ankle sprain' might not capture studies that refer to 'sprains of the ankle' or 'sprained ankles'. (Some databases, such as PubMed and the simple search in PEDro will capture either instance with the search term 'ankle sprain'.) Of course, the search term 'ankle' will be far less specific than 'ankle sprain', so the best approach might be to combine all three search terms using AND. The search 'ultrasound AND ankle AND sprain' is likely to be both sensitive and specific.

Box 4.1

Using AND and OR

In general, AND is used to mandate more than one search term, and OR is used to search for word variants or synonyms. We can illustrate how ANDs and ORs are combined using a table such as the following:

	Key term 1	AND	Key term 2	AND ...
Synonym 1				
OR				
Synonym 2				
OR ...				

To perform a search for a question about the effects of ultrasound for lateral epicondylitis, we might consider two key terms, one pertaining to ultrasound and the other pertaining to epicondylitis. There are no obvious synonyms for ultrasound, but a common synonym for 'epicondylitis' is 'tennis elbow'. Also, epicondylitis is occasionally referred to as epicondylalgia. Hence:

	Key term 1	AND	Key term 2
Synonym 1	Ultrasound		epicondyl*
OR			
Synonym 2			tennis elbow

Thus our search would be 'ultrasound AND (epicondyl* OR tennis elbow)'.[6]

In general, we specify OR when we want to broaden a search by looking for alternative key terms or synonyms for key terms. We specify AND when we want to narrow a search by mandating more than one key term. The appropriate use of ANDs and ORs can greatly increase the sensitivity and specificity of database searches. In most (not all) databases it is possible to combine multiple search terms mixing both ANDs and ORs. Box 4.1 illustrates how AND and OR can be combined in a single search.

In many databases we can also use NOT to refine our search. We use this to specify that we want to exclude studies containing specific terms. This might be a tempting way of leaving out irrelevant studies and narrowing our search. But beware, using NOT can cause you to miss important studies! Going back to the example of shoulder dislocation, we might be interested specifically in studies on shoulder dislocation in children rather than adults. So, we could search for '(shoulder AND dislocation) NOT adults'. By doing this we would leave out all studies mentioning the word 'adults'. There may be studies of shoulder dislocation in both children and adults. Such studies might be very relevant, but by searching for 'NOT adults' we would miss those studies. Using NOT to narrow your search is not recommended. Instead, try to think of another search term that should be mentioned in the study and add that to your search with AND. In this example we could add 'AND child*'.

In the rest of this chapter we shall consider specifically how to find evidence of the effects of interventions, experiences, prognosis and accuracy of diagnostic tests. We will depart from the order that we use in most of this book and consider searching for evidence of experiences last, because it is convenient first to discuss issues regarding searches for prognosis and diagnostic accuracy before discussing searches for evidence of experiences.

Finding evidence of effects of interventions

In Chapter 3 we saw that the best evidence of effects of interventions comes from randomized trials or systematic reviews of randomized trials.

Contrary to popular belief, there is an extensive literature of randomized trials and systematic reviews in physiotherapy. At the time of writing (August 2010) there are at least 13 700 randomized trials and 2500 systematic reviews relevant to physiotherapy. (For a description of the trials, see Maher et al 2008.) The rate of production of trials and systematic reviews has accelerated rapidly (Figure 4.1) so that more than one-third of all trials and over half of all systematic reviews relevant to physiotherapy have been published in the last 5 years. At the time of writing, about 14 new randomized trials and 4 new systematic reviews in physiotherapy are published each week.

---

[6]Note the use of brackets. When mixing ANDs and ORs there is potential for ambiguity, and the brackets remove the ambiguity. Can you see the difference between 'ultrasound AND (epicondyl* OR tennis elbow)' and '(ultrasound AND epicondyl*) OR tennis elbow'?

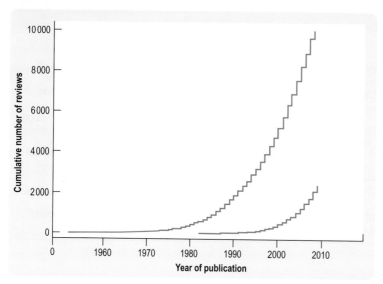

Figure 4.1 • Number of randomized trials and systematic reviews archived on the PEDro database, by year of publication (data extracted August 2010). The first trial on the database was published in 1929 (not shown on the graph), and the first systematic review was published in 1982. Since then, the number and rate of publication has increased exponentially with time. Updated and redrawn from Moseley et al (2002).

PEDro

Perhaps the first place to go looking for evidence of the effects of physiotherapy interventions is PEDro.[7] PEDro is a database of randomized trials, systematic reviews and evidence-based clinical practice guidelines in physiotherapy. In addition it provides evidence-based patient information in a subsite called Physiotherapy Choices. The database is freely available on the world wide web at http://

www.pedro.org.au/. Most of the PEDro website has been translated into Chinese, Portuguese, French and German. The most useful parts of the website are the two search pages located on the top left-hand corner of the PEDro start page. PEDro offers two search facilities: *Simple Search* and *Advanced Search*. We will begin by looking at the *Simple Search* page.

Simple Search

Let's use the *Simple Search* to find evidence about the effects of pulsed ultrasound for reducing pain and disability associated with lateral epicondylitis. (The *Simple Search* page is shown in Figure 4.2.)

---

[7]PEDro stands for Physiotherapy Evidence Database. The 'ro' at the end just gives it a more catchy name.

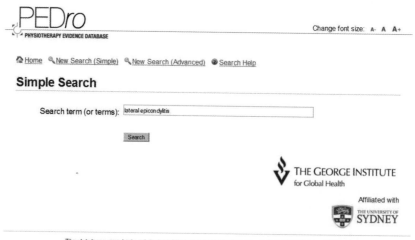

Figure 4.2 • PEDro: *Simple Search* page.

Figure 4.3 • PEDro: *Simple Search* results page.

The *Simple Search* page contains just one box in which you can type words that tell PEDro the topic of your search. When you enter a search term or multiple search terms in this box, PEDro searches for studies that contain those search terms.[8] (You can use more than one search term in *Simple Search*, but if you do you can't combine them with OR. If you enter more than one search term, PEDro will automatically find records that contain *all* the search terms you entered. That is, the *Simple Search* always combines search terms with ANDs.)

In the text box type 'ultrasound epicondylitis'[9] and click on *Search* (or just hit enter on your keyboard). PEDro returns a list of titles of all the records in the database that contain both the words 'ultrasound' and 'epicondylitis'. The top part of the search results page is shown in Figure 4.3.

You can see that, in the top right-hand corner, PEDro indicates there were 23 'hits'.[10] (By 'hits' we mean records that satisfy the search criteria.) Underneath

there is a list of the titles of the records that satisfied the search criteria; an indication of whether the record is a randomized trial, systematic review or practice guideline; a methodological quality score; and a column for selecting records. Titles of clinical practice guidelines are listed first, then titles of systematic reviews, then randomized trials. The randomized trials are listed in order of descending quality scores. So, to a rough approximation, the most useful evidence will tend to be towards the top of the list.

It is a simple matter to scroll through the list of titles looking for those that appear to be most relevant. Clicking on a title links to a *Detailed Search Results* page (Figure 4.4), which displays bibliographic details, abstracts (where available) and details of how the methodological quality score was determined (for randomized trials only). Use the Back button in your browser to go back to the list of search results. You can select articles that look relevant by clicking on the *Select* button (in the right-hand column of the *Search Results* page, or *Select this record* at the top of the *Detailed Search Results* page). This saves the record to a 'shopping basket' called *Selected Records*. You can return to your shopping basket of selected search results by clicking on *Display Selected Records* at the top of the page.[11]

---

[8]For each study, PEDro stores a range of information in containers called 'fields'. Fields include authors' names, the title and abstract, journal name and other bibliographic details, and, importantly, subject headings. Subject headings will be discussed in more detail later in this chapter. The PEDro *Simple Search* looks for records that contain all the search terms in any field.

[9]Note that, in the PEDro *Simple Search*, the AND is assumed. Do not type AND.

[10]If you are doing this search yourself, you may find you get more hits. That is because new records are continually being added to the database.

[11]The shopping basket is emptied when you click on *New Search* or *New Advanced Search*. If you want to continue searching without emptying the shopping basket, click on *Continue Searching* on the top of the page.

Change font size: A- A A+

Figure 4.4 • PEDro: *Detailed Search Results* page.

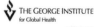

🏠 Home ✔ Select This Record ▦ Display Selected Records 🔍 New Search (Advanced) 🔍 New Search (Simple)
🔍 Continue Searching (Simple) ⦿ Search Help

Use the *Back* button in your browser to see the other results of your search or to select another record.

Detailed Search Results

Author/Association:	D'Vaz AP, Ostor AJK, Speed CA, Jenner JR, Bradley M, Prevost AT, Hazleman BL
Title:	Pulsed low-intensity ultrasound therapy for chronic lateral epicondylitis: a randomized controlled trial
Source:	Rheumatology 2006 May;45(5):566-570
Method:	clinical trial
Method Score:	7/10 [Eligibility criteria: No; Random allocation: Yes; Concealed allocation: No; Baseline comparability: No; Blind subjects: Yes; Blind therapists: Yes; Blind assessors: No; Adequate follow-up: Yes; Intention-to-treat analysis: No; Between-group comparisons: Yes; Point estimates and variability: Yes. Note: Eligibility criteria item does not contribute to total score] *This score has been confirmed*
Abstract:	Copyright release for this abstract has not been obtained.
	Abstracts and full text may be available at: http://rheumatology.oxfordjournals.org /archive/

THE GEORGE INSTITUTE
for Global Health

Affiliated with

THE UNIVERSITY OF
SYDNEY

The database was last updated on 2 August 2010 (this includes records added or amended since 5 July 2010). The next update is planned for Monday 6 September 2010. The total number of records on the database is 16,881.

Contact us   Accessibility statement   Fair use statement

It is useful to understand that PEDro searches for words in a special way. If your search terms include a particular word, PEDro will search for records containing that word or any word that starts with the same word stem as the full search term. For example, if you specify the word 'work' in your search, PEDro will return records that contain the words 'work', 'worker', 'workplace' and 'work-place'.[12] You can exploit this function when searching (see footnote 2). For example, instead of typing 'ultrasound epicondylitis' in the *Simple Search* box, we could have typed 'ultrasound epicondyl', as this will also return studies that refer to epicondylalgia.

The *Simple Search* is useful because it is easy to use, but it has some significant limitations: you need to think of the relevant text words, and they cannot be combined with OR. For some questions, such as 'Does spinal manipulative therapy reduce pain and increase function in people with acute neck pain?', this is problematic. There are many clinical trials on necks, and many more on manipulative therapy, so we really need to combine both neck-related terms and manipulative therapy-related terms in a single search to be efficient. And there are at least two important synonyms for 'neck' ('neck' and 'cervical') and several

more for 'manipulative therapy' ('manipulative therapy', 'manual therapy', 'manipulation', 'mobilization', 'adjustment', and so on). The *Simple Search* mode doesn't enable us to deal with this level of complexity. The *Advanced Search* mode gives us more flexibility.

Advanced Search

The *Advanced Search*, is located on the top left-hand corner of the PEDro start page.[13] The *Advanced Search* page is shown in Figure 4.5. The *Advanced Search* page contains 12 search fields, any of which can be used to search the database. At the top is the *Abstract & Title* field. Entering text into this field instructs PEDro to search for the search terms in the titles or abstracts of all records in the database. In addition, if you know what study you are looking for you can search by the *Author/Association, Title* or *Source* of the record.[14] You can also select subject

---

[12]In effect, PEDro automatically inserts a wild card (*) at the end of every word.

[13]From any other web page in PEDro you can click on 'Continue searching (advanced)' or 'New search (advanced)' located on the top menu.

[14]The *'Source'* refers to where the article has been published. Most of the articles on PEDro are published in journals, so the source is usually a reference to a particular journal article. But PEDro also contains clinical practice guidelines, some of which are published on the world wide web. In that case the source is a web address.

Figure 4.5 • PEDro: *Advanced Search* page.

PEDro
PHYSIOTHERAPY EVIDENCE DATABASE

Change font size: A- A A+

⌂ Home   🔍 New Search (Simple)   🔍 New Search (Advanced)   ● Search Help

Advanced Search

Abstract & Title: [   ]
Therapy: [stretching, mobilisation, manipulation, massage ▾]
Problem: [▾]
Body Part: [head or neck ▾]
Subdiscipline: [▾]
Method: [▾]
Author/Association: [   ]
Title Only: [   ]
Source: [   ]
Published Since: [   ] [YYYY]
New records added since: [   ] [MM/DD/YYYY]
Score of at least: [   ] [/10]
Return: [20 ▾] records at a time
When Searching: ● Match all search terms (AND)
                ○ Match any search term (OR)

[Start Search]

THE GEORGE INSTITUTE
for Global Health

Affiliated with
THE UNIVERSITY OF
SYDNEY

The database was last updated on 2 August 2010 (this includes records added or amended since 5 July 2010).
The next update is planned for Monday 6 September 2010. The total number of records on the database is 16,881.
Contact us   Accessibility statement   Fair use statement

headings from pull-down menus of the *Therapy*, the *Problem* or *Body Part* being treated, or the *Subdiscipline* of practice. In the *Method* search field, you can limit the search just to one study type (clinical practice guidelines, systematic reviews or clinical trials). Finally you can limit the search to those publications *Published Since or Added Since* a specific date, or (for randomized trials only) for trials of greater than a specified *Quality Score*. In *Advanced Search* mode you can search by simultaneously specifying as few or as many of these search criteria as you wish.

For our particular question on the effects of spinal manipulative therapy for neck pain we can take advantage of the subject headings to specify *Therapy* as 'stretching, mobilization, manipulation, massage' and *Body Part* as 'head or neck'. Then we combine these search criteria with an AND by checking the button at the bottom left of the screen ('Match all search terms'), and we click on *Start Search*. PEDro returns 444 records. This is too many titles to scroll through, so we could narrow the search by selecting 'systematic reviews' under *Method*. This returns 91 systematic reviews, many of which appear to be relevant to our

question.[15] We could further narrow the search by specifying that the review must have been published since 2008, which returns just nine systematic reviews. Some of them are Cochrane systematic reviews – these might be a good place to start reading!

This example illustrates one of the strengths of the *Advanced Search:* subject headings can be used as a substitute for two or more synonyms. In fact you can combine any number of subject headings and you can combine a subject heading with search terms entered as text. (So you could, if you wished, combine the text 'ultrasound' in the *Title & Abstract* field with the subject heading 'forearm and elbow' in the *Body Part* field.) However, you can select only one subject heading from each menu (so you couldn't select both 'lower leg or knee' and 'foot or ankle' from the *Body Part* menu).

PEDro has one significant limitation: either all search criteria must be combined with ANDs or they must all be combined with ORs. It is not generally

---

[15]The first nine titles are clinical practice guidelines, even though we selected 'systematic reviews'. PEDro is able to identify those clinical practice guidelines that contain systematic reviews and it returns these titles in searches for systematic reviews.

Box 4.2

Three tips for PEDro power users

1. **Backdoor ANDs and ORs I: Perform multiple searches**. PEDro won't allow you to mix ANDs and ORs. However, you can get around this problem by performing a search using AND, selecting the records that are of interest, and then repeating the search using alternative terms. For example, to search effectively for 'cystic fibrosis' AND ('flutter' OR 'PEP'), you could search for '"cystic fibrosis" AND flutter', combining these terms with the AND button, and select the relevant records by clicking on *Select*. Then repeat the search, this time for '"cystic fibrosis" and PEP', again combining these terms with the AND button, and again select the relevant records. All of the records selected from both searches can be retrieved by clicking on *Display Selected Records*.

2. **Backdoor ANDs and ORs II: Specify strings with inverted commas**. Normally PEDro treats a word string (like 'continuous passive motion') as independent words. If the whole search string is of interest, you can make PEDro treat the string as a single word by enclosing the string in inverted commas

(e.g. "continuous passive motion"; note the use of double quote marks, rather than single quote marks). By typing "continuous passive motion" in inverted commas, PEDro will look for records that contain only these three words in that order, and it will ignore studies that use the words 'continuous' and 'passive' and 'motion' in any other way. This makes it unnecessary to combine the words in the string with AND, so you could, for example, combine the terms 'continuous passive motion' and 'CPM' with the OR button like this: "continuous passive motion" cpm.

3. **Searching for ranges**. Sometimes it is handy to be able to search the *Published Since* or *Score of at Least* fields using ranges. This is done by separating the upper and lower limit of the range by '...'. For example, if you can remember a paper was published in the early 1990s you could enter '1990...1995' in the *Published Since* field. (You will need to combine this with other search criteria!) Or, to find all randomized trials published before 1950, type '0...1950'.

---

possible, in PEDro, to perform searches with combinations of ANDs and ORs. (Proficient users of PEDro might like to consult Box 4.2 for some suggestions on how to trick PEDro into effectively combining AND and OR searches.) A consequence is that, in PEDro at least, it is good policy to resist the temptation to use many search terms. Searches that employ many search terms will tend to return either many irrelevant records (when OR is used) or no records at all (when AND is used). In general, the best search strategies have few search terms. It is often possible to use just one carefully selected search term, and it is rarely necessary to use more than three.

Physiotherapy Choices is available from PEDro's start page. The Physiotherapy Choices database is designed for consumers of physiotherapy services, including the patients and their families. Reviews and studies from PEDro have been supplemented with consumer summaries in plain English. The search page is user friendly and the users can specify their own search terms or choose predefined health problems, symptoms or treatments.

The Cochrane Library

The Cochrane Library (http://www.thecochranelibrary.com) is a remarkable resource. It is a collection of databases, the most important of which are the Cochrane Database of Systematic Reviews (CDSR), the Database of Abstracts of Reviews of Effects (DARE), the Cochrane Central Register of Controlled Trials (CENTRAL) and the Health Technology Assessment Database (HTA).

We have already come across the Cochrane Database of Systematic Reviews in Chapter 3. This database contains the full text of all of the systematic reviews produced by the Cochrane Collaboration and it is updated every month. DARE and HTA, on the other hand, are produced by the Centre for Reviews and Dissemination at the University of York. DARE contains structured abstracts of systematic reviews published in the medical literature. Each abstract contains a commentary that indicates the quality of the review. HTA contains descriptive abstracts of health technology assessments, including systematic reviews and economic evaluations. CENTRAL is indisputably the world's largest database of clinical trials. It contains bibliographic details of over 600 000 clinical trials.[16]

---

[16]Most but not all of these are *randomized* trials. If, however, we take this as a rough estimate of the number of randomized trials in health care ($\approx$600 000), and we take the number of randomized trials on PEDro as an estimate of the number of randomized trials in physiotherapy ($\approx$14 000), we can estimate that approximately 2% of all randomized trials in health care are trials of physiotherapy.

Most of the physiotherapy-relevant randomized trials and systematic reviews in the Cochrane Library are also indexed in PEDro. In fact, the developers of the PEDro database regularly search the Cochrane Library to find randomized trials and systematic reviews in physiotherapy, and PEDro and the Cochrane Collaboration have a reciprocal agreement to exchange data. This means that a search of PEDro will yield most physiotherapy-relevant contents of the Cochrane Library. Nonetheless, we will describe how to search the Cochrane Library because, unlike PEDro, the Cochrane Library contains the full text of Cochrane systematic reviews. In addition, unlike PEDro, the Cochrane Library indexes randomized trials and systematic reviews in all areas of health care. Physiotherapists who are interested in the effects of medical or surgical interventions, or interventions provided by other allied health professions, will find the Cochrane Library contains a wealth of useful information.

Access to the full text of the Cochrane Library is by subscription only. Nonetheless, it is widely available. If you are a student or employee of a university or hospital you may find you can access the Cochrane Library online at http://www.thecochranelibrary.com with a password. Alternatively your nearest medical library may provide you access from a library computer. Many countries have negotiated free online access to the Cochrane Library for all their citizens, or for all health professionals. Free access is provided for people from most developing countries. (For a list of countries that have free access to the Cochrane Library, go to the Cochrane Library start page, click on 'Access' and 'Who Is Eligible for Free Online Access'.) People who do not have free online access can perform limited searches and view abstracts (not full text) of the Cochrane Database of Systematic Reviews.

When you arrive at the Cochrane Library homepage you will see a search box on the top left-hand corner. Here you can do a simple search by typing one or multiple search terms and use the drop-down menu to specify which search field you want the database to search through. You can combine search terms with AND and OR. In the rest of this chapter we will describe how to use the 'Advanced search' located below the search box. Clicking on this link takes you to the *Advanced Search* facility (Figure 4.6).[17]

Let's see what happens if we repeat our earlier search for studies of the effects of pulsed ultrasound for reducing pain and disability associated with lateral epicondylitis. Advanced searches are conducted by typing search terms into one or more of the text boxes in the left frame. The search strategy we use is similar to the strategy we used earlier in PEDro except that we type in the AND. That is, we type 'ultrasound AND epicondyl*' in the first text box. (The default option is to 'Search All Text', which is appropriate here.) Note that we also have to type an asterisk at the end of 'epicondyl' to search for different variations of the word.

Clicking on *Search* runs a search of the Cochrane Database of Systematic Reviews, as well as of the DARE, HTA and CENTRAL databases. A summary of the search results appears under the *Search Results* box. Altogether there were 53 hits.[18] Of these, 10 were in the Cochrane Database of Systematic Reviews; the titles of these records are displayed in a list. Six of the ten are completed reviews (indicated by the note 'Review' in a dark blue circle), but the titles do not look exactly relevant to our question. If any of the titles looked more relevant we could click on *Record* and we would see the full text of the review. Very handy indeed! Four of the hits are protocols (indicated by the note 'Protocol' in a light blue circle). One of the protocols is titled 'Physiotherapy and physiotherapeutical modalities for lateral epicondylitis' (Smidt et al 2008) and looks very relevant. Protocols are reviews that are not yet completed. They sometimes contain some useful information (for example, they may provide the results of a literature search), but they are not as helpful as completed reviews.

At the top of the page, under the *Search Results* heading, you can also see that our search retrieved 12 systematic reviews in DARE (described in Cochrane Library as 'Other Reviews'). By clicking on the *'Other Reviews'* heading, we find that several records appear relevant to our question, although at the time of writing one is 15 years old – probably too old to be useful now. But the most recent review, entitled 'Effectiveness of physical therapy on lateral epicondylitis', looks relevant (Kohia et al 2008), and would probably be the first choice of evidence on this topic. We can view a structured abstract of this review, with commentary, by clicking on the title.

---

[17]We will use the Cochrane Library's native 'front-end'. Other front-ends are available, notably the one produced by Ovid. The other front-ends look very different, and may differ in their search syntax.

[18]If you replicate this search you may get different results, because new records are continually being added to the databases, and because protocols eventually become reviews.

Figure 4.6 • The Cochrane Library home page.

Box 4.3

Tips for searching the Cochrane Library

1. **Use subject headings.** Subject headings (called MeSH terms) are assigned to every systematic review in the database. Often it is more efficient to search for records with specific MeSH headings than it is to search for records containing specific text words. To search by MeSH headings, click on *MeSH Search* immediately above the text box. This brings up a text box, and you are instructed to enter a MeSH term. Type in a key search term (say, 'epicondylitis') and then click on *Thesaurus*. The search engine will search the dictionary of MeSH terms and, if there is a relevant MeSH term, it will indicate below the text box what the relevant MeSH heading is. (In our example it indicates that the relevant MeSH heading is 'tennis elbow'.) Clicking on the MeSH heading takes you to a further dialogue in which you can refine how you use the MeSH heading,[19] and clicking on *Go* then applies the refined MeSH search.

2. **Use the History function to construct complex searches.** When you perform a search in the Cochrane Library, details of that search are kept in the search history. If you perform a search using the text word 'ultrasound' and then perform a second search with the MeSH term 'Tennis elbow', and then click on the *Search History* symbol in the top right-hand corner, you will see your search history:

#1. (ultrasound)	7152
#2. MeSH descriptor Tennis Elbow explode all trees	186

   (The exact wording may be a little different, depending on how you qualified MeSH headings.) You can then combine searches. For example, you could combine these two searches by typing #1 AND #2 in the search box above the search history. This yielded 23 hits.

If we had not found a relevant and recent systematic review in the Cochrane Library of Systematic Reviews, DARE or HTA, we could have looked at the CENTRAL register of clinical trials. We do that by clicking on the link to 'Clinical Trials' under the *Search Results* heading. There are 26 trials in CENTRAL that satisfied our search criteria. Again, we could scan the titles and, if a title looked interesting, we could click on Record and see bibliographic details.

The search strategy we used in this example was quite simple, but the Cochrane Library supports quite sophisticated searching. Some tips for searching the Cochrane Library are given in Box 4.3. More tips are given on the Cochrane website on the right side of every search page and in the search manual under 'Help' on Cochrane Library's start page.

Finding evidence of prognosis and diagnostic tests

In Chapter 3 we saw that best evidence of prognosis is obtained from longitudinal studies, particularly prospective cohort studies. The best evidence of the accuracy of diagnostic tests is provided by cross-sectional studies that compare the findings of the test of interest with a high-quality reference standard. Although these two sorts of question are answered by different sorts of study, the strategies for finding studies of prognosis and diagnostic tests are very similar so we will consider them together.

Finding studies of prognosis and diagnosis of physiotherapy-related questions can be difficult. A general problem with questions about prognosis is that prognostic information is sometimes buried inside clinical trials that were intended to test the effects of an intervention. The authors may not have flagged (or even appreciated) that the study contains prognostic information. Finding studies of diagnostic tests used by physiotherapists may be difficult for a different reason: there are relatively few studies. Searches for studies of diagnostic tests used by physiotherapists may be frustrated by the fact that studies relevant to a particular question do not exist.

At the time of writing there is no database dedicated to archiving studies of prognosis or diagnostic tests in physiotherapy.[20] Thus it is necessary to search general medical databases for this information. The most useful databases are MEDLINE

---

[19]In this dialogue you can add qualifiers to narrow the search. Also, you can indicate how related MeSH headings are used. MeSH terms are arranged in hierarchies (trees). Clicking on the *Explode* text box tells the search engine to look for any record that contains that MeSH term or any MeSH term located further down the tree. Clicking on *Search this term only* tells the search engine to look for any record that contains that MeSH term, but to ignore MeSH terms further down the tree. *Explode all terms* is always more sensitive; *Search this term only* is more specific.

[20]Note that search of PEDro and the Cochrane Library is likely to miss many studies of prognosis, and almost all studies of diagnostic test accuracy. Do not use PEDro or the Cochrane Library to search for studies of prognosis or diagnosis.

Box 4.4

Databases of the health literature

MEDLINE is the largest database of the medical literature. It archives about 16 million records from over 3900 journals published since 1948. Four of the top five journals identified by Maher et al (2001) as core journals exclusively in physiotherapy are indexed on MEDLINE. However, it contains few other physiotherapy-specific journals.[21] It is also likely that MEDLINE currently indexes only a small proportion of all studies on prognosis and diagnostic tests relevant to physiotherapy.[22] One of the best characteristics of MEDLINE is that it has been made freely available on the web, where it is called PubMed. The PubMed URL is http://www.pubmed.com.

Embase is nearly as big as MEDLINE. It contains about 12 million records published since 1974 in about 7000 journals. There is surprisingly little overlap between Embase and MEDLINE. However, Embase has about the same coverage of physiotherapy-specific journals as MEDLINE; it indexes 4 of 5 exclusively physiotherapy core journals. The biggest limitation of Embase is that it is available only by subscription.

CINAHL is the smallest of the four databases. It contains about 2 million records published since 1981 in about 4300 journals. Although smaller than MEDLINE and Embase, CINAHL is 'richer' because it contains many enhancements, including the full text of articles and other materials such as clinical practice guidelines, comments, book reviews and patient education (McKibbon 1999). The greatest strength of CINAHL, from a physiotherapist's perspective at least, is that it has a specific focus on nursing and allied health journals. It indexes most physiotherapy journals and all core physiotherapy journals. Unfortunately CINAHL, like Embase, is available only by subscription.

PsycINFO is a large database of the psychological literature. It contains nearly 8 million records published since 1872 in about 1900 journals. PsycINFO is an excellent place for evidence of psychological interventions, but it too is available only by subscription.

(freely available through PubMed), Embase, CINAHL and PsycINFO. Unlike PEDro and the Cochrane Library, these databases do not restrict their focus to studies of the effects of intervention. Instead they index enormously diverse literatures. Box 4.4 indicates how these databases differ.

Ideally it would be possible to search MEDLINE, Embase, CINAHL and PsycINFO simultaneously. In fact some vendors (such as Ovid) provide a service that enables such searches. However, the capacity to search across these databases is available by subscription only and not widely available, so we will not consider this further. Instead, we will focus on using PubMed to search the MEDLINE database. PubMed has two major advantages: it is freely available to anyone who has access to the internet, and it has an excellent search engine that makes searching

for studies of prognosis and diagnostic test accuracy relatively straightforward.

Many people use the main PubMed search interface to search for studies of prognosis and diagnostic accuracy. This is suboptimal. A part of PubMed, called Clinical Queries, is designed to assist people searching for such studies. Clinical Queries automatically applies search strategies that have been designed for sensitive and specific searching. If you want to conduct quick searches for studies of prognosis or diagnostic tests then you should use Clinical Queries rather than the main PubMed search page. You can find Clinical Queries by following the link from the PubMed homepage (under *'PubMed Tools'*), or by going directly to http://www.pubmed.gov/clinical.

A reproduction of the Clinical Queries home page is shown in Figure 4.7. The home page contains several buttons that allow you to search specifically for studies of therapy, prognosis, diagnosis or aetiology. You can also search for systematic reviews. We will use Clinical Queries to search for studies of prognosis and diagnostic tests.[23]

[21]The journals whose titles indicate they are specifically related to physiotherapy are the *Journal of Orthopaedic and Sports Physical Therapy, Journal of Physiotherapy, Physical Therapy, Physiotherapy, Physiotherapy Research International, Physiotherapy Theory and Practice, Physical and Occupational Therapy in Pediatrics, Pediatric Physical Therapy and Physical Therapy in Sport.*

[22]This statement is not supported by strong data. However, MEDLINE indexes only a small proportion of the randomized trials on PEDro. It is likely that a similar proportion of physiotherapy-relevant studies of prognosis and diagnostic accuracy are indexed on MEDLINE.

[23]We have not used PubMed Clinical Queries to search for studies of the effects of intervention because such searches are better conducted using PEDro or the Cochrane Library. PEDro and the Cochrane Library index many randomized trials that are not on PubMed.

Figure 4.7 • PubMed Clinical Queries home page. Source National Center for Biotechnology Information (NCBI).

You can see that there is a search box at the top and three main headings underneath: 'Clinical Studies Categories', 'Systematic Reviews' and 'Medical Genetics'. First, you need only type in search terms to specify the particular question you are interested in and then click on the 'Search' button (or simply press Enter on your keyboard). Now you are presented with a search result sorted under each of the three headings. Let's look at the heading 'Clinical Studies Categories'. Now you can refine the search further by telling Clinical Queries that you want to search specifically for studies of prognosis or diagnosis. You do this by simply choosing prognosis or diagnosis in the drop down menu called 'Category'.[24] As you choose the relevant category, you will see that the number of search results changes.

One final decision needs to be made. We need to decide whether we want to conduct a sensitive search or a specific search. Of course we would like both, but we need to tell Clinical Queries whether we are more concerned with getting every possible relevant study (emphasis on sensitivity) or with minimizing the number of irrelevant search results (emphasis on specificity). MEDLINE is a huge database, and sensitive searches often yield unmanageable numbers of hits, so we recommend that you begin by specifying a specific search. You do this by choosing 'Narrow' from the *Scope* drop-down menu. If, subsequently, you find that a specific search yields no hits, you might then try conducting a sensitive search by choosing 'Broad' from the same drop-down menu. (Alternatively you might consider trying a different set of search terms, or you might decide to give up and have a cup of coffee instead.)

Clinical Queries provides another option: you can also search for systematic reviews. (These can be systematic reviews of studies of prognosis, or of studies of diagnostic tests or, for that matter, of studies of therapy or aetiology.) However, there are few systematic reviews of prognosis and diagnostic tests, so a search for them may be fruitless. For routine searching we recommend that you don't search only for systematic reviews; if a relevant systematic review exists it will be turned up with a search that does not specifically specify systematic reviews.

Let's imagine that we are seeking an answer to the following question about prognosis: 'In a young male who has just experienced his first shoulder dislocation, what is the risk of re-dislocating within 1 year?'

In Clinical Queries we could type in 'shoulder and dislocat*'. Note that in Clinical Queries, as in Cochrane Library but unlike PEDro, the AND has to be typed in explicitly. Also, as in Cochrane

[24]The search terms used by PubMed Clinical Queries have been subjected to extensive testing and have been shown to have a high sensitivity and specificity (Haynes & Wilczynski 2004, Wilczynski & Haynes 2004).

Library, we need to use an asterix (*) to specify explicitly that we want to look at all words using the root 'dislocat' ('dislocat*' = 'dislocated OR dislocation OR dislocate OR dislocating'). A very nice feature of Clinical Queries is that it looks automatically for relevant MeSH terms and includes them in the search.[25] The search is sorted by Clinical Studies Categories and Systematic Reviews. To find studies of 'prognosis' we choose this option from the drop-down menu, and we also choose a narrow scope (for a specific search).

This search returns 177 hits. Only the first 5 hits are displayed. We must click on 'See all' to look at all 177 hits. A quick scroll through the results identifies several promising titles. However, 177 results might be a lot to scroll through. If we want to specify the search even further, we can go back to the search page and add 'and primary' to our initial search string.[26] This reduces our search results to 16 hits. Several look very relevant. For example, one (te Slaa et al 2004) is entitled: 'The prognosis following acute primary glenohumeral dislocation'. Clicking on the title displays the detailed reference of this publication. In general, you will need to screen search results by reading titles and, if the titles look relevant, by skimming the abstracts. (At the same time you could also screen for methodological quality; more on this in Chapter 5.) The abstract of the paper with the promising looking title confirms that this is a very relevant study.

Sometimes you will find a study that looks to be relevant but which, for one reason or another, turns out not to be. Or it may be that the study is relevant, but it is from an obscure journal and it is not possible to get a copy of the full paper. In that case you could look under *Find Related Data* at the right-hand margin of the search results screen. From the drop-down menu 'Database' choose *PubMed*, and from the menu 'Option' choose *Related Citations*. Finally, click on 'Find Items' underneath. This brings up a list of studies that are similar in content to the first. Once you have identified one study that is relevant to your search question, the *Related Citations* facility provides a quick and easy way to find more relevant studies.

The question we have just asked, on prognosis after primary shoulder dislocation, is quite a simple one because there are relatively few synonyms for the key search terms of shoulder and dislocation.[27] A more difficult question might be: 'How much return of hand function can we expect 6 months after a completely flaccid hemiparetic stroke?' This question is difficult because there are a number of synonyms for stroke (CVA, hemiparesis, cerebrovascular accident, etc.) and for hand function (upper limb function, manual dexterity, etc.). Clinical Queries allows us to combine many search terms using both ANDs and ORs in a single search. This allows us simultaneously to deal with synonyms (by using OR) and to require the presence of multiple key terms (using AND). For example, we could type: (Stroke OR CVA OR cerebro-vascular OR cerebrovascular OR hemipare*) AND (hand OR upper limb OR manual).[28] Then we could refine our search by choosing 'prognosis' and 'narrow'.

In this example we have used brackets to remove the ambiguity that otherwise potentially arises when we mix ANDs and ORs in a single search.[29,30] The search returns 467 hits, too many to screen quickly. So the search was refined by adding 'AND (flaccid* OR paralys*)'. This reduced the number of hits to 25, one of them entitled 'Probability of regaining dexterity in the flaccid upper limb: impact of severity of paresis and time since onset in acute stroke' (Kwakkel et al 2003). Bingo!

We shall look at one more example, this time of a search for studies of accuracy of a diagnostic test. Our question is: 'In nursing home patients, how accurate is auscultation for diagnosis of pneumonia?' The initial search strategy in PubMed Clinical Queries is

---

[25]You can see the exact search terms that Clinical Queries has applied by clicking on one of the retrieved records and examining the *Search details*. Continue by clicking on *Advanced search* on the top of the page and then on *Details*.

[26]We use the search term *primary* to define that we are interested in patients with their *first* shoulder dislocation.

[27]It is true that synonyms for shoulder could be 'gleno-humeral joint' or 'glenohumeral joint', and synonyms for dislocation could be 'subluxation' or 'instability'. Nonetheless, the synonyms are used relatively infrequently in this context, which means that a search for 'shoulder AND dislocation' is likely to be quite sensitive.

[28]Note that none of the search terms pertains to the time window we are interested in (6 months). This is because, although our question concerns a specific time window, we would usually be happy to take studies with any similar time window. Search terms relating to time may hugely reduce search sensitivity, so in general they should not be used.

[29]Can you see the problem if brackets are not used? When we type 'X AND Y OR Z' it may not be clear whether we mean '(X AND Y) OR Z' or 'X AND (Y OR Z)'. In fact there is no real ambiguity because Clinical Queries has a rule for how to deal with such apparent ambiguities. Nonetheless, the use of brackets makes it much easier to ensure that ANDs and ORs are combined in the correct way.

[30]It is also possible to use brackets in the same way in search queries of the Cochrane Library.

to conduct a specific (or narrow) search for studies of diagnosis using the terms 'auscultation AND pneumonia'. This returns 13 hits of which one, entitled 'Diagnosing pneumonia by physical examination: relevant or relic?' (Wipf et al 1999), looks nearly relevant but does not pertain specifically to nursing home patients. Clicking on *Related Citations for this specific article* yields 212 hits. This search was narrowed by combining with 'AND (nursing home OR aged care)'. (Combining searches like this requires use of the *History* function, which we introduce below under the heading of Searching PubMed for qualitative studies.) The narrower search yielded 35 hits, of which one, entitled 'Clinical findings associated with radiographic pneumonia in nursing home residents' (Mehr et al 2001), looks very relevant.

Finding evidence of experiences

If you want to find evidence about how people feel or experience certain situations, or what attitudes they have towards a phenomenon, you should look for studies that use qualitative methods. Unfortunately, finding studies of experiences might be difficult.

One of the problems is that qualitative research is indexed in many different ways. For example, it may be identifiable as qualitative research only by the method used to collect data (e.g. in-depth interviews, focus groups or observation) or only by the type of qualitative research (e.g. phenomenology, grounded theory, ethnographic research). Another problem is that the popularity of qualitative research approaches is relatively new in the health care literature and, consequently, methodological 'hedges' (search strategies used to locate particular types of study) are not yet widely available . There is no button in PubMed Clinical Queries for locating qualitative study designs; nor is there a specific PEDro-like database that indexes only qualitative research. This might make it hard to find high-quality studies relating to experiences.

Here we make some suggestions on how you can find studies of experiences with CINAHL (if you are able to access this database) or PubMed. We consider CINAHL (the Cumulative Index to Nursing and Allied Health Literature), even though it has the disadvantage of being available by subscription only, because it is one of the best databases for locating studies of attitudes and experiences. And we

consider PubMed because it also contains many relevant studies, and it is freely available.

Both CINAHL and PubMed can be searched by 'text words'. Text words are the words provided by the authors in the titles and abstracts of the original study report; these are entered into the database just as they were printed in the journals. Alternatively, the databases can be searched by subject headings. Every study in CINAHL and PubMed is assigned subject headings that have been derived from a standardized vocabulary developed by the database producers. Each database has slightly different subject headings (for example, bedsores are indexed as pressure ulcer in PubMed and CINAHL, and as decubitus in Embase. PsycINFO, being a database on mental health, does not have a specific subject heading for bedsores). Usually it is best to search both text words and subject headings.

Unfortunately, when you go looking for studies of experiences, meanings or processes you will find there are only a few subject headings in PubMed that relate to qualitative research. One exception is that, in 2003, the National Library of Medicine (makers of PubMed) introduced a new MeSH term, 'Qualitative research'. This makes searching for studies of experiences published since 2003 more straightforward. CINAHL has many subject headings related to qualitative study designs. Consequently CINAHL is one of the most useful databases for identifying qualitative studies.

The Social Sciences Citation Index is another resource that might be relevant for finding qualitative research, although again it is available by subscription only. This database provides a multidisciplinary index to the journal literature of the social sciences. It fully indexes more than 2600 journals across 55 social sciences disciplines, and it indexes individually selected, relevant items from 3500 leading scientific and technical journals. It provides access to current information and retrospective data from 1900 onward. More information can be found at http://wokinfo.com/products_tools/multidisciplinary/webofscience/ssci/.

CINAHL

Now let's consider how you could structure a search of the CINAHL database for evidence about experiences.

An efficient search might have two parts. The first part could specify the subject you are interested in and the second part could specify qualitative research and methodology. The two parts are combined with AND. This helps you find qualitative studies that are potentially relevant to your question. Both parts could contain text words or subject headings. Box 4.5 lists headings and text words relevant to qualitative research that could be used for CINAHL searches (McKibbon 1999).

Databases such as MEDLINE, CINAHL, Embase, PsycINFO and Social Science Citation Index have a number of different 'front-ends'. That is, each database may be queried using any of a number of interfaces, each of which looks different on the screen and uses slightly different ways of entering and combining search terms. In the following example we will describe how to use the EBSCO front-end to search CINAHL. EBSCO and other front-ends (such as Ovid) can be searched using similar, but not identical, strategies in MEDLINE, Embase and PsycINFO.

An example of searching CINAHL is shown in Table 4.1. The question is: 'What are immigrants' attitudes and experiences towards exercise?' Each line of the table shows a new search that introduces new

Box 4.5

Search terms for finding qualitative research in CINAHL (McKibbon 1999)

Subject headings

Qualitative studies
Ethnological research
Ethnonursing research
Focus groups
Grounded theory
Phenomenological research
Qualitative validity
Purposive sample
Theoretical sample
Semi-structured interview
Phenomenology
Cultural Anthropology
Observational methods
    Non-participant observation
    Participant observation

Text words

Lived experience
Narrative analysis
Hermeneutic

Table 4.1 Strategy for searching CINAHL with the EBSCO front-end for answers to the question: 'What are immigrants' attitudes and experiences towards exercise?'

Search	Terms	Hits
S1	(MH "Exercise+")	36 703
S2	TI exercis* or AB exercis*	36 560
S3	TI "physical activit*" or AB "physical activit*"	12 243
S4	S1 or S2 or S3	66 935
S5	(MH "Immigrants")	4 005
S6	TI emigra* or AB emigra*	200
S7	TI immigra* or AB immigra*	4 081
S8	S5 or S6 or S7	6 060
S9	S4 and S8	153
S10	(MH "Qualitative Studies+")	45 278
S11	TI qualitative or AB qualitative	28 829
S12	S10 or S11	55 130
S13	S9 and S12	37

S: Search; MH: subject heading; +: explode; TI: title; AB: abstract; *: 'wild card' (any combination of characters)

search terms or combines searches from previous lines. The first column shows the number corresponding to each search, the second column shows the search terms, and the third column shows the number of hits from each search. In this search, search terms (both text words and subject headings) for 'exercise' and 'immigrants' are combined, yielding 153 citations. Then we have combined this result with some of the relevant search terms for qualitative studies selected from those shown in Box 4.5 (both subject headings and text words), yielding 37 hits.

PubMed

When searching PubMed for qualitative research you might need to base your search more on text words because, as mentioned above, PubMed has few subject headings relevant to qualitative research. Relevant search terms (both subject headings and text words) are shown in Box 4.6.

Box 4.6

Search terms (text words) for finding qualitative studies in PubMed

Subject headings

Qualitative research
Focus Groups
Ethnology
Observation

Text words

Ethnon*
Hermeneutic
Focus group
Lived experience
Life experience
Ethnography

Table 4.2 Combining the terms for exercise and immigrants

Search	Terms	Hits
#1	'exercise'[MeSH]	50 905
#2	exercis*	206 817
#3	physical activ*	37 595
#4	#1 OR #2 OR #3	227 090
#5	'emigration and immigration' [MeSH]	20 847
#6	emigra*	26 325
#7	immigra*	31 058
#8	#5 OR #6 OR #7	34 513
#9	#4 AND #8	339

[MeSH] = medical subject heading; * = wild card; # = search

Examples of strategies for searching PubMed for studies of immigrant attitudes and experiences towards exercise are shown in Tables 4.2 and 4.3. Table 4.2 outlines the first part of the search combining the terms for exercise and immigrants. The search is performed on the main search page of PubMed (not Clinical Queries as described earlier).[31]

The search strategies we will use here are a little more complex than those we used in the earlier section where we searched PubMed Clinical Queries for studies of prognosis and accuracy of diagnostic tests. This means that it becomes awkward fitting the search terms on to one line. To be able to perform multiline searches in PubMed you have to go to 'Advanced search' and look under *Search History*. When searching this way you should search each term individually before combining them. Terms are combined by referring to the line number of the search. Thus '#1' refers to the search on line number 1, and '#2 AND #6' combines the results of searches on lines 2 and 6 with AND.

The search in Table 4.2 yields 339 studies – too many to screen efficiently. So, to narrow your search, you can combine the result with search terms for

Table 4.3 Combining exercise and immigrant terms with terms for qualitative research

Search	Terms	Hits
#1	'exercise'[MeSH]	50 905
#2	exercis*	206 817
#3	physical activ*	37 595
#4	#1 OR #2 OR #3	227 090
#5	'emigration and immigration'[MeSH]	20 847
#6	emigra*	26 325
#7	immigra*	31 058
#8	#5 OR #6 OR #7	34 513
#9	#4 AND #8	339
#10	Search "Qualitative Research"[MeSH] OR "Focus Groups"[MeSH] OR "Ethnology"[MeSH] OR "Observation"[MeSH]	21 851
#11	qualitative	88 259
#12	#10 OR #11	99 019
#13	#9 AND #12	25

---

[31]In this example we have searched for MeSH subject headings and text words separately. As mentioned in the section on 'Finding evidence of prognosis and diagnostic tests', PubMed automatically looks for relevant MeSH terms and includes them in the search. In practice, this means that you will not always have to search for the MeSH term first, and then for the text word. To see the exact search terms that PubMed has applied, look at *Search Details* on the right side of the list of search results.

qualitative studies using the *History* button (Box 4.6), as shown in Table 4.3. In our search example this yields 25 studies. You can easily screen through the 25 titles to see whether there are any relevant studies.

Note that it will not generally be useful to search using the text word 'phenomenology' in PubMed, because many articles use the term 'phenomenology' to mean the description or classification of things, and not to refer to the qualitative design or methodology of phenomenology (McKibbon 1999).

Getting full text

A search of the literature will yield the titles, bibliographic details and abstracts of relevant research reports, but this is usually not sufficient for critical appraisal. It is almost always better to have at hand the full report of the study.

Obtaining the full text of a report can be difficult, and for some physiotherapists this can be a major impediment to evidence-based practice. How can full reports be obtained?

The best way to obtain full text is electronically. Physiotherapists affiliated with large institutions (such as hospitals or universities) may have full-text electronic access to a selection of subscription-only journals by virtue of their affiliation with that institution. This makes it possible to download the selected paper to any computer that is connected to the internet.

Even physiotherapists who do not have access to subscription-only journals can access a wide range of journals electronically. An increasing number of journals are made freely available on the internet (notably, at the time of writing, the full text of the *BMJ* is free at http://www.bmj.com). Many journals make back issues (typically, issues more than 1 year old) freely available on the web. A very useful hub that provides access to all such journals is FreeMedicalJournals.com at http://www.freemedicaljournals.com/. Physiotherapists working for health institutions in more than 100 developing countries can access electronic full text of over 7000 journals through the HINARI website (http://www.who.int/hinari/en/). Some professional associations provide members access to free full text. For example, the Australian Physiotherapy Association provides its members access to approximately 450 journals through the APA Library, which members access through a members-only part of the association's website. Finally, some countries provide full-text access

to the Cochrane Library for all their citizens, or to all health professionals. (See http://www.thecochranelibrary.com/view/0/FreeAccess.html for a list of countries that provide such access.) Other countries provide full access to a range of electronic journals for health workers. Examples are the National Electronic Library for Health (http://www.library.nhs.uk/) in England, and state-based sites in Australia (New South Wales, http://www.clininfo.health.nsw.gov.au/; Queensland, http://ckn.health.qld.gov.au/; Victoria, http://www.clinicians.vic.gov.au; Western Australia, http://www.ciao.health.wa.gov.au/; South Australia, http://www.salus.sa.gov.au/).

Of course, many journals are not available as electronic full text. In that case it may be possible to obtain a copy of the paper from a local library. For some this may be straightforward, albeit a little time-consuming. But other physiotherapists will not have access to a well-stocked local library, or they may find that travel to the library is too time-consuming, or their library does not hold the particular journals that are needed. The unfortunate reality is that many physiotherapists still find it difficult to access reports of the full text of high-quality clinical research.

In the preceding sections we have looked at how to find evidence to answer questions about effects of interventions, experiences, prognosis and accuracy of diagnostic tests. Table 4.4 provides a simple summary of our recommendations concerning which databases to consult for particular questions.

Table 4.4 Which database should I use? Summary of recommendations

Question is about	Recommended database	Comments
Effects of therapy	PEDro Cochrane Library	Physiotherapy interventions only Subscription only*
Experiences	CINAHL PubMed	Subscription only
Prognosis	PubMed	Use Clinical Queries
Diagnostic tests	PubMed	Use Clinical Queries

*Many countries provide free access to the Cochrane Library. Go to http://www.thecochranelibrary.com/view/0/FreeAccess.html for details.

Ankle exercises in combination with intermittent ice and compression following an ankle sprain improves function in the short term

Synopsis

Summary of: Bleakley CM, O'Connor SR, Tully MA, Rocke LG, MacAuley D, Bradbury I, et al (2010) Effect of accelerated rehabilitation on function after ankle sprain: randomised controlled trial. *BMJ* 340: c1964 doi:10.1136/bmj.c1964 [Prepared by Margreth Grotle and Kåre Birger Hagen, CAP Editors.]

Question: What is the effect of an accelerated intervention incorporating early therapeutic exercise as compared to a standard intervention of protection, rest, ice, compression, and elevation after acute ankle sprain? *Design*: Randomised, controlled trial with blinded outcome assessment and intention-to-treat analysis. *Setting*: An emergency department and sports injury clinic in Northern Ireland. *Participants*: Men and women 16–65 years, with acute (< 7 days) grade 1 or 2 ankle sprain. Key exclusion criteria were complete (grade 3) rupture, bony ankle injury, and multiple injuries. Randomisation allocated 101 participants to an accelerated intervention incorporating early therapeutic exercises (exercise group) or a standard protection, rest, ice, compression, and elevation intervention (standard group). *Interventions*: During the first week after baseline both groups received written advice on using ice and compression. The exercise group also undertook 20 minutes of exercises three times a day focused on increasing ankle range of movement, activation and strengthening of ankle musculature, and restoring sensorimotor control. In the

following four weeks a standardised treatment consisting of ankle rehabilitation exercises was provided to both groups. *Outcome measures*: The primary outcome was subjective ankle function assessed by the lower extremity functional scale (0–80) at weeks 1 to 4. Secondary outcomes assessed were: pain at rest and pain with activity with 10-cm visual analogue scales, swelling by a modified version of the figure of eight method, and physical activity by a physical activity logger. Ankle function by the Karlsson score and rate of reinjury were also assessed at 16 week follow-up. *Results*: 15 of the 101 patients dropped out during the trial, 11 in the exercise group and 4 in the standard group. An effect was found in favour of the exercise group with the lower extremity functional scale (0–80) at week 1 (MD 5.3, 98.75% CI 0.3 to 10.3) and week 2 (MD 4.9, 95% CI 0.3 to 9.6). In addition, the exercise group was more active in the first week as measured by time spent walking (0.4 hours per day, 95% CI 0.2 to 0.6). No between-group differences were observed for pain at rest, pain with activity, or swelling. At 16 weeks there were no significant differences between the groups in the Karlsson score or reinjury rate (2 in each group). *Conclusion*: An accelerated exercise protocol during the first week after ankle sprain improved ankle function and early return to weight bearing activity.

[Between-group difference in time spent walking per day calculated by CAP editors]

Commentary

This study is the first to describe the effect of early mobilisation in combination with the standard PRICE (Protection, Rest, Ice, Compression, Elevation) treatment after an acute ankle sprain using a randomised controlled trial where, instead of rest, the intervention group performed therapeutic exercises aimed at increasing ankle movement, as well as static strengthening and stretching exercises (Knight 1995). The main finding was a significant improvement in short-term ankle function for those completing the exercise protocol during the first week following an ankle sprain. It is worth noting that the size of the effect (expressed as change in the lower extremity functional score from baseline to week 1) was smaller than the change of 9 points nominated as the clinically important change. However, as the adherence rate to the prescribed treatment was higher in the standard group compared to the exercise group (77.9% versus 67.8%), the effect for those adhering to the exercise protocol might have been higher than confirmed by the published results. The authors did not describe in detail how often the exercises should be performed during

the first week ('20 min, 3 times a day'). However, based on the study protocol previously published (Bleakley et al 2007) we assume that the exercises were prescribed daily during the first week. For general practitioners, as well as sports physicians and physiotherapists, seeing patients with acute ankle sprains in the clinic, these findings emphasise the importance of prescribing exercises in combination with the PRICE protocol in the first week after injury to optimise rehabilitation. However, the optimal dosage of treatment, including PRICE, choice of exercises, intensity and frequency of the exercise protocol, requires further investigation.

Kathrin Steffen, Agnethe Nilstad
Norwegian School of Sport Sciences, Oslo, Norway

References

Bleakley CM (2007) *BMC Musculoskelet Disord* 8: 125.

Knight KL (1995) *Champaign IL, Human Kinetics*: 220–229.

Figure 4.8 • A critically appraised paper (CAP). Reproduced with permission from the *Journal of Physiotherapy*.

Finding evidence of advances in clinical practice (browsing)

The preceding sections have described search strategies for finding answers to specific questions about the effects of intervention, experiences, prognosis and diagnosis. It is useful to supplement the process of seeking answers to specific clinical questions with 'browsing'. Browsing is reading that is not targeted at specific clinical questions. Browsing provides a mechanism by which we can keep abreast of new developments in professional practice that might otherwise pass us by.

Until recently there were few mechanisms for efficient browsing. Physiotherapists who wished to stay up-to-date with research may have stumbled across important papers while browsing recent issues of journals in the New Issues shelves at a library, or they may have exchanged key papers with colleagues. But, by and large, keeping up-to-date was a hit and miss affair.

A number of relatively new resources have greatly increased the efficiency of browsing. One example is 'pre-appraised' papers, such as those published in journals like *Evidence-Based Medicine, Evidence-Based Nursing* and the *Journal of Physiotherapy* (where they are called 'Critically Appraised Papers', or CAPs for short). A common characteristic of pre-appraised papers is that they provide easily read, short summaries of high-quality, clinically relevant research.

A CAP from the *Journal of Physiotherapy* has been reproduced in Figure 4.8. The CAP (Steffen & Nilstad 2010) describes a randomized trial of early active intervention for grade I and II ankle sprains (Bleakley et al 2010). This study, like others that are described in CAPs, was chosen by the CAP Editors because it was considered to be a high-quality study of importance to the practice of physiotherapy. The CAP has a declarative title that gives the main findings of the study, a short, structured abstract that describes how the study was conducted and what it found, and a commentary from an expert in the field giving the commentator's opinion of the implications of the study for clinical practice.

The CAPs in the *Journal of Physiotherapy*, and similar features in *Evidence-Based Medicine* and *Evidence-Based Nursing*, provide a simple way that physiotherapists can keep up-to-date. All three are available by subscription, but CAPs in past issues of the *Journal of Physiotherapy* are freely available at http://jop.physiotherapy.asn.au.

References

Bleakley, C.M., O'Connor, S.R., Tully, M.A., et al., 2010. Effect of accelerated rehabilitation on function after ankle sprain: randomised controlled trial. BMJ 340, c1964.

Haynes, R.B., Wilczynski, N.L., 2004. Optimal search strategies for retrieving scientifically strong studies of diagnosis from Medline: analytical survey. BMJ 328, 1040.

Kohia, M., Brackle, J., Byrd, K., et al., 2008. Effectiveness of physical therapy treatments on lateral epicondylitis. Journal of Sport Rehabilitation 17 (2), 119–136.

Kwakkel, G., Kollen, B.J., van der Grond, J., et al., 2003. Probability of regaining dexterity in the flaccid upper limb: impact of severity of paresis and time since onset in acute stroke. Stroke 34, 2181–2186.

McKibbon, A., 1999. PDQ. Evidence-based principles and practice. Decker BC, Hamilton, Ontario.

Maher, C., Moseley, A., Sherrington, C., et al., 2001. Core journals of evidence-based physiotherapy practice. Physiother. Theory Pract. 17, 143–151.

Maher, C.G., Moseley, A., Sherrington, C., et al., 2008. A description of the trials, reviews and practice guidelines indexed on the PEDro database. Phys. Ther. 88, 1068–1077.

Mehr, D.R., Binder, E.F., Kruse, R.L., et al., 2001. Clinical findings associated with radiographic pneumonia in nursing home residents. J. Fam. Pract. 50, 931–937.

Moseley, A.M., Herbert, R.D., Sherrington, C., et al., 2002. Evidence for physiotherapy practice. A survey of the Physiotherapy Evidence Database (PEDro). Aust. J. Physiother. 48, 43–49.

Smidt, N., Assendelft, W.J.J., Arola, H., et al., 2008. Physiotherapy and physiotherapeutical modalities for lateral epicondylitis (protocol for a Cochrane review). In: The Cochrane Library, Issue 2. Wiley, Chichester.

Steffen, K., Nilstad, A., 2010. Ankle exercises in combination with intermittent ice and compression following an ankle sprain improves function in the short term. Journal of Physiotherapy 56, 202.

te Slaa, R.L., Wijffels, M.P., Brand, R., et al., 2004. The prognosis following acute primary glenohumeral dislocation. J. Bone Joint Surg. 86-B, 58–64.

Wilczynski, N.L., Haynes, R.B., 2004. Developing optimal search strategies for detecting clinically sound prognostic studies in MEDLINE: an analytic survey. BMC Med. 2, 23.

Wipf, J.E., Lipsky, B.A., Hirschmann, J.V., et al., 1999. Diagnosing pneumonia by physical examination: relevant or relic? Arch. Intern. Med. 24, 1082–1087.

Can I trust this evidence?

5

CHAPTER CONTENTS

Overview 61
A process for critical appraisal
of evidence 62
Critical appraisal of evidence about
the effects of intervention 64
   Randomized trials 65
   Were intervention and control
   groups comparable? 65
   Was there complete or near-complete
   follow-up? 67
   Was there blinding to allocation
   of patients and assessors? 71
   Systematic reviews of
   randomized trials 77
   Was it clear which trials were to be reviewed? . . 77
   Were most relevant studies reviewed? 78
   Was the quality of the reviewed studies
   taken into account? 80
Critical appraisal of evidence about
experiences 81
   Was the sampling strategy
   appropriate? 82
   Was the data collection sufficient
   to cover the phenomena? 82
   Were the data analysed in a
   rigorous way? 83
Critical appraisal of evidence about
prognosis 84
   Individual studies of prognosis 84
   Was there representative sampling
   from a well-defined population? 84
   Was there an inception cohort? 85
   Was there complete or near-complete
   follow-up? 86
   Systematic reviews of prognosis 87

Critical appraisal of evidence about
diagnostic tests 87
   Individual studies of diagnostic tests . . . 88
   Was there comparison with an adequate
   reference standard? 88
   Was the comparison blind? 88
   Did the study sample consist of participants
   for whom there was diagnostic uncertainty? . . . 89
   Systematic reviews of diagnostic tests . . . 89
References 90

OVERVIEW

Well-designed research can produce relatively unbiased answers to clinical questions. Poorly designed research can generate biased answers. Readers of the clinical research literature need to be able to discriminate between well-designed and poorly designed research. This is best done by asking simple questions about key methodological features of the study. When reading clinical trials you should consider whether intervention and control groups were comparable, whether there was complete or near-complete follow-up, and whether there was blinding of patients and assessors. For studies of experiences you should consider whether the sampling strategy was appropriate, whether the data collection procedures were sufficient to capture the phenomenon of interest, and whether the data were analysed in a rigorous way. For studies of prognosis you should consider whether there was representative sampling from a well-defined population at a uniform point in the course of the condition. And for studies of diagnostic tests you should consider whether there was blind comparison of the test with a rigorous reference standard on participants in whom there was

diagnostic suspicion. For systematic reviews on any type of question you should consider whether it was clear which studies were to be reviewed, whether there was an adequate literature search, and whether the quality of individual studies was taken into account when drawing conclusions.

As discussed in the previous chapter, ideally the search for evidence will yield a small number of studies. If you have systematically sought out studies of the type needed to answer your question then you can begin the process of critical appraisal that we describe below. If you have happened upon a study incidentally (for example, you were given a copy from a friend), you will first need to confirm that the study has the right sort of design to answer your question (see Chapter 2).

The studies you find may or may not be well designed and executed, so they may or may not be of sufficient quality to be useful for clinical decision-making. In this chapter we consider how to decide whether a study is of sufficient quality that its findings are likely to be valid.[1] We begin with a general discussion of approaches to appraising validity and then describe specific methods for appraising validity of studies of the effects of interventions, experiences, prognosis and the accuracy of diagnostic tests.

A process for critical appraisal of evidence

Many physiotherapists experience a common frustration. When they consult the research literature for answers to clinical questions they are confronted by a range of studies with very different conclusions. Consider, for example, the findings that confront a physiotherapist who would like to know whether acupuncture protects against exercise-induced asthma. One study, by Fung et al (1986: 1419) concluded 'acupuncture provided better protection

against exercise-induced asthma than did sham acupuncture'. On the other hand, Gruber et al (2002: 222) concluded: 'acupuncture treatment offers no protection against exercise-induced bronchoconstriction'. These conclusions appear inconsistent. It seems implausible that both could be true. Situations like this, where similar studies draw contradictory conclusions, often arise.

Why is the literature apparently so inconsistent? There are several possible explanations. First, there may be important differences between studies in the type of patient included, the way in which the intervention was administered, and the way in which outcomes were measured. Simple conclusions may obscure important details about patients, interventions and outcomes. However, as we shall see later, it may be difficult to draw more precise conclusions from clinical research.

Another important cause of inconsistency is bias. Many studies are poorly designed and may therefore have seriously biased conclusions. The findings of poorly designed studies and well-controlled studies of the same interventions can differ markedly. Of the two studies of acupuncture for exercise-induced asthma cited above, only the study by Gruber et al (2002) blinded the participants and assessors of outcomes. The inconsistency of the conclusions of these studies may arise because the study by Gruber and colleagues provides a relatively unbiased estimate of the effects of acupuncture, whereas the study by Fung et al (1986) may have been subject to a range of biases.

How much of the published research is of high quality? How much research provides us with findings that we can be confident are not distorted by bias? Methodologists have conducted numerous surveys of the quality of published research and the conclusion has almost always been that much of the published research is of poor quality (see, for example, Anyanwu & Treasure 2004, Dickinson et al 2000, Kjaergard et al 2002). Systematic reviewers typically conclude the same: inspection of the abstracts of a sample of 20 systematic reviews randomly selected from the PEDro database found that 8 (40%) explicitly mentioned problems with trial quality in their conclusions. There is, however, some evidence that the quality of the research literature is slowly improving (Kjaergard et al 2002, Moher et al 2002, Moseley et al 2002, Quinones et al 2003).

Many people who are not familiar with the research process find it difficult to believe that much of the published research is potentially seriously biased. They imagine that research is usually carried

---

[1]There are several dimensions to validity. (For enlightening discussions of aspects of validity in experimental research, see the classic texts by Campbell & Stanley (1963) and Cook & Campbell (1979).) In this chapter we look at some aspects of study validity when we consider aspects of study design (as distinct from aspects of the analysis, or of the selection of participants, implementation of interventions and measurements of outcomes) that can control for bias. In studies of the effects of interventions, we could say our concern is with what Campbell & Stanley call 'internal validity', but the term internal validity is not easily applied to studies of prognosis of diagnostic tests. Other aspects of validity are considered in Chapter 6.

out by experts, that research reports are peer-reviewed by people with methodological expertise, and that research papers are therefore usually of a high standard. The reality is that much of the clinical research we read in journals is conducted by people who have little or no training in research design. Some researchers are intent on proving a point of view rather than testing hypotheses objectively. And even informed and well-intentioned researchers may be unable to conduct high-quality research because they are thwarted by practical impediments, such as difficulty recruiting adequate numbers of participants for the research. Research reports, particularly those in lower-quality journals, may be peer-reviewed by people who have little better understanding of research design than the people who conducted the research. And journal editors may be forced to publish reports of poorly designed studies to fill the pages of their journals.

> These and other factors conspire to make a substantial proportion of published research potentially seriously biased.

A quantitative estimate of the quality of randomized trials in physiotherapy is provided by the PEDro database. All trials on the database are assessed according to 10 methodological criteria. A methodological quality score is generated by counting the number of criteria that are satisfied. Figure 5.1 shows that most trials on the database satisfy some but not all of the key methodological characteristics. The typical trial satisfies 5 of the 10 criteria. (In many trials it is not possible to satisfy the criteria of blinding patients or therapists; in such trials the maximum possible score is effectively 8.) Thus a small proportion of trials are of very high quality, the typical trial is of moderate quality, and there are many trials of low quality. There are few data on the quality of typical studies of experiences and processes, prognosis, or diagnosis, but our impression is that the quality of such studies tends to be somewhat lower than that of clinical trials.

If it is true that a substantial proportion of the clinical research published in journals is poorly designed and potentially misleading, readers of clinical research must be able to distinguish between high-quality studies that potentially provide useful information for clinical decision-making and low-quality clinical research which is potentially misleading. Readers who are unable to make that distinction will be unable to make sense of the apparently contradictory clinical research literature.

This might appear to be too much to ask of readers. Surely, if many researchers and journal reviewers cannot distinguish between high-quality and low-quality research, it is unreasonable to expect readers of clinical trials to be able to do so. In fact, as recognized by the pioneers of evidence-based medicine (Department of Clinical Epidemiology and Biostatistics 1981), it is probably possible to use very simple checklists to distinguish coarsely between high-quality research and research that is likely to be biased. The assumption is that a few carefully chosen criteria can be used to discriminate between studies that are likely to produce relatively unbiased answers to clinical questions and those that are potentially

Figure 5.1 • Distribution of quality scores of randomized trials in physiotherapy (2297 trials). Reproduced with permission from Moseley et al (2002).

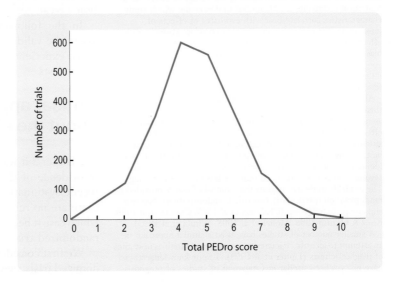

seriously biased. The value of this approach is that it puts the assessment of the quality of clinical research within the reach of readers who do not necessarily have research expertise themselves. A little bit of training (or just reading this chapter) is all that is needed to be able to discriminate coarsely between low-quality and high-quality clinical research.

What criteria should be used to discriminate between high-quality and low-quality research? How should these quality criteria be developed? The most common approach is to seek the opinions of experts. In fact there are now numerous sets of criteria based on expert opinion that have been used to assess the quality of studies of effects of intervention, and several sets of criteria based on expert opinion that have been used to assess the quality of studies of experiences, prognosis or the accuracy of diagnostic tests. One set of criteria that is of particular interest is the Delphi list of criteria for assessing the quality of clinical trials, developed by Verhagen and colleagues (1998a). These researchers asked experts to nominate criteria they felt were important and then used a formal method (the 'Delphi technique') to achieve a consensus. The Delphi list forms the basis of the PEDro scale that was introduced in Chapter 4.[2]

---

[2]An alternative approach is more empirical and less subjective. This approach (the 'meta-epidemiological approach') bases the selection of quality criteria on findings of research into characteristics of research designs that minimize bias. Most of this research has been directed at assessing the quality of studies of the effects of intervention, rather than studies of prognosis or accuracy of diagnostic tests, and the approach cannot easily be applied to studies of experiences. The usual approach with studies of the effects of intervention is to assemble large numbers of clinical trials and extract from each an estimate of the effect of intervention. Statistical techniques are then used to determine which study characteristics correlate best with estimates of effects of intervention. Study characteristics that correlate strongly with effects of intervention are thought to be those that are indicative of bias. Thus, if studies without a particular characteristic (such as concealment of allocation) tend to show larger effects of interventions, this is thought to be evidence the characteristic (concealment) reduces bias.

Although this approach is less subjective and more transparent than seeking expert opinion, it relies on the questionable assumption that study characteristics that correlate strongly with effects of intervention are indicative of bias. The design of these studies does not provide rigorous control of confounding, so it may be that this approach identifies spurious quality criteria or fails to identify important quality criteria. It is reassuring, then, that several studies have produced more or less consistent findings. The available evidence suggests that control of bias is provided by randomization (particularly concealed randomization), blinding and adequate follow-up (Chalmers et al 1983, Colditz et al 1989, Kunz & Oxman 1998, Moher et al 1998, Schulz et al 1995).

A smaller number of studies have used a similar approach in an attempt to identify characteristics that control for bias in studies of diagnostic tests (Lijmer et al 1999). To our knowledge there have not yet been similar investigations of studies of prognosis.

In this chapter we will use the approach to critical appraisal popularized in the *JAMA* Users' Guides (Guyatt & Rennie 1993) and refined by Sackett et al (2000). This approach involves first asking a small number of key questions about study design in order to distinguish between low-quality and high-quality studies, before proceeding to interpret study findings. Such questions have been called 'methodological filters' because they can be used to 'filter out' studies of low methodological quality. Most (not all) of the methodological filters we will describe are the same as those described by others.

We have made the case that readers of clinical research need to be careful to discriminate between high-quality research, which can be used for clinical decision-making, and low-quality research, which is potentially biased – but we do not wish to encourage excessively critical attitudes. Inexperienced readers of clinical research may be inclined to be very dismissive of imperfect research and apply methodological filters harshly. However, no research is perfect, so the highly critical reader will find very little research trustworthy.

> We should not demand perfection from clinical research because it is not generally attainable. Instead, we should look for studies that are *good enough* for clinical decision-making.

That is, we need to identify studies that are sufficiently well designed to give us more certainty than we could otherwise have. Usually we need to be prepared to accept the findings of good but not excellent studies, because they give us the best information we can get.

In the following sections we consider how to assess the validity of studies of effects of interventions, experiences, prognosis and accuracy of diagnostic tests.

Critical appraisal of evidence about the effects of intervention

In Chapter 3 it was argued that the preferred source of evidence of the effects of a therapy is usually a recent systematic review. But for some questions there are no relevant, recent systematic reviews, in which case it becomes necessary to consult individual randomized trials.

We first consider how to assess the validity of randomized trials, even though the reader is encouraged to look first for systematic reviews, because it is easier to understand critical appraisal of systematic reviews after having first contemplated critical appraisal of randomized trials.

Randomized trials

Readers of clinical trials can ask three questions to discriminate coarsely between those trials that are likely to be valid and those that are potentially seriously biased.

Were intervention and control groups comparable?

In Chapter 3 it was argued that we expect to obtain unbiased estimates of the effects of intervention only from studies that compare outcomes in intervention and control groups. It is essential that the groups are comparable, and comparability can be expected only when participants are randomly assigned to groups. 'Matching' of participants in the intervention and control groups cannot, on its own, ensure that the groups are comparable, regardless of how diligently the matching is carried out. The only way to ensure probable comparability is to randomize participants to intervention and control groups.

Randomization is best achieved by using a computer to generate a random allocation schedule. Alternatively, random allocation schedules can be generated by effectively random processes such as coin-tossing or the drawing of lots. Sometimes quasi-random allocation procedures are used: participants may be allocated to groups on the basis of their birth dates (for example, participants with even-numbered birth dates could be assigned to the treatment group and participants with odd-numbered birth dates assigned to the control group), or medical record numbers, or the date of entry into the trial. It is likely that, if carried out carefully, all of these procedures could assign participants to groups in a way that is effectively random in the sense that all the procedures could generate probably comparable groups. That is not to say that coin-tossing and drawing of lots is optimal (see the discussion of concealment of allocation later in this section), but it may be adequate.

Some studies match participants *and* randomly allocate participants to groups. The technical term for this is stratified random allocation. Stratification of allocation has the effect of constraining chance. It ensures that there is an even greater comparability

of groups than could be achieved by simple random allocation alone. For example, a randomized trial that compared home-made and commercially available spacers in metered-dose inhalers for children with asthma (Zar et al 1999) allocated participants to one of four groups after stratifying for severity of airways obstruction (mild or moderate/severe). The researchers constrained randomization to ensure that within each stratum of severity of airway obstruction equal numbers of participants were allocated to each group. By separately randomizing strata with and without moderate/severe airway obstruction it was possible to ensure that the two groups were 'balanced' with respect to the proportion of participants with moderate/severe airway obstruction.[3] In general, stratified random allocation ensures more similarity between groups, but usually only slightly more similarity, than would occur with simple randomization. For readers of clinical trials the important point is that it is the randomization, not the stratification, that ensures comparability of groups. Stratified random allocation ensures comparability of groups because it involves randomization. But randomization on its own is adequate.[4]

The most commonly used techniques of randomization are simple ('unconstrained') randomization and stratified randomization procedures. But there are many other ways in which participants can be randomized (or effectively randomized) to groups (Herbert 2005). The details of these procedures need not concern readers of randomized trials. The essential issue is whether randomization occurred, because it is random allocation that ensures probable comparability of groups.

---

[3]Usually, if allocation is to one of two groups the stratum is evenly numbered in size; if allocation is to one of three groups the size of the stratum is a multiple of three, etc. Random allocation is then conducted in a way that ensures participants in each stratum are allocated to equally sized groups. (The strata are referred to as 'blocks'; blocked random allocation is analogous to repeatedly randomly drawing lots without replacement). Stratification without blocking does not ensure greater comparability of groups than simple randomization alone (Herbert 2005, Lavori et al 1983).

[4]At this stage some readers may want to object to the assertion that randomization ensures comparability. They might argue that randomization ensures comparability only when sample sizes are sufficiently large. In one sense that is true: the groups will be more similar, on average, when the sample size is large. The consequence is that trials with larger samples provide more precise estimates of effects of intervention; we will consider precision at greater length later in this chapter. But there is another way of looking at comparability. Comparability can also be thought of as a lack of bias. Insofar as 'bias' refers to a *long-run tendency* to overestimate or underestimate the true value of a parameter, randomization removes bias regardless of sample size.

It is usually a very easy matter to determine whether a clinical trial was randomized or not. Reports of randomized trials will usually explain that participants were 'randomly allocated to groups'.[5] This might appear in the title of the paper, or in the abstract, or in the Methods section.

One concern is that particularly naive authors may refer to 'random allocation' when describing *haphazard* allocation to groups. These authors might believe that if they made no particular effort to ensure that participants were in one group or the other (for example, if participants or their therapists, but not the researchers, determined whether the treatment or control condition was received) then they could call the allocation process 'random'. This, of course, is potentially seriously misleading, because there is no guarantee in such trials that the groups are comparable in the sense that they differ only by chance; these sorts of process should not be referred to as random allocation. The term 'random allocation' should be reserved strictly for allocation procedures that use random number generators or, perhaps, random processes such as coin-tossing or the drawing of lots. As there is always the concern that the term 'random allocation' has been used in an inappropriate way, it is reassuring when the trial report describes the randomization procedure, so that the reader can know that the allocation procedure was truly random rather than just haphazard. An example of a clear description of the randomization is provided in the report of a trial of community-based physiotherapy for people with chronic stroke (Green et al 2002). The authors reported that: 'Randomization was achieved by numbered, sealed, opaque envelopes prepared from random number tables . . .'.

Some readers would like to see evidence, in reports of randomized trials, that randomization 'worked'. That is, they would like to see data that demonstrate randomization produced groups that were comparable at the time they were randomized ('baseline comparability'). Often the authors of reports of randomized trials oblige by providing a table that compares the baseline characteristics of participants in intervention and control groups. The report may state that the groups appeared similar (or dissimilar) at baseline, or statistical tests may

be used to demonstrate that the groups did not (or did) differ at baseline by more than could be attributed to chance alone. Some authors go one step further: if they detect differences between groups at baseline they use statistical procedures to 'adjust' estimates of the effect of intervention for baseline imbalances.[6] However, such procedures are, arguably, unnecessary and illogical. In a properly randomized trial, differences at baseline are due only to chance, so it does not make sense to conduct statistical tests to determine whether differences at baseline are greater than could be attributed to chance alone (Pocock et al 2002).[7] The confidence intervals that we discuss in Chapter 6 properly account for the uncertainty in estimates of effects of intervention caused by random baseline imbalances, so further adjustments are not necessary. Moreover, the process of adjusting treatment effects to account for baseline imbalances is known to be biased (Raab et al 2000). For these reasons we advise readers of reports of randomized trials to focus on the allocation procedure, not similarity of groups at baseline. If it is clear that allocation was truly random then dissimilarities at baseline can usually be safely ignored. In trials with true random allocation, we would prefer to see unadjusted estimates of effects of intervention.

True randomization can be ensured only when randomization is concealed.[8] This means that the researcher is not aware, at the time a decision is made about eligibility of a person to participate in the trial, whether that person will subsequently be randomized to the intervention or the control group. Concealment is important because, even though most trials specify inclusion and exclusion criteria that determine who is and who is not eligible to participate in the trial, there is sometimes uncertainty about whether a particular patient satisfies those criteria, and often the researcher responsible for entering new patients into the trial has some latitude in such decisions. It could seriously bias the trial's findings if the researcher's decisions about who was and was not entered into the trial were influenced

---

[5]Some studies will state that participants were 'randomly *selected*' for treatment or control groups, when they really mean participants were randomly *allocated* to treatment or control groups. The term 'selection' is best reserved for describing the methods used to determine who participated in the trial, not which groups participants were allocated to.

[6]These tests are sometimes called analysis of covariance or ANCOVA. In the contemporary parlance, estimates are adjusted by including the unbalanced baseline variables as covariates in a linear model.

[7]For a stridently different view, see Berger (2005).

[8]Concealment of allocation is commonly misunderstood to mean blinding. Blinding and concealment are quite different features of clinical trials. It would probably be clearer if concealment of allocation were called concealment of recruitment.

by knowledge of which group patients would subsequently be assigned to. For example, a researcher who favoured the hypothesis that intervention was effective might be reluctant to admit patients with a particularly severe case if he or she knew that the next patient entered into the trial was to be allocated to the control group. (This might occur if the researcher did not claim equipoise, and was concerned that this patient received the best possible treatment.) In that case, allocation would no longer be random even if the allocation sequence itself was truly random, because participants with the most severe cases could be allocated only to the treatment group. Consequently the groups would not differ only by chance, and they would no longer be 'comparable'. Similar reasons necessitate that potential *participants* are not aware, at the time they decide whether to participate in the trial, whether they would subsequently be randomized to the intervention or control group. Foreknowledge about which group they are to be allocated to could influence the patient's decision about whether to participate in the trial, potentially producing serious allocation bias. Lack of concealment potentially leads to non-random allocation.

How can the allocation be concealed? The simplest way is for a person not otherwise involved in entering participants into the trial to draw up the random allocation schedule. Then each participant's allocation is placed in a sealed envelope. The allocation schedule is concealed from the researcher who enters participants into the trial, and from potential participants, so that neither the researcher nor potential participant knows, at the time a decision is made about participation in the trial, which group the participant would subsequently be allocated to. Then, when the researcher is satisfied that the participant has met the criteria for participation in the trial and the participant has given informed consent to participate, the envelope corresponding to that participant's number is opened and the allocation revealed. Once the envelope is opened, the participant is considered to have entered the trial. This simple procedure ensures that allocation is concealed.

An alternative procedure involves holding the allocation schedule off-site. Then, when the researcher is satisfied a patient is eligible to participate in the trial and the patient has given informed consent, the researcher contacts the off-site holder of the allocation schedule and asks for the allocation. Again, once the researcher is informed of the allocation, the patient is considered to have entered the trial. This procedure also ensures concealment of allocation.

There are other, less satisfactory, ways to conceal random allocation. Allocation could be concealed if, once the researcher was satisfied that a patient was eligible to enter a trial and had given informed consent, allocation was determined by the toss of a coin ('heads' = treatment group, 'tails' = control group) or by the drawing of lots. Theoretically this would provide an allocation schedule that was both effectively random and concealed. The problem with coin-tossing and the drawing of lots is that the process is easily corrupted.[9] For example, the researcher could toss the coin or draw lots *before* making a final decision about the patient's eligibility for the trial. Alternatively if either the patient or the researcher was unhappy with the coin toss or the lot that was drawn, it might be tempting to repeat the toss or draw lots again until the preferred allocation was achieved. The benefit of using sealed envelopes or contacting a central allocation registry is that the randomization process can be audited, and corruption of the allocation schedule is more difficult.

Some reports of clinical trials will explicitly state that allocation was concealed. Usually statements about concealment of allocation are made in the part of the Methods section that describes the allocation procedures. More often, trial reports do not explicitly state that allocation was concealed, but they describe methods such as the use of sealed envelopes or contacting a central registry that probably ensured concealment. Unfortunately, most trials do not either explicitly state that allocation was concealed or describe methods that would have ensured concealment. Some (perhaps most) of these trials may have used concealed allocation (Soares et al 2004), but we cannot know which trials did.[10]

Was there complete or near-complete follow-up?

Doing clinical trials is hard and often mundane work. One of the difficulties is ensuring that the trial protocol is adhered to. And one of the hardest parts of

---

[9]Schulz & Grimes (2002) argue that, unless mechanisms are put in place to prevent corruption of allocation schedules, corruption of allocation is likely to occur.

[10]Systematic reviewers often write to the authors of papers to seek clarification of the exact methods used in the study, but this is not usually practical for readers of trials. Consequently, it is often not possible for readers of clinical trials to determine whether there was concealed allocation or not.

the trial protocol to adhere to is the planned measurement of outcomes ('follow-up').

Most clinical trials involve interventions that are implemented over days or weeks or months. Outcomes are usually assessed at the end of the intervention, and they are often also assessed one or several times after the intervention has ceased. Trials of chronic conditions may assess outcomes several years after the intervention period has ceased.

A problem that arises in most trials is that it is not always possible to obtain outcome measures as planned. Occasionally participants die. Others become too sick to measure, or they move out of town, or go on long holidays. Some may lose interest in participating in the study or simply be too busy to attend for follow-up appointments. For these and a myriad of other reasons it may be impossible for the researchers to obtain outcome measures from all participants as planned, no matter how hard the researchers try to obtain follow-up measures from all participants. This phenomenon of real-life clinical trials is termed 'loss to follow-up'. Subjects lost to follow-up are sometimes called 'dropouts'.[11]

Loss to follow-up would be of little concern if it occurred at random. But in practice loss to follow-up may be non-random, and this can produce bias. Bias occurs when dropouts from one group differ systematically from dropouts in the other group. When this occurs (it can only occur when the experimental intervention has an effect, one way or the other, on rate of loss to follow-up), differences between groups are no longer attributable just to the intervention and chance. Randomization is undone. Estimates of the effect of treatment potentially become contaminated by differences between groups due to loss to follow-up.

It is quite plausible that the people lost to follow-up from one group will differ systematically from people lost to follow-up in the other group. This is because it is quite plausible that participants' experiences of the intervention or its outcomes will influence whether they attend for follow-up.[12] Imagine a hypothetical trial of treatment for cervical headache. The trial compares the effect of six sessions of manual therapy with a no-intervention control condition, and outcomes in both groups are assessed 2 weeks after randomization. Some participants in the control group may experience little resolution of their symptoms. Understandably, these participants may become dissatisfied with participation in the trial and may be reluctant to return for outcome assessment after not having received any intervention. The consequence is that there may be a tendency for those participants in the control group with the worst outcomes to be lost to follow-up, more so than in the intervention group. In that case, estimates of the effects of intervention (the difference between the outcomes of intervention and control groups) are likely to be biased and the treatment will appear less effective than it really is.

We could imagine many such scenarios that would illustrate that loss to follow-up can bias estimates of the effects of intervention in either direction. Unfortunately, although statistical techniques have been formulated to try to reduce the bias associated with loss to follow-up (Raghunathan 2004), none is completely satisfactory. All involve estimating, in one way or another, values of missing data. But, because the missing data are not available, it is never possible to check how accurate these estimates are. Ultimately it will always be true that trials with missing data are potentially biased.

The potential for bias is low if few participants drop out. When only a small proportion of participants are lost to follow-up, the findings of the trial can depend relatively little on the pattern of loss to follow-up in such participants. On the other hand, large numbers of dropouts can seriously bias the findings of a study. The more participants lost to follow-up, the greater the potential for bias.

How much loss to follow-up is required seriously to threaten the validity of a study's findings? Many statisticians would not be seriously concerned with dropouts of as much as 10% of the sample. On the other hand, if more than 20% of the sample were lost to follow-up there would be grounds for concern about the possibility of serious bias. A rough rule of thumb might be that, if greater than 15% of the sample is lost to follow-up then the findings of the trial could be considered to be in doubt. (This is an arbitrary threshold. Some experts recommend a threshold of 20%; van Tulder et al 2003. However, a threshold of 10% might also be reasonable.) Of course this 'rule' ought to be applied judiciously: where trialists can provide data to show that losses to follow-up of greater than 15% were due largely to

---

[11]Note that a participant is *not* a dropout if he or she discontinues therapy, or does not comply with the allocated intervention, provided that follow-up data are available for that participant.

[12]In some trials it may be *others'* experiences of the intervention or its outcomes that influence loss to follow-up. For example, if the participant is dependent on a carer and the participant's carer is unhappy with therapy, the carer may be reluctant to attend follow-up and the participant may be lost to follow-up.

factors that were clearly not related to intervention, we may be prepared to accept the findings of the trial. On the other hand, where loss to follow-up is much greater in one group than in the other (clear evidence that loss to follow-up is due to intervention), or where loss to follow-up is clearly dependent on the intervention, we may be suspicious of the findings of trials that have loss to follow-up of less than 15%.

In some trials, particularly trials of the management of chronic conditions, the outcomes of most interest are those at long-term follow-up. But follow-up becomes progressively more difficult with time, so long-term follow-ups are often plagued by large losses. Consequently, many studies have adequate short-term follow-up but inadequate long-term follow-up. Such studies may provide strong evidence of short-term effects of intervention but weak evidence of long-term effects.

Some clinical trial reports clearly describe loss to follow-up. It is particularly helpful when the trial

report provides a flow diagram (as recommended in the CONSORT (Consolidated Standards of Reporting Trials) statement; Moher et al 2001) that describes the number of participants randomized to each group and the number of participants from whom outcomes could be obtained at each occasion of follow-up. An example is shown in Figure 5.2. Flow diagrams such as this make it relatively easy for the reader to assess whether follow-up was adequate.

More often, trial reports do not explicitly supply data on loss to follow-up. In that case the reader must calculate loss to follow-up from the data that are supplied. Two pieces of information are required. It is necessary to know both the number of participants randomized to groups (i.e. the number of participants in the trial) and the number of participants from whom outcome measures are available at each time point. These numbers are sometimes given in the text. Alternatively it may be possible to find these data in tables of results, or in summaries of

Figure 5.2 • An example of a flow diagram, showing how participants progress through the trial or are lost to follow-up. Redrawn from Hinman et al (2003), with permission from BMJ Publishing.

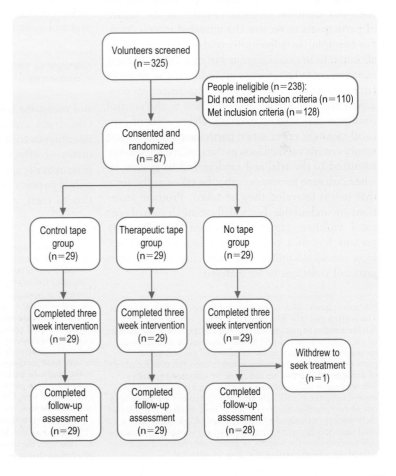

statistical analyses.[13] A degree of detective work is sometimes required to extract these data. Calculation of loss to follow-up is straightforward: the percentage lost to follow-up = 100 × number lost to follow-up/number randomized.

Some trial reports commit a special crime: they provide no clues about loss to follow-up, even for the most cunning detective. In such studies there may, of course, have been no loss to follow-up. But it is unusual to have no loss to follow-up. The more likely explanation, particularly in trials with long follow-up periods, is that loss to follow-up occurred but was not reported.

> Studies that do not provide data on loss to follow-up and that do not explicitly state that there was no loss to follow-up should be considered potentially biased.

A problem that is closely related to loss to follow-up is the problem of protocol violation. Protocol violations occur when the trial is not carried out as planned. In trials of physiotherapy interventions, the most common protocol violation is the failure of participants to receive the intended intervention. For example, participants in a trial of exercise may be allocated to an exercise group but may fail to do their exercises, or fail to exercise according to the protocol (this is sometimes called 'non-compliance' or 'non-adherence'), or participants allocated to the control condition may take up exercise. Other sorts of protocol violation occur when participants who do not satisfy criteria for inclusion in the trial are mistakenly admitted to the trial and randomized to groups, or when outcome measures cannot be taken at the time that it was intended they be taken. Protocol violations are undesirable, but usually some degree of protocol violation cannot be avoided. Usually they present less of a problem than loss to follow-up. How would we prefer data from clinical trials with protocol violations to be analysed?

One alternative would be to discard data from participants for whom there were protocol violations. Readers should be suspicious of studies that discard data because, insofar as protocol violations are influenced by the intervention, discarding data biases results. (This is because, once a participant's data are discarded, that participant is, as far as interpretation is concerned, effectively lost to follow-up.) Another unsatisfactory 'solution' is sometimes applied when there has been non-compliance with intervention. Some trialists analyse data from non-complying intervention group participants as though these participants had been allocated to the control group. This is sometimes called a 'per protocol' analysis. Per-protocol analyses potentially produce even greater bias than discarding data of non-compliant participants.[14] The most satisfactory solution is the least obvious one. It involves ignoring the protocol violations and analysing the data of all participants in the groups to which they were allocated. This is called 'analysis by intention to treat'.[15]

Analysis by intention to treat has properties that make it better than other approaches to dealing with protocol violations. Most importantly,

> analysis by intention to treat preserves the benefits of randomization

and maintains the comparability of groups. In addition, from a pragmatic point of view, analysis by intention to treat provides the most meaningful estimates of effects of intervention. This is because, pragmatically speaking, interventions can be effective only if patients comply.[16] When analysis is by intention to treat, non-compliance reduces estimates of

---

[13]A good place to look is the column headers in tables of results. These often give '$n = X$'. (Even then, it may not be clear whether X is the number of participants that entered the trial or the number of participants followed up.) When outcomes of dichotomous measures are expressed as the number *and* percentage of participants experiencing some outcome then the total number of participants followed up can easily be calculated (number followed up = 100 × number experiencing event/percentage experiencing the event). (Dichotomous outcomes are those with one of two possible outcomes, such as lived or died. We consider dichotomous outcomes further in Chapter 6.) Readers with a good understanding of tests based on t, F or χ^2 distributions may be able to determine the number of participants followed up from quoted degrees of freedom of t, F or χ^2 statistics.

[14]In trials with equally sized groups, the bias produced by crossing non-compliant intervention group participants over to the control group is twice that produced by omitting data of non-compliant participants.

[15]With the intention-to-treat approach, protocol violations are ignored in both the conduct and the analysis of the trial. Follow-up measurements are obtained from all participants, wherever possible, even if there were serious protocol violations. For example, participants are followed up, wherever possible, even if they were incorrectly admitted to the trial, or even if, as soon as they were randomized, they decided not to participate further in the study. In trials that do not use an intention-to-treat approach, these participants may not be followed up, in which case they become lost to follow-up. So the intention-to-treat approach has two benefits: it minimizes loss to follow-up and provides a coherent method for dealing with protocol violations.

[16]This assumes that the response to exercise continues to increase with the amount of exercise, at least up to the amount of exercise that is prescribed.

the magnitude of treatment effects. To the pragmatist, this is as it should be. We consider the issue of pragmatic interpretation of clinical trials in more detail later in this chapter.

It will usually be apparent that a trial has analysed by intention to treat only when the authors of the trial report refer explicitly to 'analysis by intention to treat'. However, analysis by intention to treat is often not reported, even when the trial was analysed by intention to treat (Soares et al 2004).[17]

Was there blinding to allocation of patients and assessors?

> There is reason to prefer that, in clinical trials, participants are unaware of whether they received the intervention or control condition. This is called blinding of participants.[18] Blinding of participants is considered important primarily because it provides a means of controlling for placebo effects.

In the following paragraphs we define placebo effects and discuss in more detail why and how blinding of participants is used. Then we present an alternative point of view which holds that blinding of participants may be relatively unimportant.

Placebo effects are effects of intervention attributable to patients' expectations of a beneficial effect of therapy. The placebo effect is demonstrated when patients benefit from interventions that could have no direct physiological effects, such as detuned ultrasound. That is, the placebo is an effect of the ritual of administration of the intervention, rather than of the intervention itself. Although the mechanisms are unknown, some have speculated that expectation or conditioning could trigger beneficial biochemical responses (Brody 2000). Placebo effects of one kind or another are widely believed to accompany most interventions. The effects, it is thought, can be very large – placebo can be more effective than many established interventions. Many good clinicians seek to exploit the placebo effect by maximizing the credibility of interventions in the belief that this will give the best possible outcomes for their patients.

Although there have been many well-controlled studies demonstrating placebo effects, most have been conducted in laboratory settings. Relatively few well-controlled studies have examined placebo effects of real clinical interventions on meaningful clinical outcomes in clinical populations. One of the best clinical studies was conducted by Kaptchuk and colleagues (2008). They randomized 262 adults with irritable bowel syndrome to one of three groups. The Wait group received no intervention, the Limited group received sham acupuncture with minimal interaction with the acupuncturist, and the Augmented group received sham acupuncture from an acupuncturist who displayed warmth, interest in the patient's well-being, and professional confidence. (The sham acupuncture employed a retractable needle that did not pierce the skin.) After 3 weeks, outcomes were assessed on a 7-point scale of global improvement (3 = slightly worse, 4 = no change, 5 = slightly improved) and by asking participants whether they had experienced 'adequate relief' of their symptoms over the last week. Mean global improvement scores were, respectively, 3.8, 4.3 and 5.0, and the proportions experiencing adequate relief of symptoms were, respectively, 28%, 44% and 62%. Comparison of outcomes of the Limited and Wait groups demonstrated that the ritual of provision of (sham) therapy had a beneficial effect, even when the (sham) therapy had no specific therapeutic effects. Comparison of outcomes of the Augmented and Limited groups demonstrated that the practitioner's warmth, attentiveness and confidence also had a beneficial effect. It should be noted, however, that the effects in this well-controlled study were small: the individual effects of both the ritual of provision of therapy and of practitioner warmth, attentiveness and confidence improved outcomes by about half a point on the 7-point global improvement scale (half of a slight effect!) and produced adequate symptom relief in 1 in every 6 patients.

A goal of many trials is to determine what effects intervention has over and above those effects due to placebo. Blinding is instituted in an attempt to do just that. Blinding means that participants in intervention and control groups do not know which group they were allocated to. Blinded participants can only guess whether they received the intervention or control condition. In the absence of any information about which group they were in, the guesses of participants in intervention and control groups will be, on average, similar. In some circumstances this will ensure that estimates of the effects

---

[17]Occasionally the opposite is true: some trialists may state they analysed by intention to treat even though the description of their methods indicated they did not.

[18]Sometimes 'blinding' is referred to as 'masking'.

of intervention are not substantially biased by placebo effects.[19]

How is it possible to blind patients to allocation? How can participants not know whether they received the intervention or the control? The general approach (nicely illustrated in the study conducted by Kaptchuk and colleagues) involves giving a 'sham' intervention to the control group. Sham interventions are those that look, feel, sound, smell and taste like the intervention but could not affect the presumed mechanism of the intervention. The clearest examples in physiotherapy come from studies of electrotherapies. Several clinical trials (for example, Ebenbichler et al 1999, McLachlan et al 1991, van der Heijden et al 1999) have used sham interventions in studies of pulsed ultrasound. In these studies the ultrasound machine is adapted so that it either emits pulsed ultrasound (intervention) or does not (sham intervention). In the study by McLachlan et al (1991), the sham ultrasound transducer was designed to become warm when turned on, so the patient was unable to distinguish between intervention and sham. The intervention and sham could not be distinguished by the patient, and yet the sham could not affect the presumed specific therapeutic mechanisms of ultrasound therapy because no ultrasound was emitted. Consequently this is a near-perfect sham. Other near-perfect shams used in clinical trials of physiotherapy interventions include the use of coloured light as sham low-level laser therapy (for example, de Bie et al 1998), and the use of specially constructed collapsing needles in studies of acupuncture (Kaptchuk et al 2008, Kleinhenz et al 1999).

Often it is not possible to apply sham interventions that are truly indistinguishable from the intervention. It is hard to imagine, for example, how one might apply a convincing sham stretch for ankle plantarflexor contractures, or sham gait training for people with Parkinson's disease, or a community-based rehabilitation programme after stroke. In these circumstances the highest degree of control is supplied by a quasi-sham intervention that is similar to the intervention (rather than indistinguishable from the intervention) yet could have no specific therapeutic effect. One example comes from a study of motor training of sitting balance after stroke. Dean & Shepherd (1997) trained participants in the intervention group by asking them to perform challenging reaching tasks in sitting; participants in the sham control group performed similar tasks but did not reach beyond arm's length. Another example comes from a recent trial of advice for management of low back pain. Subjects in the intervention ('advice') group received specific advice on self-management strategies from physiotherapists, whereas participants in the control ('ventilation') group talked to a physiotherapist who refrained from providing specific advice (Pengel 2004). In these examples the sham control is similar to but distinguishable from the intervention; nonetheless the sham probably provides quite a high degree of control for potential placebo effects.

In many physiotherapy trials there is no real possibility of applying a sham intervention because it is not possible to construct an ineffective therapy that even moderately resembles the true intervention. In that case, some control of placebo effects may be achieved by providing a control intervention that, like a sham, has no direct therapeutic effect, but that, unlike a sham, does not resemble the true intervention at all. In this case, as the control condition does not resemble the true intervention, it probably should not be called a sham. It may, nonetheless, still provide some control of placebo effects. This strategy has been used in trials of manipulative physiotherapy. It is difficult to apply sham manipulative therapy, so several trials have compared the effects of manipulative physiotherapy with de-tuned ultrasound (for example, Schiller 2001). De-tuned ultrasound has no direct therapeutic effects, but it does not resemble manipulative therapy. These *partially* blinded trials may provide some control for placebo effects,[20] but they provide less control than studies that use true shams.

---

[19]This is a methodological issue that has not been well investigated and is currently an area of active research. It can be shown that even when blinding confers similar perceptions of allocation in intervention and control groups there may still be, in some circumstances, bias associated with perceptions of allocation. The bias associated with perceptions of allocation is likely to be least when (a) most participants are uncertain about whether they were allocated to the intervention or control group, (b) perceptions of allocation have little effect on measured outcome, and (c) there are similar distributions of belief about allocation in the intervention and control groups (E. Mathieu, A. Barrett, K. McGeechan & R. Herbert, unpublished findings).

[20]In some studies the sham therapy may be very unconvincing to patients; that is, the sham may be an obviously ineffective therapy. It is possible that such studies accentuate, rather than control for, placebo effects. It is reassuring, in clinical trials employing sham therapies, to read that participants were asked whether they believed they received the experimental or the sham therapy. If the sham was convincing, similar proportions of participants in the treated and sham groups should say they thought they were given the experimental intervention.

We have seen that some studies employ true shams that are indistinguishable from the true intervention. And other studies employ shams that are similar to but not indistinguishable from the true intervention, or use control interventions that do not have direct therapeutic effects but do not resemble the true intervention. Some studies compare two active therapies, and yet other studies compare an active therapy to no-treatment controls. These latter studies are particularly exposed to potential bias from placebo effects. We will consider the seriousness of this bias further below.

Although the primary purpose of applying sham interventions is usually to control for placebo effects, there is a potentially useful secondary effect. In Chapter 3 we introduced the idea that polite patients can make interventions appear more effective than they truly are. When outcomes in clinical trials are self-reported, participants in the intervention group may exaggerate perceived improvements in outcome because they feel that is the socially appropriate thing to do, and patients in the control group may provide pessimistic reports of outcomes because they perceive that is what the investigators want to hear. Blinding of participants means that participants in intervention and control groups should have similar beliefs about whether they received intervention or control conditions, so trials with blinded participants are less likely to be biased by polite patients.

The preceding paragraphs have presented a conventional view of the value of blinding of participants in randomized trials. But there is another point of view that says blinding of participants may not be necessary.

The first argument against the need for blinding participants is that, from a pragmatic view, it does not matter whether the effects of therapy are direct effects of therapy or effects of placebo (Vickers & de Craen 2000). In this pragmatic view, the purpose of clinical trials is to help therapists determine which of two alternatives (intervention or control conditions) produces the better outcome. The intervention that produces the better clinical outcome is the better choice, even if its effects are due only to placebo. Therefore, it is argued, therapists need not be concerned whether an effect of intervention is due to placebo. They need only determine whether the intervention produces better outcomes. (Box 5.2, at the end of this section, summarizes the differences between pragmatic and explanatory perspectives of clinical trials.)

This point of view has some merit, but is not without problems. Perhaps the strongest counterargument is that it could be considered unethical to administer interventions whose only effects were placebo effects, because administration of placebo interventions would usually involve some sort of deception. The administration or endorsement of the intervention by a health professional might imply, either implicitly or explicitly, that there was some effect other than a placebo effect.[21] Another problem with applying interventions whose only effects are due to placebo is that this may stall the development of alternative interventions that have more scope for becoming more effective therapies. Lastly, even if it can be argued that it is not necessary to control for placebo effects, it is always desirable to control for polite patient effects. Blinding of participants with a sham intervention is always desirable, if for that reason alone.

A more radical argument against the need for blinding of participants in clinical trials is that the placebo effect may not be important in randomized trials. The placebo effect may be lessened in randomized trials, compared with its effect in routine clinical practice, for several reasons. One is that it is usually necessary, for ethical reasons, to inform potential participants in randomized trials that, should they choose to participate in the trial, they will be allocated to groups that will receive either the real intervention or a sham. That might be expected to reduce any placebo effect of intervention. What evidence is there that placebos can have measurable effects within the context of randomized trials?

An early stimulus for the now near-universal belief in the placebo effect was a literature review by Beecher (1955), aptly entitled 'The powerful placebo'. Beecher summarized the results of 15 'illustrative' clinical trials of a total of 1082 patients in which sham drugs (usually saline or lactose) were used to treat a range of conditions, including wound pain, angina pain, headache and cough. He concluded that 'placebos are found to have an average significant effectiveness of $35.2 \pm 2.2\%$' (Beecher 1955: 1603). Until recently Beecher's methods have not been seriously challenged and his conclusions became widely accepted as true.

But Beecher's data do not provide strong support for the existence of a placebo effect because they are based on an inappropriate methodology (Kienle & Kiene 1997). Beecher focused on the magnitude

---

[21] It would be interesting to know what patients receiving the intervention thought of this issue.

of the reduction in pain experienced by people receiving placebo analgesia. Even though these data were extracted from randomized trials, they did not involve comparison with a control condition. The effects observed in patients treated with placebo analgesia may have been partly due to placebo, but any such effects were almost certainly confounded by natural recovery, statistical regression,[22] polite patient effects and other biases. It is unremarkable to observe that many patients who receive placebo therapy experience recovery, because the recovery may not have been due to the placebo.

To determine the effects of placebo we need to examine randomized controlled studies that compare outcomes of people treated with sham interventions to outcomes of people who receive no intervention. In fact such comparisons are often made incidentally in clinical trials. This is because there are many randomized trials that compare intervention, sham control and no-intervention control. These trials provide estimates of the total effects of therapy (the difference between outcomes of the intervention and no-intervention groups), and also allow for the total effect of therapy to be partitioned into direct effects of therapy (the difference between outcomes of the intervention and sham intervention groups) and effects of placebo and polite patients (the difference between outcomes of the sham intervention and no-intervention groups).

In a landmark study, Hrobjartsson & Götsche (2001) systematically reviewed the evidence for effects of placebo in randomized trials. They found 114 randomized trials, distributed across all areas of health care, comparing intervention, sham intervention and no-intervention groups. To ascertain the effects of placebo they conducted a meta-analysis of the difference in outcomes of sham intervention and no-intervention groups. They found little or no effect of placebo on binary outcomes.[23] However, there was evidence of a small effect of placebo on continuous outcomes.[24] (The magnitude of this

effect was about one-quarter of one standard deviation[25] of the outcomes.) Subgroup analyses found the effect was apparent in trials that measured subjective outcomes but not in trials that measured objective outcomes.[26] The 27 trials that employed pain as an outcome showed a small effect (again, the magnitude was about one-quarter of one standard deviation; this corresponds to a pain reduction of 6.5 mm on a 100-mm visual analogue scale). The magnitude of this effect was less in trials with larger sample sizes, suggesting that the effect could be inflated by bias in small trials. An important limitation of the review is that it included trials that had imperfect shams; consequently it provided an assessment of the value of attempting to blind participants, but not necessarily of the effect of blinding participants. These findings are provocative because they suggest that placebo effects may have been exaggerated, and that the concept of the powerful placebo is a myth built on the artefact of poorly designed research. Incidentally, the review's findings also indicated that, in the typical randomized trial, bias caused by polite patients was small or negligible. The implication of Hrobjartsson & Götsche's fascinating study is that it is not important to blind participants in randomized trials.

Although the need for blinding of *participants* is, therefore, arguable, there are compelling reasons to want to see blinding of *assessors* in randomized trials.

> Wherever possible, assessors (the people who measure outcomes in clinical trials) should be unaware, at the time they take each measurement of outcome, whether the measurement is being made on someone who received the intervention or control condition.

This is because blinding of assessors protects against measurement bias. In the context of clinical trials, measurement bias is the tendency for measurements to be influenced by allocation. For example, measurements obtained from participants in the intervention group might tend to be slightly optimistic, or measures obtained from participants in the control group might tend to be slightly pessimistic, or both. This would bias (inflate) estimates of the effect of intervention.

---

[22]The concept of statistical regression, as it pertains to clinical trials, is explained in Chapter 3.

[23]Binary outcomes are events (such as lived/died, or returned to work/did not return to work). Typically binary outcomes are relatively 'hard' (objective) outcomes. We look at examples of binary outcomes in more detail in Chapter 6.

[24]Continuous outcomes are those that have a measurable magnitude, such as pain intensity or degree of disability. We look at examples of continuous outcomes in more detail in Chapter 6.

[25]The standard deviation is a measure of variability of a set of scores. It is calculated by taking the square root of the average squared deviation of the scores from the mean.

[26]We shall see, later in this chapter, that subgroup analyses are potentially misleading and should be interpreted cautiously.

Potential for measurement bias occurs whenever the measurement procedures are subjective. In practice there are very few clinical measurement procedures that do not involve some subjectivity. (By subjectivity we mean operator dependency.) Even measurement procedures that look quite objective, such as measurements of range of motion, strength or exercise capacity, probably involve some subjectivity. Indeed, the history of scientific research suggests that even relatively objective measures are prone to measurement bias.[27] Fortunately, measurement bias is often easily prevented by asking a blinded assessor to measure outcomes. In the words of Leland Wilkinson and the American Psychological Association's Task Force on Statistical Inference (1999: 596), 'An author's self-awareness, experience, or resolve does not eliminate experimenter bias. In short, there are no valid excuses, financial or otherwise, for avoiding an opportunity to double-blind.'

This statement might imply that blinding of assessors is easier than it really is. There *is* one circumstance that often prevents the use of blind assessors: in many trials outcomes are self-reported. In that case the assessor is the participant, and assessors are blinded only if participants are blinded. This is often overlooked by readers of clinical trials. The trial may employ blinded assessors to measure some outcomes, but self-reported outcomes cannot be considered assessor blinded unless the participants themselves are blinded. An example is the trial by Powell et al (2002) that examined whether a community-based rehabilitation programme could reduce the disability of patients with severe head injury. The authors ensured that, as far as possible, the researcher performing assessments was blinded to allocation.[28] However, one of the primary outcomes was assessed 'by the research assessor based on a combination of limited observation and interview with the client and, if applicable, carers'. The other outcome, a questionnaire, was completed 'by patients who were able to do so without assistance [*or*] on their behalf by a primary carer (where applicable)' (Powell et al 2002: 195). Patients and carers

were not (and could not be) blinded, so this trial was not assessor blinded.

There are other participants in clinical trials whom we would also like to be blind to allocation. Ideally, the providers of care (physiotherapists or anyone else involved in the delivery of the intervention) would also be blinded, because care providers may find it difficult to administer experimental and control therapies with equal enthusiasm, and care providers' enthusiasm may influence outcomes. We would prefer that the effects of therapy were not confounded by differences in the degree of enthusiasm offered by care providers when treating experimental and control groups. Unfortunately, it is even harder to blind care providers than it is to blind patients. Thus only a small proportion of trials, notably those investigating the effects of some electrotherapeutic modalities such as low-energy laser or pulsed ultrasound, are able to blind care providers. An example is the randomized trial, by de Bie and colleagues (1998), of low-level laser therapy for treatment of ankle sprains. In this trial, people with ankle sprains were treated with either laser therapy or sham laser therapy. The output of the machines was controlled by inputting a code that was concealed from patients and physiotherapists, so that both patients and physiotherapists were blind to allocation.[29] In most trials, blinding of care providers is not possible, so readers have to accept that many trials may be biased to some degree by care provider effects.[30]

Some trials also blind the statistician who analyses the results of the trial. This is because the methods used to analyse most trials cannot usually be specified completely prior to the conduct of the trial; some decisions can be made only after inspection of the data. It is preferable that decisions about methods of analysis are made without regard to the effect they would have on the conclusions of the trial. This can be achieved by blinding the statistician.

---

[27]For an excellent example, and a ripping good read, see Steven Jay Gould's account of nineteenth century craniometry (Gould 1997).

[28]The authors mention that 'Inevitably, however, some patients who had been treated by outreach, despite being instructed not to do so, inadvertently gave information [about their allocation] to the assessor during the interview assessment' (Powell et al 2002: 194–195). This is a common experience of clinical trialists!

[29]The authors reported that 'The additional 904 nm [*laser therapy*] was similar in all three groups except for the dose ... Laser dose at skin level was 0.5 J/cm^2 in the low-dose group, 5 J/cm^2 in the high-dose group, and 0 J/cm^2 in the placebo group ... Blinding of the treatment setting was ensured by randomizing the three settings (high, low or placebo) over 21 treatment codes (7 for each group) ... Both the patient and therapist were fully blinded. In all three groups, the laser apparatus produced a soft sound and the display read 'Warning: laser beam active!', Both patients and therapists also wore protective glasses. In addition, 904-nm laser light is invisible to the human eye' (de Bie et al 1998: 1416).

[30]Moseley and colleagues (2002) found that only 5% of all trials on the PEDro database used blinded therapists.

Statisticians can easily be blinded by presenting them with coded data – the statistician is given a spreadsheet that indicates participants are in the Apple group and the Orange group, rather than intervention and control group. Blinding of statisticians is rarely done, but it is easily done, and arguably should be routine practice.

Reports of clinical trials frequently refer to 'double-blinding'. This is a source of some confusion because, as we have seen, there are several parties who could be blinded in clinical trials (participants, the person recruiting participants, therapists, assessors and statisticians). For this reason the term 'double-blind' is uninformative and should be avoided.[31]

To summarize this section, readers of clinical trials should routinely appraise the trial validity. This can be done quickly and efficiently by considering whether treatment and control groups were comparable (that is, whether there was concealed random allocation), whether there was sufficiently complete follow-up, and whether patients and assessors were blinded (Box 5.1).

Box 5.1

Assessing validity of clinical trials of effects of intervention

Were intervention and control groups comparable?

Look for evidence that participants were assigned to groups using a concealed random allocation procedure.

Was there complete or near-complete follow-up?

Look for information about the proportion of participants for whom follow-up data were available at key time points. You may need to calculate loss to follow-up yourself from numbers of participants randomized and numbers followed up.

Was there blinding to allocation of patients and assessors?

Look for evidence of the use of a sham therapy (blinding of patients or therapists) and an explicit statement of blinding of assessors. Remember that when outcomes are self-reported, blinding of assessors requires blinding of participants.

Box 5.2

Pragmatic and explanatory trials

The distinction between 'explanatory' and 'pragmatic' clinical trials, first made by Schwartz & Lellouch (1967), is subtle but important, and is the source of much confusion amongst readers of clinical trials.[32] (An accessible and contemporary interpretation of the distinction between explanatory and pragmatic trials is given by McMahon (2002) and a more detailed discussion is provided by Herbert (2009)). An example might illustrate the distinction between the two approaches.

Imagine you are a clinical trialist who has decided to investigate whether a programme of exercise reduces pain and increases function in patients with subacute non-specific neck pain. You could adopt a pragmatic or an explanatory approach.

If your primary interest was about the *potential effects of the exercise* you would adopt the explanatory approach. You would carefully select from the pool of potential participants those expected to comply with the exercise programme,[33] reasoning that it will be possible to learn of the effects of exercise only if the participants actually do their exercises. You are fastidious about ensuring the exercises are carried out exactly according to the protocol because your aim is to find out about the effects of precisely that exercise protocol. You design the trial so that participants in the control group perform sham exercise, and you ensure that control group participants do exercises of a kind that could not be considered to have therapeutic effects, and that they exercise as frequently and as intensely as

---

[31]This leads to an obvious recommendation for authors of reports of clinical trials: avoid reference to double-blind and instead refer explicitly to blinded participants, blinded therapists, blinded assessors and blinded statisticians.

[32]Some authors refer to 'efficacy' trials and 'effectiveness' trials (e.g. Nathan et al 2000). The distinction between efficacy and effectiveness trials is similar to the distinction between explanatory and pragmatic trials (Box 5.2). Efficacy refers to the effects of an intervention under idealized conditions (as determined by trials with carefully selected patients, carefully supervised protocols, and per-protocol analysis) and effectiveness refers to the effects of an intervention under 'real-world' clinical conditions (as determined by trials with participants from a typical clinical spectrum, clinical

levels of protocol supervision, and intention-to-treat analysis). Thus efficacy trials have much in common with explanatory trials and effectiveness trials have much in common with pragmatic trials. It would appear that the most logical sequence would be for efficacy trials to be performed before effectiveness trials. If efficacy trials demonstrate that an intervention *may* have clinically worthwhile effects, effectiveness trials can be conducted to determine whether the intervention *does* have clinically worthwhile effects.

[33]A common practice, in explanatory trials, is to have a 'run-in' period prior to randomization. Only participants who comply with the trial protocol in the run-in period are subsequently randomized (that is, only participants who comply are given the opportunity to participate in the trial).

Box 5.2

Pragmatic and explanatory trials—cont'd

participants in the experimental group. In this way you can determine specifically the effects of the exercise over and above the effects (such as placebo effects) of the ritual of intervention. If there were protocol deviations then you would be tempted, when analysing the data, to analyse on a per-protocol basis. You seek to verify subjective outcomes with objective measures wherever possible.

Alternatively, your interest could be in the more clinical decision about *whether prescription of an exercise programme produces better clinical outcomes*, in which case you could adopt a more relaxed, pragmatic approach. Instead of recruiting only those participants expected to comply with the intervention, you recruit those participants who might reasonably be treated with this intervention in the course of normal clinical practice. As a pragmatist you are less choosy about who participates in the trial because your aim is to learn of the effects of prescribing exercise for the clinical spectrum that might reasonably be treated with this intervention, not on a subset of patients carefully selected because they comply unusually well. Even pragmatists like to see the exercise protocol complied with (all clinicians do), but as a pragmatist you see no point in going to unusual ends to ensure compliance – you want to know what the effects of exercise are when it is administered in the way it would be administered in everyday clinical practice. You specify that the control group receives no treatment, rather than a sham treatment, because you reason that this is the appropriate comparison group when the aim is to know

whether people will fare better when given exercise than when they are not given exercise. You are not interested in determining whether better outcomes in exercised participants are due to the exercise itself or to placebo effects; either way, from your perspective, you have achieved what you want to achieve. And as a pragmatist you analyse the data by intention to treat because you want to know the effects of therapy on the people to whom it is applied, not the effects of therapy on the selected group that comply (and, anyhow, analysis by intention to treat may be less biased than per-protocol analysis). In your pragmatic view, a therapy cannot be effective if most people do not comply with it. You are happy to base your conclusions on patients' perceptions of outcomes because your view is that the role of intervention is to make patients perceive that their condition has improved.

This example shows just some of the critical differences between explanatory and pragmatic approaches to clinical trials. The important point is that both perspectives, explanatory and pragmatic, are useful.[34] Both can tell us something worth knowing about. Nonetheless, readers of clinical trials often come to the literature with an interest in either an explanatory question or a pragmatic question. In that case they should look for trials with designs that are consistent with their focus. This is not always easy, because often the authors themselves are not clear on whether the trial has an explanatory or pragmatic focus, and often trials mix features of explanatory and pragmatic designs.

Systematic reviews of randomized trials

If a systematic review is to produce valid conclusions it must identify most of the relevant studies that exist and produce a balanced synthesis of their findings. To determine whether this goal has been achieved, readers can ask three questions.

Was it clear which trials were to be reviewed?

When we read systematic reviews we need to be satisfied that the reviewer has not selectively reviewed those trials that support his or her own point of view. One of the strengths of properly conducted systematic reviews is that the possibility of selective reviewing is reduced.

To reduce the possibility of selective reviewing, reviewers should clearly define the scope of the review prior to undertaking a search for relevant

trials. The best way to do this is to describe clearly the criteria that are used to decide what sorts of trial will be included in the review, and perhaps also which trials will not. The inclusion and exclusion criteria usually refer to the population, interventions and outcomes of interest.

An example of a systematic review that provides clear inclusion and exclusion criteria is the review by Green et al (1998) of interventions for shoulder pain. In their review the authors indicated that they 'identified trials independently according to predetermined criteria (that the trial be randomized, that the outcome assessment be blinded, and that the intervention was one of those under review). Randomized controlled trials which investigated common interventions for shoulder pain in adults (age greater than or equal to 18 years) were included provided

---

[34]But explanatory trials are hard; explanatory trialists have gastric ulcers and high blood pressure.

that there was a blinded assessment of outcome' (Green et al 1998: 354).

Systematic reviews that specify clear inclusion and exclusion criteria provide stronger evidence of effects of therapy than those that do not.

Were most relevant studies reviewed?

Well-conducted reviews identify most trials relevant to the review question.

There are two reasons why it is important that reviews identify most relevant trials. First, if the review does not identify all relevant trials it may conclude that there is less evidence than there really is.[35] More seriously, when not all relevant trials are found there is the possibility that those trials that were not found had systematically different conclusions from those included in the review. In that case the review findings could be seriously biased. For these reasons it is important that systematic reviews search for and locate most relevant trials.

Locating all relevant trials is not an easy task. As we saw in Chapter 4, randomized trials in physiotherapy are indexed across a range of partially overlapping major medical literature databases such as MEDLINE, Embase, CINAHL, AMED, and PsycINFO. The Cochrane Collaboration's Register of Clinical Trials and the Centre for Evidence-Based Physiotherapy's PEDro database attempt to provide more complete indexes of the clinical trial literature, but they rely on other databases to locate trials. Some trials are not indexed on any databases, or are so poorly indexed that they are unlikely ever to be found. So even the most thorough systematic reviews may sometimes miss relevant trials.

Health information scientists have developed optimal search strategies for the major medical literature databases. (See Box 5.3 for an example of an optimized search strategy for finding controlled trials in PubMed.) These search strategies are designed to assist reviewers to locate as many relevant clinical trials as possible.[36]

A substantial number of trials may not be indexed on major health literature databases; they may be published in obscure journals, or they may not have been published at all. Some high-quality systematic reviews

---

Box 5.3

An optimized search strategy for finding randomized trials in PubMed (Robinson & Dickersin 2002)

These search terms would be combined with subject-specific search terms to complete the search strategy for a particular systematic review:

(randomized controlled trial [pt] OR controlled clinical trial [pt] OR randomized controlled trials [mh] OR random allocation [mh] OR double-blind method [mh] OR single-blind method [mh] OR clinical trial [pt] OR clinical trials [mh] OR ('clinical trial' [tw]) OR ((singl* [tw] OR doubl* [tw] OR trebl* [tw] OR tripl* [tw]) AND (mask* [tw] OR blind* [tw])) OR ('latin square' [tw]) OR placebos [mh] OR placebo* [tw] OR random* [tw] OR research design [mh: noexp] OR comparative study [mh] OR evaluation studies [mh] OR follow-up studies [mh] OR prospective studies [mh] OR cross-over studies [mh] OR control* [tw] OR prospectiv* [tw] OR volunteer* [tw]) NOT (animal [mh] NOT human [mh])

---

supplement optimized searches of health literature databases with other strategies designed to find trials that are not indexed. An example is shown in Box 5.4.

These heroic searches are enormously time consuming, but they are thought to be justified because there is evidence that the trials that are most difficult to locate tend to have different conclusions from those of more easily located trials. It has been shown that unpublished studies and studies published in languages other than English tend to have more negative estimates of the effects of interventions than trials published in English (for example, Easterbrook et al 1991, Egger et al 1997, Stern & Simes 1997). Hence systematic reviews that search only for published trials are said to be exposed to 'publication bias', and systematic reviews that search only for trials reported in English are said to be exposed to 'language bias'. Reviewers perform exhaustive searches because they believe this will minimize publication bias and language bias.[37] However, it is possible that exhaustive searches create a greater problem than they solve. The studies that are hardest to find may also be, on average, lower-quality trials that are potentially more biased than trials that are

---

[35]If a meta-analysis is conducted, it may provide less precise estimates of effects of intervention.

[36]The search strategies are designed for maximum sensitivity, so they are not appropriate for use by clinicians seeking answers to clinical questions. That is why, in Chapter 4, we used simpler search strategies to find evidence.

[37]As we shall see in Chapter 7, clinical guidelines may involve the production of multiple systematic reviews, so they can be multiply heroic. The time-consuming nature of literature searches in systematic reviews is one reason why clinical guidelines tend to be developed at a national level.

Box 5.4

Example of a comprehensive search strategy in a systematic review of ventilation with lower tidal volumes versus traditional tidal volumes in adults with acute lung injury and acute respiratory distress syndrome (reproduced in Petrucci & Iacovelli 2003)

We searched the Cochrane Central Register of Controlled Trials (CENTRAL), *The Cochrane Library* issue 4, 2003, MEDLINE (January 1966 to October 2003), EMBASE and CINAHL (1982 to October 2003) using a combination of MeSH and text words. The standard methods of the Cochrane Anaesthesia Review Group were employed. No language restrictions were applied.

The MeSH headings and text words applied (MEDLINE) were:

Condition MeSH: 'respiratory distress syndrome, adult'. Text words: 'Adult Respiratory Distress Syndrome', 'Acute Lung Injury', 'Acute Respiratory Distress Syndrome', 'ARDS', 'ALI'

Intervention MeSH: 'respiration, artificial'. Text words: 'lower tidal volume', 'protective ventilation', 'LPVS', 'pressure-limited'

The search was adapted for each database (EMBASE, CINAHL).

The Cochrane MEDLINE filter for randomized controlled trials was used (Dickersin et al 1994); see additional Table 04. A randomized controlled trial filter was also used for EMBASE (Lefebvre et al 2008). All the searches were limited to patients 16 years and older.

An additional hand search was focused on:
- references lists
- abstracts and proceedings of scientific meetings held on the subject.

In particular, proceedings of the Annual Congress of the European Society of Intensive Care Medicine (ESICM) and of the American Thoracic Society (ATS) were searched over the last 10 years.

The following databases were also searched:
- Biological abstracts
- ISI web of science
- Current Contents.

Data from unpublished trials and 'grey' literature were sought by:
- The System for Information on Grey Literature in Europe (SIGLE)
- The Index to Scientific and Technical Proceedings (from the Institute for Scientific Information, accessing via BIDS)
- Dissertation abstracts (DA). This database includes: CDI – Comprehensive Dissertation Index, DAI – Dissertation Abstracts International, MAI – Master Abstract International, ADD – American Doctoral Dissertation
- Index to Theses of Great Britain and Ireland
- Current Research in Britain (CRIB). This database also includes Nederlanse Onderzoek Databank (NOD), the Dutch current research database
- Web Resources: the meta Register of Controlled Trials (mRCT) (www.controlled-trials.com).

An informal inquiry was made through equipment manufacturers (Siemens, Puritan-Bennet, Comesa) in order to obtain any clinical studies performed before the implementation and marketing of new ventilatory modes on ventilators.

The original author(s) were contacted for clarification about content, study design and missing data, if needed.

---

easier to find (Egger et al 2003). Exhaustive searches may substitute one sort of bias for another.

What constitutes an adequate search? How much searching must reviewers do to satisfy us that they have reviewed a nearly complete and sufficiently representative selection of relevant trials? It is clearly insufficient to search only MEDLINE: a review of studies of the sensitivity of MEDLINE searches for randomized trials found that MEDLINE searches, even those conducted by trained searchers, identified only a relatively small proportion of the trials known to exist (range 17–82%, mean 51%; Dickersin et al 1994). It is desirable that the reviewers perform sensitive searches of several medical literature databases (say, at least two of MEDLINE, Embase, CINAHL and PsychINFO) and at least one of the specialist

databases such as the Cochrane Collaboration's Central Register of Clinical Trials (CENTRAL) or PEDro.

A further consideration is the recency of the review. Systematic reviews tend to date rather quickly because, in most fields of physiotherapy, new trials are being published all the time (Maher et al 2008, Moseley et al 2002). The recency of reviews is particularly critical in fields that are being very actively researched. In actively researched fields, a systematic review that involved a comprehensive search but that was published 5 years ago is unlikely to provide a comprehensive overview of the findings of all relevant trials. In fact, there is often a lag of several years between when a search was conducted and the review was eventually published, so the search may be considerably older than the year of publication of the review suggests.

The year in which the search was conducted is usually given in the Methods section of the review. For example, the systematic review of spinal manipulation for chronic headache by Bronfort and colleagues, published in 2001, was based on literature searches conducted up to 1998. In general, if the search in a systematic review was published more than a few years ago it may be better to use a more recent systematic review or, if a more recent review is not available, to supplement the systematic review by locating individual randomized trials published since the review.

Was the quality of the reviewed studies taken into account?

Many randomized trials are poorly designed and provide potentially seriously biased estimates of the effects of intervention. Consequently, if a systematic review is to obtain an unbiased estimate of the effects of intervention, it must ignore those studies that are exposed to a high risk of bias.[38]

The simplest way to incorporate quality assessments into the findings of a systematic review is to list minimum quality criteria for trials that are to be considered in a review. Most (but not all) reviews specify that trials must be randomized. The consequence is that non-randomized trials are effectively ignored.

Excluding non-randomized trials protects against the allocation bias that potentially distorts findings of non-randomized trials. However, as we have seen, randomization alone does not guarantee protection from bias. Even randomized trials are exposed to other sources of bias, so it is not sufficient to require only that trials be randomized; it is necessary to apply additional quality criteria. Some systematic reviewers stipulate that a trial must also be participant- and assessor-blinded if it is to be considered in the review. An example of this is the review of spinal manipulation by Ernst & Harkness (2001). This review considered only randomized 'double-blind' trials.[39]

An alternative way to take into account trial quality in a review is to assess the quality of the trial using a checklist or scale. Earlier in this chapter we mentioned that there are now many such checklists and scales of trial quality, derived both from expert opinion and from empirical research about what best discriminates biased and unbiased studies. This diversity reflects the fact that we do not yet know the best way to assess trial quality. The most popular methods used to assess trial quality in systematic reviews of physiotherapy are the methods described by the Cochrane Collaboration (Higgins & Green 2009) and the Cochrane Back Review Group (van Tulder et al 2003), the Jadad scale (Jadad et al 1996), the Maastricht scale (Verhagen et al 1998b), and the PEDro scale (Maher et al 2003). Two of these, the Maastricht scale and the PEDro scale, generate a quality score (that is, they are scales), and the others do not (they are checklists). There is a high degree of consistency of the criteria used in four scales: the scales with more extensive criteria include all of the criteria in the less extensive scales.

In well-conducted reviews, assessments of trial quality are considered when drawing conclusions: the findings of high-quality trials are weighted more heavily than the findings of low-quality trials, and the degree of confidence expressed in the review's conclusions is determined, at least in part, by consideration of the quality of the trials.

If a scale has been used to assess quality, the quality score can be used to set a quality threshold. Trials with quality scores below this threshold are not used to draw conclusions. For example, in their systematic review of the effects of stretching before sport on muscle soreness and injury risk, Herbert & Gabriel (2002) indicated that only those trials with scores of at least 3 on the PEDro scale were considered in the initial analysis. This is an extension of the approach of specifying minimum criteria for inclusion in the trial. Another common alternative is to use a less formal approach, and simply comment on the quality of trials when drawing conclusions from them.[40]

We do not yet know which of these approaches is best. There is the risk that quality thresholds are too low (biased trials are still given too much weight) or too high (important trials are ignored), or that quality criteria do not really discriminate between biased and unbiased trials (so the conclusion becomes a lottery). However, it seems reasonable to insist that trial quality should be taken into account in some way.

[38]In the following pages we will call studies that are exposed to a low risk of bias 'high-quality studies' and studies that are exposed to a high risk of bias 'low-quality studies'. We will refer to the analysis of risk of bias as 'quality assessment'.

[39]See the comment in footnote 31 regarding problems with interpretation of the term 'double-blinding'.

[40]Detsky et al (1992) discuss four ways of incorporating quality in systematic reviews: using threshold score as an inclusion criterion; use of quality score as a weight in statistical pooling; plotting effect size against quality score; and sequential combination of trial results based on quality score.

Box 5.5

Assessing validity of systematic reviews

Was it clear which studies were to be reviewed?

Look for a list of inclusion and exclusion criteria (that defines, for example, the patients or population, intervention and outcomes of interest).

Were most relevant studies reviewed?

Look for evidence that several key databases were searched with sensitive search strategies, and that the search was conducted recently.

Was the quality of the reviewed studies taken into account?

Did the trials have to satisfy minimum quality criteria to be considered in the review? Alternatively, was trial quality assessed using a scale or checklist, and were quality assessments taken into account when conclusions were drawn?

Some reviews do not consider trial quality at all, and others assess trial quality but do not use these assessments in any way when drawing conclusions. Such reviews potentially base their findings on biased studies. Readers of systematic reviews should check that trial quality was taken into account when formulating a review's conclusions.

In conclusion, when appraising the validity of a systematic review, readers should consider whether the review clearly defined the scope and type of studies to be reviewed, whether an adequate search was conducted, and whether the quality of trials was taken into account when formulating conclusions (Box 5.5). When not all criteria are satisfied, the reader needs to weigh up the magnitude of the threats to validity.

Critical appraisal of evidence about experiences

So far in this chapter we have considered the appraisal of studies of effects of interventions. Such studies use quantitative methods. But we saw in Chapter 3 that it is necessary to use qualitative methods to answer other sorts of question. Both quantitative and qualitative studies make useful contributions to knowledge and should be regarded as complementary rather than conflicting (Herbert & Higgs 2004).

The particular strength of qualitative research is that it 'offers empirically based insight about social and personal experiences, which necessarily have a more strongly subjective – but no less real – nature than biomedical phenomena' (Giacomini and Cook 2002: p431).

In this section we consider appraisal of qualitative research of experiences. As pointed out in Chapter 3, we use the term 'experiences' as a shorthand way of referring to the phenomena that qualitative research might explore, which also include attitudes, meanings, beliefs, interactions and processes.

Before beginning the process of appraisal it is first necessary to ask whether an appropriate method has been used to address the research question. If the aim of the study was to explore social or human phenomena, or to gain deep insight into experiences or processes, then a qualitative methodology is appropriate.

In all kinds of research, no matter which method is used, it is necessary to observe phenomena in a systematic way and to describe and reflect upon the research findings. This applies equally well to qualitative research: insight emerges from systematic observations and their competent interpretation. Just as with quantitative research of effects of therapy, qualitative research is not uniformly of high quality. Although the adequacy of checklists and guidelines has been vigorously debated, and although it has been claimed that qualitative research cannot be assessed by a 'cookbook approach', scientific standards and checklists do exist (Giacomini and Cook 2002, Greenhalgh 2001, Kitto et al 2008, Malterud 2001, Seers 1999). The framework we will use for critical appraisal of qualitative studies is drawn from those sources. All sources emphasize that there is no definitive set of criteria for appraisal, and that the criteria should be continually revised. Consequently we see these criteria as a guide that we expect to change with time.

Qualitative research uses methods that are substantively different from most quantitative research. The methods differ with regard to sampling techniques, data collection methods and data analysis. Consequently, the criteria used to appraise qualitative research must differ from those used to appraise quantitative research. When critically appraising the methodological quality of qualitative research, you need to ask questions that focus on elements and issues other than those that are relevant to research, which includes numbers and graphs. Appraisal should focus on the trustworthiness, credibility and dependability of the study's findings – the qualitative parallels of validity and reliability (Gibson & Martin 2003). As qualitative research often seeks to discern subjective realities, interpretation of the research is frequently greatly influenced by the researcher's perspective. Consequently, a clear account of the process of collecting and interpreting data is needed. This is sometimes referred to as a decision trail (Seers 1999). Subjectivity is thus accounte for, though not eliminated. Subjectivity becomes problematic only when the perspective of the researcher is ignored (Malterud 2001).

When readers look to reports of qualitative research to answer clinical questions about experiences, we suggest they routinely consider the following three issues.

Was the sampling strategy appropriate?

Why was this sample selected? How was the sample selected? Were the participants' characteristics defined?

In qualitative research we are not interested in an 'on average' view of a population. We want to gain an in-depth understanding of the experience of particular individuals or groups. The characteristics of individual study participants are therefore of particular interest.

The sample in qualitative research is often made up of individual people, but it can also consist of situations, social settings, social interactions or documents. The sample is usually strategically selected to contain participants with relevant roles, perspectives or experiences.

> The methods of sampling randomly from populations, or sampling consecutive patients satisfying explicit criteria, common in quantitative research, are replaced in qualitative research by a process of conscious selection of a small number of individuals meeting particular criteria – a process called purposive sampling (Giacomini and Cook 2002).

People may be selected because they are typical or atypical, because they have some important relationship, or just because they are the most available participants. Sometimes sampling occurs in an opportunistic way: one person leads the researcher to another person, and that person to one more, and so on. This is called snowball sampling (Seers 1999). Often the goal of sampling is to obtain as many perspectives as possible. The author should explain and justify why the participants in the study were the most appropriate to provide access to the type of knowledge sought in the study. If there

were any problems with recruitment (for example, many people who were invited to participate chose not to take part), this should be reported. As the aim is to gain in-depth and rich insight, the number of observations need not be predetermined. Instead, data collection may continue until all phenomena have emerged. Nonetheless, readers should expect to see an explanation of the number of observations or people included in the study and why it is thought that this number was sufficient (Seers 1999).

Was the data collection sufficient to cover the phenomena?

Was the method used to collect data relevant? Were the data detailed enough to interpret what was being researched?

A range of very different methods is used to collect data in qualitative research. These vary from, for example, participant observations, to in-depth interviews, to focus groups, to document analysis. The data collection method should be relevant and address the questions raised, and should be justified in the research report. A common method in physiotherapy research involves the use of observations or in-depth interviews to explore communication and interactions of physiotherapists and patients. In-depth interviews are also used to explore experiences, meanings, attitudes, views and beliefs, for example the experiences of being a patient or of having a certain condition, as in a study that explored stroke patients' motivation for rehabilitation (Maclean et al 2000). Focus groups might be a relevant method of identifying barriers and facilitators to lifestyle changes or understanding attitudes and behaviours, as demonstrated by Steen & Haugli (2001), who conducted focus groups to explore the significance of group participation for people with chronic musculoskeletal pain.

Sometimes qualitative research uses more than one data collection method to obtain a broader or deeper understanding of what is being studied. The use of more than one method of data collection can help to confirm or extend the analysis of different facets of the experience being studied. For example, the data from observations of a mother playing with her child with cerebral palsy might be supplemented by interviewing the mother about her attitudes and experiences.

In observations or interviews, the researcher becomes the link between the participants and the data. Consequently, the information collected is likely to be influenced by what the interviewer or researcher believes or has experienced. A rigorous study clearly describes where the data collection took place, the context of data collection, and why this context was chosen. A declaration of the researcher's point of view and perspectives is important, as these might influence both data collection and analysis. A critical reflection on the potential implications of influence and role should follow.

Data collection should be comprehensive enough in both breadth (type of observations) and depth (extent of each type of observation) to generate and support the interpretations. That means that as many data as possible should be collected. Often a first round of data collection suggests whether it is necessary to continue sampling in order to confirm the preliminary findings. A sufficient number of participants should be interviewed or reinterviewed so that emerging theories are either confirmed or refuted and no new views are obtained. This is often called saturation (Seers 1999). The point of saturation is the point at which the sample size becomes sufficient. A description of saturation reassures the reader that sufficient data were collected.

Another important question to ask about data collection is whether ethical issues have been taken into consideration. The ethics of a study do not have a direct bearing on the study's validity but may, nonetheless, influence a reader's willingness to read and use the findings of the study. In qualitative research, people's feelings and deeper thoughts are revealed and it is therefore important that issues around informed consent and confidentiality are clarified. In such situations we would like to see the authors describe how they have handled the effects on the participants during and after the study. This issue was raised after the publication of a project that explored interactions between two physiotherapists and their patients. The authors were criticized because they had characterized one physiotherapist as competent and caring and the other as incompetent and non-empathic. This conclusion was criticized on ethical grounds, and raised the importance of careful explanation of the study aim to the participants, and also how the results are to be presented. One good way of handling this is to invite participants to read a draft of the research report.[41] Having participants verify that the researcher's interpretation is accurate and representative is also a common method for checking trustworthiness of the analysis (Gibson & Martin 2003).

---

[41]This is controversial. Very few researchers ask participants to read a draft of the research report.

Were the data analysed in a rigorous way?

Was the analytical path described? Was it clear how the researchers derived categories or themes from the data, and how they arrived at the conclusion? Did the researchers reflect on their roles in analysing the data?

The process of analysis in qualitative research should be rigorous. This is a challenging, complex and time-consuming job. The aim of this process is often to make sense of an enormous amount of text, tape recordings or video materials by reducing, summarizing and interpreting the data. The researchers often extend their conceptual frameworks into themes, patterns, hypotheses or theories; but ultimately they must communicate what their data mean. An in-depth description of the decision trail gives the reader a chance to follow the interpretations that have been made and to assess these interpretations in the light of the data.

An indication of a rigorous analysis is that the data are presented in a way that is clearly separated from the interpretation of the data. There should be sufficient data (such as transcripts) to justify the interpretation. Sometimes the data and the interpretation of the data are conflated, and then it can be difficult to know what is the author's view and what is a reflection of a participant. Separation of these elements makes it possible for the reader to draw his or her own interpretations from the data. The reader should be satisfied that sufficient data were presented to support the findings.

In the analysis phase, researchers should reflect upon their own roles and influences in data selection and analysis. The reader needs to consider that the researcher may have presented a selection of the data that primarily reflects the researcher's pre-existing personal views. It is helpful if, when analysing and reporting the study, the investigator distinguishes between the knowledge of the participants, the knowledge that the researcher originally brought to the project, and the insights the researcher has gained along the way. The data can be considered to be more trustworthy when the researcher considers contradictory data and findings that do not support a defined theory or pattern, and discusses the strengths and weaknesses of each finding.

There are several features that can strengthen a reader's trust in the findings of a study. As noted above, one is the use by the researchers of more than one source for information when studying the phenomena, for example the use of both observation and interviews. This is often called triangulation.

Box 5.6

Assessing validity of individual studies of experiences

Was the sampling/recruitment strategy appropriate?

Why was this sample selected? How was the sample selected? Were the participants' characteristics defined?

Was the data collection sufficient to cover the phenomena?

Was the method used to collect data relevant? Were the data detailed enough to interpret what was being researched?

Were the data analysed in a rigorous way?

Was the analytical path described? Was it clear how the researcher derived categories or themes from the data, and how they arrived at the conclusion? Did the researcher reflect on his or her role in analysing the data?

Triangulation might involve the use of more than one method, more than one researcher or analyst, or more than one theory. The use of more than one investigator to collect and analyse the raw data (multiple coders) also strengthens the study. This means that findings emerge through consensus between multiple investigators, and it ensures that themes are not missed (Seers 1999).

Box 5.6 summarizes this section.

Critical appraisal of evidence about prognosis

In Chapter 2 we considered two sorts of question about prognosis: questions about what a person's outcome will be, and questions about how much we should modify our estimates of prognosis on the basis of particular prognostic characteristics.

Subsequently, in Chapter 3, we considered the types of study that are likely to provide us with the best information about prognosis and prognostic factors. We can obtain information about prognosis from studies that identify patients with the condition of interest and monitor their outcomes. The best information is likely to come from cohort studies or, occasionally, from systematic reviews of cohort studies, but sometimes we can also get useful information from clinical trials.

In this section we consider how we can assess whether studies of prognosis are likely to be valid. We begin by considering individual studies of

prognosis and then consider, very briefly, systematic reviews of prognosis.

Individual studies of prognosis

Was there representative sampling from a well-defined population?

If we are to derive useful information about prognoses from clinical research, we must be able to use the findings of the research to make inferences about prognoses of a population. We can only do this if the people participating in the research (the 'sample') are representative of the population we are interested in.

When we read studies of prognosis we first need to know population for which the study is seeking to provide a prognosis (the 'target population'). The target population is defined by the criteria used to determine who was eligible to participate in the study. Most studies of prognosis describe a list of inclusion and exclusion criteria that clearly identify the target population. For example, Coste et al (1994) conducted an inception cohort study of the prognosis of people presenting for primary medical care for acute low back pain. They stated that 'all consecutive patients aged 18 and over, self-referring to participating doctors ($n = 39$) for a primary complaint of back pain between 1 June and 7 November 1991 were eligible. Only patients with pain lasting less than 72 hours and without radiation below the gluteal fold were included. Patients with malignancies, infections, spondylarthropathies, vertebral fractures, neurological signs, and low back pain during the previous 3 months were excluded, as were non-French speaking and illiterate patients' (Coste et al 1994: 577). The target population for this study is clear.

A closely related issue concerns how participants entered the study. This is critical because it determines whether the sample is representative of the target population.[42] In the clinical populations that are of most

---

[42]There are two ways to claim representativeness. The first approach is to define clearly the population of interest and then to sample from that population in a representative way, or in as representative a way as possible. The alternative approach is to sample in a non-representative way and then use the characteristics of the sample to dictate about whom inferences can be made. With the former approach, inferences can be made about the sorts of people who satisfy the study's inclusion and exclusion criteria. With the latter approach, inferences are made about people with characteristics like the study sample's characteristics. Of the two approaches, the first is preferable because it provides samples that are representative of the real population from which they were drawn. The second approach provides samples that are representative of virtual populations from which the sample could be imagined to have been drawn.

interest to physiotherapists, representativeness is usually best achieved by selecting a recruitment site or sites and then recruiting into the study, as far as is possible, all participants presenting to that site who satisfy the inclusion criteria. Recruitment of *all* eligible participants ensures that the sample is representative. Studies in which all (or nearly all) eligible participants enter the study are sometimes said to have sampled 'consecutive cases'. Where not all people who satisfy the inclusion criteria enter the study, it is possible that those who do not enter the study will have systematically different prognoses from the participants who do enter the study. In that case the study will provide a biased estimate of prognosis in the target population. When a study recruits 'all' participants or 'consecutive cases' that satisfy inclusion criteria (as in the study by Coste, cited in the last paragraph) we can be relatively confident that the findings of the study apply to a defined population. The greater the proportion of eligible participants that participates in the study, the more representative the sample is likely to be.

Researchers may find it difficult to gather data from consecutive cases, particularly when participation in the study requires extra measurements be made over and above those that would normally be made as part of routine clinical practice. An example of a study that did not sample in a representative way is a study of the 'outcomes' (prognosis) of children with developmental torticollis (Taylor & Norton 1997). The researchers sampled 'twenty-three children (14 male, nine female) . . . diagnosed with developmental torticollis by a physician. . . . Most of the children (74%) were referred to physical therapy by pediatricians . . . Data were collected retrospectively from the initial physical therapy evaluations of the 23 children whose parents agreed to a follow-up evaluation' (Taylor & Norton 1997: 174). Such samples may not always be representative; they may comprise participants with particularly good or particularly bad prognoses. Consequently, samples of convenience can provide biased prognoses for the target population.

It was noted in Chapter 3 that clinical trials (randomized or otherwise) involve monitoring of outcomes in a sample of patients with the condition of interest, and so clinical trials potentially provide information about prognosis. However, the main purpose of clinical trials is to determine the effects of intervention, and in many trials that purpose takes precedence over incidental findings about prognosis. Moreover, participation in clinical trials often places considerable demand on participants: participants in randomized trials must consent to be assigned intervention based on chance, and participation often requires the collection of large amounts of data on multiple occasions, which may be inconvenient or tedious. For this reason many trials include only a small proportion of potential participants; that is, the sample typically does not consist of consecutive cases. When anything less than a large proportion of potentially eligible patients consents to participate in a clinical trial, the trial is unlikely to consist of a sample that is representative of an easily identifiable population, and it is therefore unlikely to provide a useful estimate of prognosis. In general, therefore, clinical trials provide a less satisfactory source of information about prognosis than cohort studies.

Failures to sample in a representative way (i.e. to sample consecutive cases) or to sample from a population that is well defined (absence of clear inclusion and exclusion criteria) commonly threaten the validity of studies of prognosis.

> When you read studies looking for information about prognosis, start by looking to see whether the study recruited 'all' patients or 'consecutive cases'. If it did not, the study may provide biased estimates of the true prognosis.

Was there an inception cohort?

At any point in time, many people may have the condition of interest. Some will have just developed the condition, and others may have had the condition for a very long period of time.

A study of prognosis could sample from the population of people who currently have the condition of interest. But samples obtained from the population of people who currently have the condition (called 'survivor cohorts') will tend to consist largely of people who have had the condition for a long time, and that introduces a potential bias. The bias arises because the prognosis of people with chronic conditions is likely to be quite different from the prognosis of people who have just developed the condition. With many conditions, the people with longstanding disease are those who fared badly; they have not yet recovered. For this reason, survivor cohorts can tend to generate unrealistically bad prognoses. With life-threatening diseases the opposite may be true: the people who have longstanding disease are the survivors; they may have a better prognosis than those who died quickly, so survivor cohorts of life-threatening diseases might generate unrealistically good prognoses. Either way, survivor cohorts provide biased estimates of prognosis.

The solution is to recruit participants at a uniform (usually early) point in the course of the disease.[43] Studies that recruit participants in this way are said to recruit 'inception cohorts' because participants were identified as closely as possible to the inception of the condition. The advantage of inception cohorts is that they are not exposed to the biases inherent in studies of survivor cohorts.

We have already seen examples of prognostic studies that used survivor cohorts and inception cohorts. In the study of prognosis of developmental muscular torticollis (Taylor & Norton 1997), the age of children with torticollis at the time of initial evaluation ranged from 3 weeks to 10.5 months. Clearly those children attending for assessments at 10.5 months are survivors, and their prognoses are likely to be worse than average. In contrast, Coste et al (1994) obtained their estimates of the prognosis of low back pain from an inception cohort of participants who developed their current episode of back pain within the preceding 72 hours. Consequently, the study by Coste and co-workers is able to provide a relatively unbiased estimate of the prognosis of people with acute low back pain, at least among those who visit a general medical practitioner with that condition.

Readers of studies of prognosis should routinely look for evidence of recruitment of an inception cohort.

> Studies that recruit inception cohorts may provide less biased estimates of prognosis than studies that recruit survivor cohorts.

Although many studies provide good evidence of the prognosis of acute conditions, relatively few provide good evidence of the prognosis of chronic conditions. This is because the dual requirements of sampling *consecutive* cases from an *inception cohort* are frequently not satisfied in studies of chronic conditions. One way around this problem is to follow an inception cohort of patients with the acute condition. Some will recover, or perhaps die, but a subset of the initial cohort will go on to satisfy the definition of chronicity. If that subset of participants can be monitored from the time that they satisfy the definition for chronicity, they can become an inception

cohort of patients with the chronic condition. An example is a cohort study of the prognosis of chronic low back conducted by Menezes Costa et al (2009). That study followed an inception cohort of 973 patients presenting for the first time to primary care with acute low back pain of less than 2 weeks' duration. Of the original cohort of 973 patients, 406 still had pain 3 months after onset of their back pain, whereupon they were considered to have developed chronic pain. Those 406 patients in this subcohort constituted an inception cohort of patients with chronic low back pain. So, by following these patients for 1 year, it was possible to study an inception cohort of patients with chronic low back pain. This design, though robust, is difficult to implement, particularly for uncommon conditions or conditions that rarely become chronic.

Was there complete or near-complete follow-up?

Like clinical trials of effects of therapy, prognostic studies can be biased by loss to follow-up. Bias occurs when those lost to follow-up have, on average, different outcomes to those who were followed up.

It is easy to imagine how this might happen. A study of the prognosis of low back pain might incompletely follow up participants whose pain has resolved, perhaps because these participants feel well and are disinclined to return for follow-up assessment. Such a study would necessarily base estimates of prognosis on the participants who could be followed up. These participants would have, on average, worse outcomes, and so such a study would provide a biased (unduly pessimistic) estimate of prognosis. In contrast, a study of the prognosis of motor function following stroke might only follow up participants discharged to home, perhaps because of difficulties following up participants discharged to nursing homes. The participants followed up are likely to have better prognoses, on average, than those who were not followed up, so this study would provide a biased (unduly optimistic) estimate of prognosis.

How much of a loss to follow-up can be tolerated? As with clinical trials, losses to follow-up of less than 10% are unlikely seriously to distort estimates of prognoses,[44] and losses to follow-up of greater than 20% are usually of concern, particularly if there is any possibility that outcomes influenced follow-up.

---

[43]Subjects recruited at the point of disease onset are sometimes called 'incident cases'.

[44]Unless the probability of loss to follow-up is highly correlated with outcome.

It may be reasonable to apply the same 85% rule that we applied to clinical trials of the effects of therapy: as a rough rule of thumb, the study is unlikely to be seriously biased by loss to follow-up if follow-up is at least 85%.

An example of a study with a high degree of follow-up is the study of the prognosis of pregnancy-related pelvic pain by Albert et al (2001). These researchers followed 405 women who reported pelvic pain when presenting to an obstetric clinic during pregnancy. It was possible to verify the presence or absence of post-partum pain in all but 18 women, giving a post-partum loss to follow-up of just 4%. Such a low rate of loss to follow-up is unlikely to be associated with significant bias. On the other hand, Jette et al (1987) conducted a randomized trial to compare the effects of intensive rehabilitation and standard care on functional recovery over the 12 months following hip fracture. This study incidentally provided information about prognosis following hip fracture. However, loss to follow-up in the standard care group at 3, 6 and 12 months was 35%, 53% and 57%, respectively. The prognosis provided by this study is potentially seriously biased by a large loss to follow-up.

In large studies with long follow-up periods, or studies of serious disease, or studies of elderly participants, it is likely that a substantial proportion of participants will die during the follow-up period. (For example, in Allerbring & Haegerstam's (2004) study of orofacial pain 13 of 74 patients had died at the 9–19-year follow-up, and in Jette et al's (1987) study of hip fracture 29% of participants died within 12 months). Should these participants be counted as lost to follow-up? For all practical purposes the answer is 'no'. If we know a participant has died, we know that participant's outcome: this particular form of loss to follow-up is informative, and does not bias estimates of prognosis. We can consider death an outcome, which means that risk of death is considered as part of the prognosis, or we could focus on prognosis in survivors.

It is relatively easy to identify losses to follow-up in clinical trials and prospective cohort studies. In retrospective studies of prognosis it can be more difficult to ascertain the proportion lost to follow-up because it is not always clear who was entered into the study. In retrospective studies, loss to follow-up should be calculated as the proportion of all *eligible* participants for whom follow-up data were available.

See Box 5.7 for a summary of this section.

Box 5.7

Assessing validity of individual studies of prognosis

Was there representative sampling from a well-defined population?

Did the study sample consecutive cases that satisfied clear inclusion criteria?

Was there an inception cohort?

Were participants entered into the study at an early and uniform point in the course of the condition?

Was there complete or near-complete follow-up?

Look for information about the proportion of participants for whom follow-up data were available at key time points. Alternatively, calculate loss to follow-up from numbers of participants entered into the study and the numbers followed up.

Systematic reviews of prognosis

In Chapter 3 we pointed out that the preferred source of information about prognosis is systematic reviews. Systematic reviews of prognosis differ from systematic reviews of therapy in several ways. They need to employ different search strategies to find different sorts of study, and they need to employ different criteria to assess the quality of the studies included in the review. Nonetheless, the methods of systematic reviews of prognosis are fundamentally similar to the methods of systematic reviews of the effects of therapy, so the process of assessing the validity of systematic reviews of prognosis is essentially the same as evaluating the validity of systematic reviews of therapy. That is, it is useful to ask whether it was clear which trials were to be reviewed, whether most relevant studies were reviewed, and whether the quality of the reviewed studies was taken into account. As these characteristics of systematic reviews have already been considered in detail, we shall not elaborate on them further here.

Critical appraisal of evidence about diagnostic tests

Chapter 3 argued that questions about diagnostic accuracy are best answered by cross-sectional studies that compare the findings of the test in question with the findings of a reference standard. What features of such studies confer validity?

Individual studies of diagnostic tests

Was there comparison with an adequate reference standard?

Interpretation of studies of diagnostic accuracy is most straightforward when the reference standard is perfectly accurate, or close to it. But it is difficult to know whether the reference standard is accurate. Assessment of the accuracy of the reference standard would require comparing its findings with another reference standard, and we would then need to know *its* accuracy. So, realistically, we have to live with imperfect knowledge of the reference standard. Claims of the adequacy of a reference standard cannot be based on data. Instead they must rely on face validity; that is, ultimately our assessments of the adequacy of the reference standard must rely on our assessment of whether the reference standard appears to be the sort of measurement that would be more-or-less perfectly accurate.

An example of a reference standard that has apparent face validity is open surgical or arthroscopic confirmation of a complete tear of the anterior cruciate ligament. It is reasonable to believe that the diagnosis of a complete tear could be made unambiguously at surgery. On the other hand, the diagnosis of partial tears is more difficult, and the surgical presentation may be ambiguous. Thus, open surgical exploration and arthroscopic examination are excellent reference standards for diagnosis of complete tears, but less satisfactory reference standards for partial tears.

When the reference standard is imperfect, the accuracy of the diagnostic test of interest will tend to be underestimated. This is because when the reference standard is imperfect we are asking the clinical test to do something that is impossible: if the test is to perform well, its findings must correspond with the incorrect findings of the reference standard as well as the correct ones.[45] Readers of studies of the accuracy of diagnostic tests that use imperfect reference standards should recognize that the true

accuracy of the test may be higher than the observed accuracy.[46]

Was the comparison blind?

Studies of the accuracy of diagnostic tests can be biased in just the same way as randomized trials by the expectations of the person taking the measurements. If the person administering the diagnostic test (the 'assessor') is aware of the findings of the reference standard then, when the test's findings are difficult to interpret, he or she may be more inclined to interpret the test in a way that is consistent with the reference standard. In theory this could also happen in the other direction. When the reference standard is difficult to interpret, the assessor of the reference standard may be more inclined to interpret the findings in a way that is consistent with the diagnostic test. Either way, the consequence is the same: the effect will be to bias (inflate) estimates of diagnostic test accuracy.

It is relatively straightforward for the researcher to reduce the possibility of this bias. The simple

---

[45]Some statistical techniques have been developed to correct estimates of the accuracy of diagnostic tests when there is error in the reference standard, but these techniques require knowledge of the degree of error in the reference standard or necessitate tenuous assumptions. They are not widely used in studies of diagnostic test accuracy.

[46]Two special problems arise in the studies of the accuracy of diagnostic tests used by physiotherapists. The first is that, although it is sometimes quite straightforward to determine whether a test can accurately detect the presence or absence of a particular pathology, it may be difficult to determine whether the test can accurately detect whether that pathology is the cause of the person's symptoms. Consider the clinical question about whether, in people with stiff painful shoulders, O'Brien's test accurately discriminates between people with and without complete tears of rotator cuff muscles. An answer to this question could be provided by a study that compared the findings of O'Brien's test and arthroscopic investigation. If, however, the question was whether O'Brien's test accurately discriminates between people *whose symptoms are or are not due to* complete tears of rotator cuff muscles, it would be necessary for the reference standard to ascertain whether a patient's symptoms were due to the rotator cuff tear. Many older people have rotator cuff tears that are asymptomatic, so the arthroscopic finding of the presence of a rotator cuff tear cannot necessarily be interpreted as indicating that the person's symptoms are due to the tear. There is no reference standard for determining whether symptoms are due to a rotator cuff tear, so we cannot ascertain whether O'Brien's test can accurately determine whether a rotator cuff tear is a cause of a person's symptoms.

A second problem arises in the diagnosis of conditions that are defined by a simple clinical presentation. For example, sciatica is defined by the presence of pain radiating down the leg. As the condition is defined in terms of pain radiating down the leg, there can be no reference standard beyond asking the patient where he or she experiences the pain. So it is generally not useful to ask questions about the diagnostic accuracy of tests for sciatica. There is no need to know the accuracy of tests for sciatica because it is obvious whether someone has sciatica from the clinical presentation. More generally, there is no point in testing the accuracy of a test for a diagnosis that is obvious without testing.

solution is to ensure that the assessor is unaware, at the time he or she administers the diagnostic test, of the findings of the reference standard. If the assessor is unaware of the findings of the reference standard then the estimate of diagnostic accuracy cannot be inflated by assessor bias.

> Readers of studies of the accuracy of diagnostic tests should determine whether the clinical test and reference standard were conducted independently. That is, readers should ascertain whether each test was conducted blind to the results of the other test.

Confirmation of the independence of the tests implies that estimates of diagnostic test accuracy from these trials were probably not distorted by assessor bias. The findings of studies that provide no evidence of the independence of tests should be considered potentially suspect.

A reasonably frequent scenario is that the diagnostic test is administered prior to the administration of the reference standard. When this is the case, the assessment of the diagnostic test is blind to the reference standard. This is more important than blinding the reference standard to the diagnostic test because the tester will usually feel less inclined to modify interpretation of the reference standard on the basis of a finding from the diagnostic test than he or she might feel inclined to modify interpretation of the diagnostic test on the basis of a finding on the reference standard. Consequently studies in which the diagnostic test is consistently recorded prior to administration of the reference standard need not be a cause for serious concern.

Did the study sample consist of participants for whom there was diagnostic uncertainty?

The last criterion we will consider is the least obvious, and yet there is some evidence that it is the criterion that best discriminates between biased and unbiased studies of diagnostic test accuracy.

In Chapter 3 we saw that there were two sorts of design used in studies of the accuracy of diagnostic tests. The first type, sometimes called a cohort study, samples participants who are suspected of having, but are not known to have, the condition that is being tested for. That is, cohort studies sample from the population that we would usually test in clinical practice. In clinical practice we only test people who we suspect of having the condition; we don't test if the

diagnosis is not suspected, nor do we test if the diagnosis has been confirmed.

> Cohort studies provide the best way to evaluate diagnostic accuracy because they involve testing the discriminative accuracy of the diagnostic test in the same spectrum of patients that the test would be applied to in the course of clinical practice.

Such studies provide us with the best estimates of diagnostic test accuracy.

The alternative to the cohort design is the case–control design. Case–control studies recruit samples of participants who clearly do and clearly do not have the diagnosis of interest. In Chapter 3 we saw the example of a study of the accuracy of Phalen's test for diagnosis of carpal tunnel syndrome that recruited one group of participants (cases) with clinically and electromyographically confirmed carpal tunnel syndrome and another group (controls) who did not complain of any hand symptoms. The advantage of the case–control design is that it makes it relatively easy to obtain an adequate number of participants with and without the diagnosis of interest. But there is a methodological cost: in case–control studies the test is subject to relatively gentle scrutiny. Case–control studies require the test to discriminate only between people who obviously do and obviously do not have the condition of interest. That is an easier task than the real clinical challenge of making accurate diagnoses on people who are suspected of having the diagnosis. Only cohort studies can tell us about the ability of a test to do that.

Analyses by Lijmer et al (1999) suggest that the strongest determinant of bias in studies of diagnostic test accuracy is the use of case–control designs.

> Readers should probably be suspicious of the findings of case–control studies of diagnostic test accuracy.

See Box 5.8 for a summary of this section.

Systematic reviews of diagnostic tests

The same criteria can be used to assess systematic reviews of diagnostic tests as were used to assess systematic reviews of the effects of interventions or systematic reviews of prognosis. Consequently we shall not elaborate further on appraisal of systematic reviews of studies of diagnostic test accuracy.

Box 5.8

Assessing validity of individual studies of diagnostic tests

Was there comparison with an adequate reference standard?

Were the findings of the test compared with the findings of a reference standard that is considered to have near-perfect accuracy?

Was the comparison blind?

Were the clinicians who applied the clinical tests unaware of the findings of the reference standard?

Did the study sample consist of participants for whom there was diagnostic uncertainty?

Was there sampling of consecutive cases satisfying clear inclusion and exclusion criteria?

References

Albert, H., Godskesen, M., Westergaard, J., 2001. Prognosis in four syndromes of pregnancy-related pelvic pain. Acta Obstet. Gynecol. Scand. 80, 505–510.

Allerbring, M., Haegerstam, G., 2004. Chronic idiopathic orofacial pain. A long term follow-up study. Acta Odontol. Scand. 62, 66–69.

Anyanwu, A.C., Treasure, T., 2004. Surgical research revisited: clinical trials in the cardiothoracic surgical literature. Eur. J. Cardiothorac. Surg. 25, 299–303.

Beecher, H.K., 1955. The powerful placebo. JAMA 159, 1602–1606.

Berger, V.W., 2005. Selection bias and covariate imbalances in randomized clinical trials. Wiley, Chichester.

Brody, H., 2000. The placebo response: recent research and implications for family medicine. J. Fam. Pract. 49, 649–654.

Bronfort, G., Assendelft, W.J., Evans, R., et al., 2001. Efficacy of spinal manipulation for chronic headache: a systematic review. J. Manipulative Physiol. Ther. 24, 457–466.

Campbell, D., Stanley, J., 1963. Experimental and quasi-experimental designs for research. Rand-McNally, Chicago.

Chalmers, T.C., Celano, P., Sacks, H.S., et al., 1983. Bias in treatment assignment in controlled clinical trials. N. Engl. J. Med. 309, 1358–1361.

Colditz, G.A., Miller, J.N., Mosteller, F., 1989. How study design affects outcomes in comparisons of therapy. I: Medical. Stat. Med. 8, 441–454.

Cook, T.D., Campbell, D.T., 1979. Quasi-experimentation: design and analysis issues for field settings. Houghton Mifflin, Boston.

Coste, J., Delecoeuillerie, G., Cohen de Lara, A., et al., 1994. Clinical course and prognostic factors in acute low back pain: an inception cohort study in primary care practice. BMJ 308, 577–580.

Dean, C.M., Shepherd, R.B., 1997. Task-related training improves performance of seated reaching tasks after stroke. A randomized controlled trial. Stroke 28, 722–728.

de Bie, R.A., de Vet, H.C., Lenssen, T.F., et al., 1998. Low-level laser therapy in ankle sprains: a randomized clinical trial. Arch. Phys. Med. Rehabil. 79, 1415–1420.

Department of Clinical Epidemiology and Biostatistics, 1981. How to read clinical journals: I. why to read them and how to start reading them critically. Can. Med. Assoc. J. 124, 555–558.

Detsky, A.S., Naylor, C.D., O'Rourke, K., et al., 1992. Incorporating variations in the quality of individual randomized trials into meta-analysis. J. Clin. Epidemiol. 45, 255–265.

Dickersin, K., Scherer, R., Lefebvre, C., 1994. Systematic reviews: identifying relevant studies for systematic reviews. BMJ 309, 1286–1291.

Dickinson, K., Bunn, F., Wentz, R., et al., 2000. Size and quality of randomised controlled trials in head injury: review of published studies. BMJ 320, 1308–1311.

Easterbrook, P.J., Berlin, J.A., Gopalan, R., et al., 1991. Publication bias in clinical research. Lancet 337, 867–872.

Ebenbichler, G.R., Erdogmus, C.B., Resch, K.L., et al., 1999. Ultrasound therapy for calcific tendinitis of the shoulder. N. Engl. J. Med. 340, 1533–1538.

Egger, M., Zellweger-Zahner, T., Schneider, M., et al., 1997. Language bias in randomised controlled trials in English and German. Lancet 347, 326–329.

Egger, M., Bartlett, C., Holenstein, F., et al., 2003. How important are comprehensive literature searches and the assessment of trial quality in systematic reviews? Empirical study. Health Technol. Assess. 7, 1–76.

Ernst, E., Harkness, E., 2001. Spinal manipulation: a systematic review of sham controlled, double-blind, randomized clinical trials. J. Pain Symptom Manage. 22, 879–889.

Fung, K.P., Chow, O.K., So, S.Y., 1986. Attenuation of exercise-induced asthma by acupuncture. Lancet 330, 1419–1422.

Giacomini, M., Cook, D., 2002. Qualitative research. In: Guyatt, G., Rennie, D. the Evidence-Based Medicine Working Group, (Eds.), Users' guide to the medical literature. A manual for evidence-based physiotherapy practice. American Medical Association, Chicago, pp. 433–438.

Gibson, B., Martin, D., 2003. Qualitative research and evidence-based physiotherapy practice. Physiotherapy 89, 350–358.

Gould, S.J., 1997. The mismeasure of man. Penguin, London.

Green, J., Forster, A., Bogle, S., 2002. Physiotherapy for patients with mobility problems more than 1 year after stroke: a randomised controlled trial. Lancet 359, 199–203.

Green, S., Buchbinder, R., Glazier, R., et al., 1998. Systematic review of randomised controlled trials of interventions for painful shoulder: selection criteria, outcome assessment, and efficacy. BMJ 316, 354–360.

Greenhalgh, T., 2001. How to read a paper. BMJ Books, London.

Gruber, W., Eber, E., Malle-Scheid, D., 2002. Laser acupuncture in children and adolescents with exercise induced asthma. Thorax 57, 222–225.

Guyatt, G.H., Rennie, D., 1993. Users' guides to the medical literature. JAMA 270, 2096–2097.

Herbert, R., 2009. Explanatory and pragmatic clinical trials. In: Gad, S.C. (Ed.), Clinical trials handbook. John Wiley, Chichester, pp. 1081–1098.

Herbert, R.D., 2005. Randomisation in clinical trials. Aust. J. Physiother. 51 (1), 58–60.

Herbert, R.D., Gabriel, M., 2002. Effects of pre- and post-exercise stretching on muscle soreness, risk of injury and athletic performance: a systematic review. BMJ 325, 468–472.

Herbert, R.D., Higgs, J., 2004. Complementary research paradigms. Aust. J. Physiother. 50 (2), 63–64.

Higgins, J.P.T., Green, S. (Eds.), 2009. Cochrane handbook for systematic reviews of interventions, version 5.0.2. In: The Cochrane Collaboration, Online. Available: http://www.cochrane-handbook.org/ 6 Nov 2010.

Hinman, R.S., Crossley, K.M., McConnell, J., et al., 2003. Efficacy of knee tape in the management of osteoarthritis of the knee: blinded randomised controlled trial. BMJ 327, 135.

Hrobjartsson, A., Götsche, P.C., 2001. Is the placebo powerless? An analysis of clinical trials comparing placebo with no treatment. N. Engl. J. Med. 344, 1594–1602.

Jadad, A.R., Moore, R.A., Carroll, D., et al., 1996. Assessing the quality of reports of randomized clinical trials: is blinding necessary? Control. Clin. Trials 17, 1–12.

Jette, A.M., Harris, B.A., Cleary, P.D., et al., 1987. Functional recovery after hip fracture. Arch. Phys. Med. Rehabil. 68, 735–740.

Kaptchuk, T.J., Kelley, J.M., Conboy, L.A., et al., 2008. Components of placebo effect: randomised controlled trial in patients with irritable bowel syndrome. BMJ 336, 999–1003.

Kienle, G.S., Kiene, H., 1997. The powerful placebo effect: fact or fiction? J. Clin. Epidemiol. 50, 1311–1318.

Kitto, S.C., Chesters, J., Grbich, C., 2008. Quality in qualitative research. Med. J. Aust. 188 (4), 243–246.

Kjaergard, L.L., Frederiksen, S.L., Gluud, C., 2002. Validity of randomized clinical trials in gastroenterology from 1964–2000. Gastroenterology 122, 1157–1160.

Kleinhenz, J., Streitberger, K., Windeler, J., et al., 1999. Randomised clinical trial comparing the effects of acupuncture and a newly designed placebo needle in rotator cuff tendinitis. Pain 83, 235–241.

Kunz, R., Oxman, A.D., 1998. The unpredictability paradox: review of empirical comparisons of randomised and non-randomised clinical trials. BMJ 317, 1185–1190.

Lavori, P.W., Louis, T.A., Bailar, J.C., et al., 1983. Designs for experiments: parallel comparisons of treatment. N. Engl. J. Med. 309, 1291–1299.

Lijmer, J.G., Mol, B.W., Heisterkamp, S., et al., 1999. Empirical evidence of design-related bias in studies of diagnostic tests. JAMA 282, 1061–1066.

Maclean, N., Pound, P., Wolfe, C., et al., 2000. Qualitative analysis of stroke patients' motivation for rehabilitation. BMJ 321, 1051–1054.

Maher, C.G., Sherrington, C., Herbert, R.D., et al., 2003. Reliability of the PEDro scale for rating quality of randomized controlled trials. Phys. Ther. 83, 713–721.

Maher, C.G., Moseley, A., Sherrington, C., et al., 2008. A description of the trials, reviews and practice guidelines indexed on the PEDro database. Phys. Ther. 88, 1068–1077.

Malterud, K., 2001. Qualitative research: standards, challenges and guidelines. Lancet 358, 483–489.

McLachlan, Z., Milne, E.J., Lumley, J., et al., 1991. Ultrasound treatment for breast engorgement: a randomised double blind trial. Aust. J. Physiother. 37, 23–28.

McMahon, A.D., 2002. Study control, violators, inclusion criteria and defining explanatory and pragmatic trials. Stat. Med. 21, 1365–1376.

Menezes Costa, L.d.C., Maher, C.G., McAuley, J.H., et al., 2009. Prognosis for patients with chronic low back pain: inception cohort study. BMJ 339, b3829.

Moher, D., Pham, B., Cook, D., et al., 1998. Does quality of reports of randomised trials affect estimates of intervention efficacy reported in meta-analyses? Lancet 352, 609–613.

Moher, D., Schulz, K.F., Altman, D.G., 2001. The CONSORT statement: revised recommendations for improving the quality of reports of parallel group randomized trials. BMC Med. Res. Methodol. 1, 2.

Moher, D., Sampson, M., Campbell, K., et al., 2002. Assessing the quality of reports of randomized trials in pediatric complementary and alternative medicine. BMC Pediatr. 2, 2.

Moseley, A.M., Herbert, R.D., Sherrington, C., et al., 2002. Evidence for physiotherapy practice: a survey of the Physiotherapy Evidence Database (PEDro). Aust. J. Physiother. 48, 43–49.

Nathan, P.E., Stuart, S.P., Dolan, S.L., 2000. Research on psychotherapy efficacy and effectiveness: between Scylla and Charybdis? Psychol. Bull. 126, 964–981.

Pengel, H.L., 2004. Outcome of recent onset low back pain. PhD thesis, School of Physiotherapy, University of Sydney.

Petrucci, N., Iacovelli, W., 2003. Ventilation with lower tidal volumes versus traditional tidal volumes in adults for acute lung injury and acute respiratory distress syndrome (Cochrane review). In: The Cochrane Library, Issue 3. Wiley, Chichester.

Pocock, S.J., Assmann, S.E., Enos, L.E., et al., 2002. Subgroup analysis, covariate adjustment and baseline comparisons in clinical trial reporting: current practice and problems. Stat. Med. 21, 2917–2930.

Powell, J., Heslin, J., Greenwood, R., 2002. Community based rehabilitation after severe traumatic brain injury: a randomised controlled trial. J. Neurol. Neurosurg. Psychiatry 72, 193–202.

Quinones, D., Llorca, J., Dierssen, T., et al., 2003. Quality of published clinical trials on asthma. J. Asthma 40, 709–719.

Raab, G.M., Day, S., Sales, J., 2000. How to select covariates to include in the analysis of a clinical trial. Control. Clin. Trials 21, 330–342.

Raghunathan, T.E., 2004. What do we do with missing data? Some options for analysis of incomplete data. Annu. Rev. Public Health 25, 99–117.

Robinson, K.A., Dickersin, K., 2002. Development of a highly sensitive search strategy for the retrieval of reports of controlled trials using PubMed. Int. J. Epidemiol. 31, 150–153.

Sackett, D.L., Straus, S.E., Richardson, W.S., et al., 2000. Evidence-based medicine. How to practice and teach EBM, second ed Churchill Livingstone, Edinburgh.

Schiller, L., 2001. Effectiveness of spinal manipulative therapy in the treatment of mechanical thoracic spine pain: a pilot randomized clinical trial. J. Manipulative Physiol. Ther. 24, 394–401.

Schulz, K., Chalmers, I., Hayes, R., et al., 1995. Empirical evidence of bias: dimensions of methodological quality associated with estimates of treatment effects in controlled trials. JAMA 273, 408–412.

Schulz, K.F., Grimes, D.A., 2002. Allocation concealment in randomised trials: defending against deciphering. Lancet 359, 614–618.

Schwartz, D., Lellouch, J., 1967. Explanatory and pragmatic attitudes in therapeutical trials. J. Chronic Dis. 20, 637–648.

Seers, K., 1999. Qualitative research. In: Dawes, M., Davies, P., Gray, A. et al., (Eds.), Evidence-based practice. A primer for health care professionals. Churchill Livingstone, London, pp. 111–126.

Soares, H.P., Daniels, S., Kumar, A., et al., 2004. Bad reporting does not mean bad methods for randomised trials: observational study of randomised controlled trials performed by the Radiation Therapy Oncology Group. BMJ 328, 22–24.

Steen, E., Haugli, L., 2001. From pain to self-awareness: a qualitative analysis of the significance of group participation for persons with chronic musculoskeletal pain. Patient Educ. Couns. 42, 35–46.

Stern, J.M., Simes, R.J., 1997. Publication bias: evidence of delayed publication in a cohort study of clinical research projects. BMJ 315, 640–645.

Taylor, J.L., Norton, E.S., 1997. Developmental muscular torticollis: outcomes in young children treated by physical therapy. Pediatr. Phys. Ther. 9, 173–178.

van der Heijden, G.J., Leffers, P., Wolters, P.J., et al., 1999. No effect of bipolar interferential electrotherapy and pulsed ultrasound for soft tissue shoulder disorders: a randomised controlled trial. Ann. Rheum. Dis. 58, 530–540.

van Tulder, M., Furlan, A., Bombardier, C., et al., 2003. Updated method guidelines for systematic reviews in the Cochrane Collaboration Back Review Group. Spine 28, 1290–1299.

Verhagen, A.P., de Vet, H.C., de Bie, R. A., et al., 1998a. The Delphi list: a criteria list for quality assessment of randomized clinical trials for conducting systematic reviews developed by Delphi consensus. J. Clin. Epidemiol. 51, 1235–1241.

Verhagen, A.P., de Vet, H.C., de Bie, R.A., et al., 1998b. Balneotherapy and quality assessment: interobserver reliability of the Maastricht criteria list and the need for blinded quality assessment. J. Clin. Epidemiol. 51, 335–341.

Vickers, A.J., de Craen, A.J.M., 2000. Why use placebos in clinical trials? A narrative review of the methodological literature. J. Clin. Epidemiol. 53, 157–161.

Zar, H.J., Brown, G., Donson, H., et al., 1999. Home-made spacers for bronchodilator therapy in children with acute asthma: a randomised trial. Lancet 354, 979–982.

What does this evidence mean for my practice?

6

CHAPTER CONTENTS

Overview 93

What does this randomized trial mean
for my practice? 93

  Is the evidence relevant to me and
  my patient/s? 93

  Are the participants in the study similar
  to the patients to whom I wish to apply
  the study's findings? 94

  Were interventions applied appropriately? . . 96

  Are the outcomes useful? 97

  What does the evidence say? 99

    Continuous outcomes 100

    Dichotomous outcomes 107

What does this systematic review of effects
of intervention mean for my practice? 114

  Is the evidence relevant to me and
  my patient/s? 114

  What does the evidence say? 115

What does this study of experiences
mean for my practice? 122

  Was there a clear statement of findings? . 122

  How valuable is the research? 123

What does this study of prognosis mean
for my practice? 124

  Is the study relevant to me and
  my patient/s? 124

  What does the evidence say? 125

What does this study of the accuracy of
a diagnostic test mean for my practice? . . 127

  Is the evidence relevant to me and
  my patient/s? 128

  What does the evidence say? 128

    Likelihood ratios 128

References 132

OVERVIEW

Interpretation of clinical research involves assessing, firstly, the relevance of the research. This may involve consideration of the type of participants and outcomes in the study, as well as the way in which the intervention was applied (for studies of the effectiveness of an intervention), or the context of the phenomena being studied (for studies of experience), or the way in which the test was administered (for studies of the accuracy of a diagnostic test). Relevant studies can provide answers to clinical questions. Estimates of the average effects of interventions can be obtained from the difference in outcomes of intervention and control groups. Answers to questions about experiences might be in the form of descriptions or theoretical insights or theories. Prognoses may be quantitative estimates of the expected magnitude of an outcome or the probability of an event. The accuracy of diagnostic tests is best expressed in terms of likelihood ratios.

What does this randomized trial mean for my practice?

Is the evidence relevant to me and my patient/s?

If, having asked the questions about validity in Chapter 5, we are satisfied that the evidence is likely to be valid, we can proceed to the second step of critical appraisal. This involves assessing the relevance (or 'generalizability', or 'applicability' or 'external validity') of the evidence. This is an important step. Indeed, one of the major criticisms of randomized trials and systematic reviews of effects of therapies has been that they often do not address the questions asked by physiotherapists and patients.

Readers should ask the following three questions about relevance.

Are the participants in the study similar to the patients to whom I wish to apply the study's findings?

We read clinical trials and systematic reviews because we want to use their findings to assist clinical decision-making. This can be done only if we are prepared to make inferences about what will happen to *our* patients on the basis of outcomes in *other* patients (the participants in clinical trials). How reasonable is it to use clinical trials to make inferences about effects of therapy on our patients?

The process of using trials to make inferences about our patients is convoluted. First, we use the sample to make inferences about a hypothetical population: the universe of all people from which the sample could be considered to have been randomly selected (Efron & Tibshirani 1993). This is the role of inferential statistics; we will consider this step in detail in the next section. Then we 'particularize' (Lilford & Royston 1998) from the hypothetical population to individual patients or particular sets of patients. That is, we make inferences about individual patients from our understanding of how hypothetical populations behave. We will consider this second step a little further.

We can most confidently use clinical trials to make inferences about the effects of therapy on our own patients when the patients and interventions in those trials are similar to the patients and interventions we wish to make inferences about. Obviously, the more similar the patients in a trial are to our patients, and the more similar the interventions in a trial are to the interventions we are interested in, the more confidently we can use those trials to inform our clinical decisions. In this section we consider the issue of making inferences about particular patients: how similar must patients in a trial be to the particular patients we are interested in? How can we decide whether patients are similar enough to reasonably make such inferences?

Immediately we run into a problem. On what dimensions do we measure similarity? What characteristics of participants are we most concerned about? Is it critical that the patients have the same diagnosis, or the same disease severity, or the same

access to social support, or the same attitudes to therapy? Or do they need to be similar in all these dimensions? To answer these questions we need to know, or at least have some feeling for, the major 'effect modifiers'. That is, we need to know what factors most influence how patients respond to a particular therapy. We would like major effect modifiers of participants in a clinical trial to be similar to the patients we want to make inferences about. But, as we shall see below, it is very difficult to obtain objective evidence about effect modifiers. Consequently, when we make decisions about whether participants in a trial are sufficiently similar to the patients we wish to make inferences about, we must base our decisions on our personal impressions of the importance of particular factors.

One factor that sometimes generates particular controversy is the diagnosis. First, diagnostic labels are often applied inconsistently. One physiotherapist's complex regional pain syndrome is another physiotherapist's reflex sympathetic dystrophy (or shoulder–hand syndrome, or algodystrophy) and one physiotherapist's posterior tibial compartment syndrome is another physiotherapist's tibial stress syndrome. The precise clinical presentation of patients in a clinical trial may not be clear from descriptions of their diagnoses. When this is the case it may be difficult to know precisely to whom the trial findings can be applied. A greater problem arises when several diagnostic taxonomies coexist or overlap, because readers may want the diagnosis to be based on a taxonomy that is not reported. Thus, a trial of manipulation for low back pain might report that participants have acute non-specific low back pain (a taxonomy based on duration of symptoms), but some readers will ask whether these patients had disc lesions or facet lesions (they are interested in a pathological taxonomy); others will ask whether the patients had stiff joints (their taxonomy is based on palpation findings); and others will ask whether the patients had a derangement syndrome (they use a taxonomy based on McKenzie's theory of low back pain). There are many taxonomies for classifying low back pain, and patients cannot be (or never are) classified according to all taxonomies. The reason we have many taxonomies is that we do not know which taxonomies best differentiate prognosis or responses to therapy. That is, we do not know which taxonomy is the strongest effect modifier. A consequence of the diversity of taxonomies is that readers of clinical trials are frequently not satisfied that the patients in a trial are 'similar enough' to the patients about whom they wish to make inferences.

But there is a paradox here. Readers of clinical trials may be least prepared to use the findings of clinical trials when they most need them. For some interventions there is an enormous diversity in the indications for therapy applied by different therapists. A case in point is manipulation for neck pain (Jull 2002). A small number of physiotherapists, and many chiropractors, would routinely manipulate people with neck pain. Others may restrict manipulation to only those patients with non-irritable symptoms who do not respond to gentler mobilization techniques. Yet other physiotherapists never manipulate necks, under any circumstances. Conscientious and informed physiotherapists sit at either end of the spectrum. This diversity of practice suggests that at least some therapists, possibly all, are not applying therapy to an optimal spectrum of cases. We just do not have precise information on who is best treated with manipulation. That is, we do not know with any certainty what the important effect modifiers are for treatment of neck pain with manipulation. Under these circumstances, when there is a diversity of practice with regard to indications for therapy, the readers of a clinical trial may not be prepared to accept the trial's findings because the participants in the trial did not necessarily satisfy the reader's impressions of appropriate indications for therapy. When we least know who best to apply therapy to, physiotherapists are most reluctant to accept the findings of clinical trials. The paradox is that, when readers most need information from clinical trials, they may be most prepared to ignore them.

A simplistic solution to the problem of identifying subgroups of patients who would most benefit from therapy might involve more detailed analysis of trial data. Readers could look for analyses designed to see whether subgroups of patients, patients with certain characteristics, respond particularly well or particularly badly to therapy. This information could inform decisions about whether appropriate inclusion and exclusion criteria were used in subsequent clinical trials. Unfortunately, it is usually very difficult to identify subgroups of responders and non-responders with subgroup analyses. This is because subgroup analyses are typically exposed to a high risk of statistical errors: they will typically fail to detect true differences between subgroups when they exist *and* they may be prone to identify spurious differences between subgroups

as well.[1,2] One of the consequences is that subgroup analyses must usually be considered to be exploratory rather than definitive. Usually the best estimate of the effect of an intervention is the estimate of the average effect of the intervention in the whole population (Yusuf et al 1991).

> The best that a clinical trial can tell us about the effects of an intervention on patients with particular characteristics is the average effect of the intervention on the heterogeneous population from which that patient was drawn.

[1]These issues have been studied intensively. Accessible treatments of this subject are those by Yusuf et al (1991), Moyé (2000) and Brookes et al (2004). Alternatively, readers might prefer to consult the light-hearted and equally illuminating reports of the effects of DICE therapy (Counsell et al 1994) and the analysis of effects of astrological star sign in the ISIS II trial (Second International Study of Infarct Survival Collaborative Group 1988).

[2]Since the first edition of this book, physiotherapy researchers have increasingly used clinical trial data to identify patients who respond best to therapy. In our opinion much of that research is potentially seriously misleading. A common problem has been that researchers have generated 'clinical prediction rules' (algorithms to identify 'effect modifiers' or characteristics of treatment responders) using data from uncontrolled trials. For example, Flynn et al (2002) studied a cohort of 75 patients with low back pain treated with a standardized spinal manipulation protocol. They found that patients with short duration of symptoms, greater hip internal rotation range of motion, lumbar hypomobility, no symptoms distal to the knee and low fear avoidance beliefs were much more likely to experience large reductions in disability than patients who did not have most of these characteristics. They concluded that therapists could use these characteristics to identify patients who respond to manipulation. The approach they used is potentially seriously misleading for several reasons. Most importantly, cohort studies may be capable of identifying people who are likely to have good *outcomes*, but they cannot provide rigorous evidence of who *responds to intervention*. To identify people who respond best to intervention it is necessary to determine the effects of intervention, and this can be done rigorously only in the context of a randomized trial.

The best way to identify people who will respond well (or badly) to intervention is to examine the interactions between patient characteristics and the effects of intervention in randomized controlled trials. However, such investigations are technically difficult and prone to over-interpretation. They need large sample sizes (at least four times those needed for a conventional analysis of treatment effects; Brookes et al 2004) to be adequately powered. Great care must be taken to reduce the risk of identifying spurious effect modifiers. To reduce the risk of identifying spurious effect modifiers, researchers should explicitly nominate a small number of candidate effect modifiers prior to conducting the analysis. If statistical methods are used to select effect modifiers then those methods should take into account the number of effect modifiers that were considered. Clinical prediction rules are only useful if they can identify people with substantially greater (or substantially lower) than average probabilities of responding to intervention, so researchers should provide evidence that their clinical prediction rules can substantially modify those probabilities. Hancock et al (2009) provide a more extended discussion of these issues. Regardless of how carefully subgroup analyses are conducted, we caution readers to be sceptical about the findings of subgroup analyses until these have been replicated in other randomized trials.

That said, common sense must prevail. Some characteristics of participants in trials could well be important. For example, trials of motor training for patients with acute stroke may well not be relevant to patients with chronic stroke because the mechanisms of recovery in these two groups could be quite different. Occasionally, trials sample from populations for whom the intervention is patently not indicated. Such trials should not be used to assess the effectiveness of the therapy. The reader must assess whether participants in a trial *could* be those for whom therapy is indicated, or *could* be similar enough to those patients they want to make inferences about, given the current understanding of the mechanisms of therapy.

There is a simple conclusion from this rather philosophical discussion. It is difficult to know with any certainty which patients an intervention is likely to benefit most. Consequently, readers of clinical trials should not be too fussy about the characteristics of participants in a clinical trial.

> If patients in a trial are broadly representative of the patients we want to make inferences about, we should be prepared to use the findings of the trial for clinical decision-making. It is only when there are strong grounds to believe that the patients in a trial are clearly different to those for whom therapy is indicated that we should be dismissive of a trial's findings on the basis of the participants in the trial.

To some, this approach seems to ignore everything that theory and clinical experience can tell us about who will respond most to therapy. The reader appears to be faced with a choice between accepting the findings of clinical trials without considering the characteristics of patients in the trial, or ignoring clinical trials altogether. That is, there appears to be a choice between the unbiased but possibly irrelevant conclusions of high-quality clinical trials and relevant but possibly biased clinical intuition. This suggests a compromise: a sensible way to proceed is to use estimates of the effects of therapy as a starting point, but to modify these estimates on the basis of clinical intuition. We will return to this idea in more detail later in the chapter.

Were interventions applied appropriately?

We have just considered how the selection of patients in a clinical trial may affect our decision about the trial's relevance to our patients. Exactly the same considerations apply to the way in which interventions were applied. Just as some readers will choose to ignore clinical trials whose participants differ in some way from the patients about whom the reader wishes

to make inferences, we could choose to ignore clinical trials that apply the intervention in a way that differs from the way that we might apply it.

A specific example concerns electrotherapy. There have now been a large number of clinical trials in electrotherapy (at the time of writing, around 700 randomized trials). For the most part they are not very flattering. Most of the relevant high-quality trials suggest that electrotherapies have little clinically worthwhile effect. Nonetheless, Laakso and colleagues (2002) have argued that it would not be appropriate to dismiss electrotherapies as ineffective because not all possible permutations of doses and methods of administration have yet been subjected to clinical trials. They argue that trials may not yet have investigated the optimal modes for administering interventions and that future clinical trials may identify optimally effective modes of administration that produce clinically worthwhile effects.

The counterargument mirrors that in the preceding section. It is very difficult to identify precise characteristics of optimally administered therapy. Indeed, it would seem impossible to expect that we could know with any certainty about how *best* to apply a therapy before we have first established with some certainty that the therapy is generally effective. As there are usually many ways an intervention could be applied, it will usually be impossibly inefficient to examine all possible ways of administering the therapy in randomized trials. The same paradox applies: when we don't know how best to apply a therapy there is likely to be diversity of practice, and when there is diversity of practice readers are least inclined to accept the findings of clinical trials because, they argue, therapy was not applied in the way they consider to be optimal. But this is not a workable approach: when we do not know the best way to apply therapy we cannot be too fussy about how therapy is applied in a clinical trial.

On the other hand, where theory provides clear guidelines about how a therapy ought to be administered, there is no point in basing clinical decisions on trials that have clearly applied therapy in an inappropriate way. Several clinical trials have investigated the effects of inspiratory muscle training on dyspnoea in people with chronic airway disease (reviewed by Lotters et al 2002). But many of these trials (30 of 57 identified by Lotters et al) utilized training intensities of less than 30% of maximal inspiratory pressure. Laboratory research suggests that much higher training intensities (perhaps more than 60% of maximal force) are required to increase strength, at least in appendicular muscles (McDonagh & Davies 1984). So it would be inappropriate to base conclusions about the effects of inspiratory muscle training on studies which use low training intensities.

What practical recommendations can be made?

A sensible approach to critical appraisal of clinical trials might be to consider whether the intervention was administered in a theoretically reasonable way. We should choose to disregard clinical trials that apply therapy in a way that is clearly and unambiguously inappropriate. However, where there is uncertainty about how best to apply a therapy we should be prepared to accept the findings of the trial, even if the therapy was administered in a way that differs from the way we may have chosen to provide the therapy, at least until better evidence becomes available.

We conclude this section by considering how trial design influences what can be inferred about intervention. In Chapter 3 we indicated that there are three broad types of contrast in controlled clinical trials: trials can either compare an intervention with no intervention, with standard intervention plus a new intervention with standard intervention alone, or with two interventions. The nature of the contrast between groups determines what inferences can be drawn from the trial. Thus, a trial that randomizes participants to receive either an exercise programme or no intervention can be used to make inferences about how much more effective exercise is than no intervention, whereas a trial that randomizes participants to receive either advice to remain active and an exercise programme or advice alone can be used to make inferences about how much more effective exercise and advice are than advice alone. In one sense, both trials tell us about the effects of an exercise programme, but they tell us something slightly different: the former tells us about the effects of exercise in isolation, whereas the latter tells us about the supplementary effects of exercise, over and above the effects of advice. The two may differ if there is an interaction between the co-interventions. (In this example, we might expect that the effects of exercise would be smaller if all participants received advice to remain active.)

Are the outcomes useful?

Good therapeutic interventions are those that make people's lives better.[3] When we ask questions about the effects of an intervention, we most need to know

whether the therapy improves the quality of people's lives.

What is a 'better' life? Is it a life free from suffering, or a happy life, a life filled with satisfaction, or something else? If clinical trials are to tell us about the effects of an intervention, what are they to measure? Clinical trials may provide indirect measures of people's suffering, but they rarely report the effects of therapy on happiness or satisfaction. The closest clinical trials get to telling us about outcomes that are really worth knowing about is probably 'health-related quality of life'. Health-related quality of life is usually assessed with patient-administered questionnaires.

In principle there are two sorts of measure of health-related quality of life: generic measures, designed to allow comparison across disease types, and disease-specific measures (Guyatt et al 1993). Two examples of generic measures of quality of life are the Short Form 36 (SF-36) and the EuroQol. Examples of specific measures of quality of life are those designed for people suffering from respiratory disease (the Chronic Respiratory Disease Questionnaire; Guyatt et al 1987) and rheumatoid arthritis (the RAQol; e.g. Tijhuis et al 2001). Disease-specific measures of quality of life focus on the dimensions of quality of life that most affect people with that disease, so they tend to be more sensitive and they usually provide more useful information for clinical decision-making.

But many clinical trials, probably a majority, do not attempt to directly measure quality of life. Instead they measure variables that are thought to directly relate to, or are a component of, quality of life. Examples include measures of pain, disability or function, dyspnoea and exercise capacity. Insofar as these measures are related to quality of life, they can help us make decisions about intervention.

Sometimes the variables that relate most closely to quality of life cannot be measured easily. A work-around used in many trials is to measure more easily measured outcomes that are known to be related to the construct of interest. The measured outcome (sometimes referred to as a 'surrogate' measure) acts as a proxy for the construct of real interest. An example arises in trials of the effects of an exercise programme for post-menopausal women with osteoporosis. Exercise programmes are offered to post-menopausal women with or at risk of osteoporosis, with the aim of reducing fracture risk. But it is very difficult to conduct trials that assess the effects of exercise on fracture risk. Such trials must monitor

---

[3]Good interventions might also make lives longer. But relatively few physiotherapy interventions are designed to increase length of life, so we will focus here on the aim of increasing quality of life.

very large numbers of people for long periods of time in order to observe enough fractures.[4] The easier alternative is to assess the effects of exercise on bone density. Many trials have measured the effects of exercise programmes on bone density because the effects of exercise on bone density can be assessed in much smaller trials. Other examples of surrogate measures in clinical trials in physiotherapy are measures of postural sway (sometimes used as a surrogate for falls risk in trials of falls prevention programmes; Sherrington et al 2004) and measurement of performance on lung function tests (used as a surrogate for respiratory morbidity in trials of interventions for cystic fibrosis; McIlwaine et al 2001).

Trials that measure surrogate measures potentially provide us with answers to our clinical questions. However, there are two reasons why such trials may appear to be more useful than they really are. First, our primary interest in clinical trials stems from their potential to provide us with clinically useful estimates of the effects of intervention (more on this in the next section), yet it may be very difficult to get a sense for the effect of an intervention by looking at surrogate measures. It is easier to interpret a trial that tells us exercise reduces 1-year fracture risk from 5% to 3% than a trial that tells us exercise increases bone density by 6 mg/cm^3 at 1 year.[5] A more serious concern is that the surrogate and the construct of interest may become uncoupled as a result of intervention. That is, it may be that the surrogate measure and the outcome of interest respond differently to intervention. There have been notorious examples from medicine in which drugs that had been shown to have beneficial effects on surrogate outcomes were subsequently shown to produce harmful effects on clinically important outcomes. For example, encainide and flecainide were known to reduce ventricular ectopy (a surrogate outcome) following myocardial infarction, but a randomized trial (Echt et al 1991) showed that these drugs substantially increased mortality[6] (a clinically important

outcome). We can rarely be sure that surrogate measures provide us with valid indications of the effect of therapy on the constructs we are truly interested in (de Gruttola et al 2001).

One of the reasons that not all clinical trials measure quality of life is the concern that such measures may not be sensitive to effects of intervention. Indeed, some trialists believe that generic quality of life measures such as the SF-36 are generally not useful in clinical trials because they may change little, even when there are apparent changes in a patient's condition. It is true that outcome measures in clinical trials are only useful if they are sensitive to clinically important change. However, there may be circumstances in which interventions produce effects that are clinically evident but not clinically important. An example might be an intervention that increases capacity for voluntary muscle activity in the hemiparetic hand after stroke, but which does not produce appreciable improvements in hand function. Outcome measures in clinical trials must be capable of detecting changes that are important to patients,[7] but they need not always be sensitive to clinically evident change.

Some clinical trials do not measure outcomes that matter to patients. This may be because the trialists are interested in questions about the mechanisms by which interventions have their effects, rather than in whether the intervention is worth applying in clinical practice. For example, Meyer et al (2003) randomized participants with reduced ventricular function to either a 2-month high-intensity residential exercise training programme or to a control group. They measured indices of ventilatory gas exchange, blood lactate and arterial blood gas levels, cardiac output, and pulmonary artery and wedge pressures. The effect of exercise on these outcomes may be of considerable interest because it is important to know the physiological effects of exercise in the presence of ventricular failure. However, the outcomes have no intrinsic importance to patients, so the trial cannot tell us whether the intervention has effects that will make it worth implementing. Trials such as this tell us about mechanisms of therapy, but they give us little

[4]For example, according to the usual conventions, if the 1-year fracture risk in control participants was 5% and we wanted to be able reliably to detect reductions in risk of 2% or more, we would need to see 3000 participants in the trial.

[5]The best way to make sense of this result would be to look at well-designed epidemiological studies that try to quantify the effects of bone density on fracture risk.

[6]Over the mean 10-month follow-up in this trial, 23 of 743 participants receiving placebo therapy, and 64 of 746 patients receiving encainide or flecainide died. As we shall see later in this chapter, this implies that encainide and flecainide killed 1 in every 18 patients to whom they were administered.

[7]This does not mean that the outcome measure must be sensitive to change in *individual* patients. One factor that limits sensitivity to change of measures on individual patients is random measurement error. Random measurement error can be quantified with a range of indices, including the minimal change detectable with 90% certainty, or MDC$_{90}$. But random errors can be of less concern in clinical trials because they average out across participants. Some trials, particularly trials with large sample sizes, can detect average effects of intervention that are smaller than the smallest change detectable on individuals.

information that can help us decide whether the therapy is worth applying. These trials are of use to theoreticians interested in developing ways of providing therapy, but they do not help clinicians decide whether they should use the therapy in clinical practice.

> In summary, when critically appraising a clinical trial it is sensible to consider whether the trial measures outcomes that matter to patients. If not, the trial is unlikely to be able to guide clinical decision-making.

What does the evidence say?[8]

The third and last part of the process of critical appraisal of studies of the effects of interventions involves assessing whether the therapy does more good than harm.

Does the intervention do more good than harm?

In controlled clinical trials, attention is often focused on the 'p value' of the difference between groups. The p value is used to determine whether the difference between groups is likely to represent a real effect of intervention or could have occurred simply by chance: 'p' is the probability of the observed difference in groups occurring by chance alone. A small probability (conventionally $p < 5\%$) means that it is unlikely that the difference would have occurred by chance alone, so it is said to constitute evidence of an effect of intervention.[9] Higher probabilities (conventionally, probabilities $\geq 5\%$) indicate that the effect could have occurred by chance alone. High p values are usually interpreted as a lack of evidence of an effect of intervention.

A consequence of this tortuous logic is to distract readers from the most important piece of information that a trial can provide, that is, information about the magnitude of the intervention's effects. If clinical trials are to influence clinical practice they must determine more than simply whether the intervention has an effect. They must, in addition, ascertain how big the effect of the intervention is. Good clinical trials provide unbiased estimates of the size of the effect of an intervention. Such estimates can be used to determine whether the intervention has a large enough effect to be clinically worthwhile.

What is a clinically worthwhile effect? That depends on the costs and risks of the intervention. Costs most obviously include monetary costs (to the patient, health provider or funder), but they also include the inconvenience, discomfort and side-effects of the intervention. When costs are conceived of in this way it is apparent that all interventions come at some cost. If an intervention is to be clinically worthwhile its positive effects must exceed its costs; it must do more good than harm. Clinical trials often provide information about the size of effects of interventions, but they rarely provide information about all of the costs of intervention.

> Thus the evaluation of whether an intervention provides a clinically worthwhile effect usually requires weighing evidence about beneficial effects of the intervention (provided by clinical trials) against subjective impressions of the costs and risks of the intervention.

Continuous and dichotomous outcomes

In subsequent sections we will consider how we can use clinical trials to tell us about what the effects of a particular intervention are likely to be. We will go about this in a slightly different way, depending on whether outcomes are measured on continuous or dichotomous scales.[10] Outcomes can be considered

---

[8]This section is reproduced, with only minor changes, from Herbert (2000a,b). We are grateful to the publishers of the *Australian Journal of Physiotherapy* (now called the *Journal of Physiotherapy*) for granting permission to reproduce this material.

[9]This is a conventional interpretation of p values. However, critics argue that this interpretation is incorrect. The contemporary view is not consistent with either the Fisherian or Neyman–Pearson approaches to statistical inference (Gigerenzer et al 1989). Moreover, there are some powerful arguments supporting the view that p should not provide a measure of the strength of evidence or belief for or against a hypothesis. In the internally consistent Neyman–Pearson view of statistical inference, p serves no other function than to act as a criterion for optimally accepting or rejecting hypotheses. The strength of the evidence supporting one hypothesis over another is given by the ratio of their likelihoods, not by p values. And the strength of belief for or against a hypothesis requires consideration of prior probabilities. Readers interested in exploring these ideas further could consult the marvellous expositions of these ideas by Barnett (1982) and Royall (1997). An accessible treatment of the interpretation of p is given by Nickerson (2000).

[10]Purists will object to classification of outcomes as either continuous or dichotomous. Their first objection might be that we should add further classes of outcome. Some outcomes are 'polytomous': they can have more than two values (like continuous variables) but can only take on discrete values (like dichotomous variables). An example is the walking item of the Motor Assessment Scale, which can have integer values of 1–6. For our purposes we can treat most polytomous outcomes (all with more than a few levels on their scale) as if they were continuous outcomes. Another class of outcome is 'time-to-event' outcomes. As the name suggests, measurement of time-to-event outcomes involves determining the time taken until an event (such as injury) occurs. Yet another form of outcome is counts of events. Clinical trials that report time-to-event data or count data often provide the data in a form that enables the reader to extract dichotomous data. We will not consider polytomous, time-to-event or count data any further here.

to be measured on continuous scales when it is the *amount* of the outcome that has been measured on each patient. Examples of outcomes measured on continuous scales are pain intensity measured on a visual analogue scale, disability measured on an Oswestry scale, exercise capacity measured as 12-minute walking distance, or shoulder subluxation measured in millimetres. These contrast with dichotomous outcomes, which can have only one of two values. Dichotomous variables are usually *events* that either happen or do not happen to each participant. Examples of dichotomous variables are death, respiratory complications, ability to walk independently, ankle sprains, and so on.

We will first consider how to obtain estimates of the size of the effects of intervention from clinical trials with continuous outcomes. Then we will consider how to obtain estimates of the effect of intervention on dichotomous outcomes.

Continuous outcomes

All interventions have variable effects. With all interventions, some patients benefit from the intervention but others experience no effect, or even harmful effects. Thus, strictly speaking, we cannot talk of 'the effect' of an intervention. Most clinical trials can provide an estimate of only the *average* effect of intervention – they cannot tell us about how *all* patients, or any *individual* patient, will respond to intervention.[11]

> Fortunately, the *average* effect of intervention is usually the *most likely* or *expected* effect of intervention.[12]

Thus, although clinical trials cannot tell us about what the effect of an intervention will be for a particular patient, we can still use estimates of effects of

intervention provided by clinical trials to aid clinical decision-making.

A sensible way to use estimates, from clinical trials, of the effects of intervention is to consider them as a starting point for predicting the effect of intervention on any particular patient. The estimate can then be modified up or down depending on the characteristics of the particular patients to whom the intervention is to be applied.[13] For example, Cambach et al (1997) found that a 3-month community-based pulmonary rehabilitation programme produced modest effects on 6-minute walking distance (39 metres) and quality of life (17 points on the 100-point Chronic Respiratory Disease Questionnaire). We could reasonably anticipate larger effects than this among people who have very supportive home environments and access to good exercise facilities, and we might expect relatively poor effects among people who have co-morbidities, such as rheumatoid arthritis, that make exercise more difficult.

The advantage of this approach is that it combines the objectivity of clinical trials (which provide unbiased estimates of average effects of intervention) with the richness of clinical acumen (which may be able to distinguish between probable good and poor responders to intervention).[14] Of course, care must be taken when using clinical reasoning to modify estimates of effects provided by clinical trials. A conservative approach would be to ensure that the estimate of the effect of intervention was modified downwards as often as it was modified upwards, although it might be reasonable to depart from this approach if the patients in the trial differed markedly, on average, from the clinical population being treated. Particular caution ought to be applied when a clinical trial provides evidence of no effect of intervention.

Weighing benefit and harm: is the effect clinically worthwhile?

The easiest way to make decisions about whether an intervention has a clinically worthwhile effect is first to nominate the smallest effect that is clinically worthwhile. This is a subjective decision that involves

---

[11]The same limitation applies to all sources of information about effects of intervention – this is not a unique limitation of clinical trials.

[12]This bold statement is true in one sense but not in another. It is true in the sense that the mean effect in the population is the *expectation* of the effect (Armitage & Berry 1994). The difficulty arises because we can only estimate, and cannot know, the population mean. The mean effect of the intervention observed in the study sample is a 'maximum likelihood estimator' of the mean effect in the hypothetical population from which the sample could be considered to have been randomly drawn (Barnett 1982). This implies that the estimated mean effect would have been most likely to have been observed if the mean effect in the population were equal to the estimated mean effect. But this is *not* equivalent to saying that the mean effect observed in the sample is the most likely value of the mean effect in the population.

[13]Later in this chapter we will see that there are complementary statistical techniques for modifying estimates of treatment effects on the basis of baseline severity or risk.

[14]Some of our colleagues object to this approach on the grounds that clinical acumen is not all it is cracked up to be. It would be very interesting to see some empirical tests of the accuracy of clinical judgements of who will respond most and least to intervention.

consideration of patients' perceptions of both the benefits and costs of intervention. Then we can use estimates of the effects of intervention to decide whether intervention will do more good than harm.

The process of weighing benefit and harm can be done in two ways. Individual therapists can develop personal 'policies' about particular interventions. Such policies might stipulate that particular interventions will, or will not, be offered routinely to patients with certain conditions. For example, some therapists have a personal policy not to offer ultrasound therapy to people with ankle sprains. This policy can be defended on the grounds that, on average, ultrasound does not appear to produce benefits that most patients would consider minimally worthwhile (e.g. van der Windt et al 2004). To make this decision, the physiotherapist has to anticipate patient preferences and make decisions that he or she believes are in the patients' best interests.

Alternatively, decisions about therapy can be negotiated individually with patients. This involves exploring what individual patients want from therapy, and what their values and preferences are (see the section titled *Estimating the smallest worthwhile effect of intervention*). Some patients are intervention averse, and will be interested in intervention only if it makes a big difference to their quality of life. Others are intervention tolerant (or even intervention hungry!) and are prepared to try interventions that are expected to have little effect. As an example, there is quite strong evidence that electrical stimulation of rotator cuff muscles can prevent glenohumeral subluxation after hemiparetic stroke (Ada & Foongchomcheay 2002), but this does not mean that all patients with hemiparetic stroke should be given electrical stimulation. Instead, the benefits (a mean reduction of subluxation by 6.5 mm) should be weighed against 'costs' (application of a moderately uncomfortable modality for several hours each day for several weeks). Some patients will consider the expected benefit of therapy worthwhile and others will not. This provides a legitimate basis for variations in practice. Quite different decisions about interventions might be made for patients with similar clinical presentations but different values and preferences. The physiotherapist's role is to elicit patient preferences and assist in the process of making decisions about intervention, as discussed in Chapter 1.

To illustrate this process we will consider whether the application of a pneumatic compression pump produces clinically worthwhile reductions in post-mastectomy lymphoedema. We might begin by nominating the smallest reduction in lymphoedema that would make the costs of the compression therapy worthwhile. Most therapists, and perhaps even most patients, would agree that a short course of daily compression therapy would be clinically worthwhile if it produced a sustained 75% reduction in oedema. Most would also agree that a 15% decrease was not clinically worthwhile. Somewhere in between these values lies the smallest worthwhile effect. This value is best arrived at by discussion with the particular patients for whom the intervention is intended. Let us assume for the moment that a particular patient (or a typical patient) considers the smallest reduction in oedema that would make therapy worthwhile is around 40%.

Does compression therapy produce reductions in lymphoedema of this magnitude? Perhaps the best answer to this question comes from a randomized trial by Dini et al (1998) that compared 2 weeks (10 days) of daily intermittent pneumatic compression with a control (no treatment) condition. We will use the findings of this trial to estimate what the effect of compression therapy is likely to be.

Estimating the size of an intervention's effects

For continuous outcomes, the best estimate of the effect of an intervention is simply the difference in the means (or, in some trials, the medians) of the intervention and control groups. In the trial by Dini et al (1998), oedema was measured by measuring arm circumference at seven locations, summing the measures, and then taking the difference of the summed circumference of affected and unaffected arms (positive numbers indicate that the affected arm had a larger circumference than the unaffected arm). After the 2-week experimental period the oedema was 14 cm (SD 6 cm) in both the control group and the intervention group. Thus the best estimate of the effect of intervention (compared with no intervention) is that it has no effect on oedema. Clearly the effect is smaller than the smallest worthwhile effect, which we had decided might be about 40%. Our expectation should be that when pressure therapy is applied to this population in the manner described by Dini and colleagues, there will be little effect. Our best guess is that the effect of the intervention will be, on average, not clinically worthwhile.

Another example comes from a trial by O'Sullivan and co-workers (1997). These authors examined the effects of specific segmental exercise for people with painful spondylolysis or spondylolisthesis. Participants in the trial were allocated randomly to groups that received either a 10-week programme of training of the deep spinal stabilizing muscles (10–15 minutes of exercise daily) or routine care from a medical practitioner. Pain intensity was measured after the intervention period on a 100-mm visual analogue scale (maximum score 100).

To interpret the findings of this study we could begin by nominating the smallest worthwhile effect. Patients with spondylolisthesis often experience chronic pain or recurrent episodes of pain, so they may be satisfied with the intervention even if it had relatively modest effects: a 20% reduction in pain intensity, if sustained, may be perceived as worthwhile. The trial found that, after intervention, mean pain in the intervention group was 19 mm and mean pain in the control group was 48 mm, indicating that the effect of specific muscle training was, on average, 29 mm (or 29/48 = 60% of the pain level in the control group). Effects of this magnitude are considerably greater than the 20% threshold that we nominated as the smallest worthwhile effect and are likely to be perceived as worthwhile by most patients. Of course, some patients may perceive that therapy would be worthwhile only if it gave them complete relief of symptoms; these patients would consider the treatment effect too small to be worthwhile.

In the two examples just used, outcomes were measured in terms of the amount of oedema and the degree of pain intensity *at the end of the experimental period*. Some trials, instead, report the *change* in outcome variables over the intervention period. In such trials the measure of the effect of intervention is still the difference of the means (this time of the difference of the mean *change*) in intervention and control groups.[15]

---

[15]Some readers will wonder why we do not always use change scores rather than end scores to estimate the effects of intervention. At first glance, change scores seem to take account of differences between groups at baseline, whereas end scores do not. It is true that change scores may be preferred over end scores, but not because they take better account of baseline differences. When the correlation between baseline scores and end scores is greater than 0.5 (as is usually the case), change scores will have less variability than end scores, so that (as we shall see shortly) when these conditions are satisfied we can get more precise estimates of the effect of intervention from change scores than end scores (Cohen 1988). (In fact, even change scores are not optimally efficient. Covariate-adjusted scores will always be more efficient again, so covariate-adjusted scores are preferred wherever they are available.) But change scores do not account better for baseline differences, at least not in the sense of removing bias due to baseline differences. In randomized trials, baseline differences are due to chance alone. Averaged across many trials, baseline differences will be zero. So, averaged across many trials, analyses of change scores and analyses of end scores will give the same result. Both give unbiased estimates of the average effect of intervention.

Estimating the smallest worthwhile effect of intervention

In the preceding section we argued that, if we are to make sense of the findings of randomized controlled trials, we need to determine whether the estimated effects of intervention are large enough to make intervention worthwhile. We suggested that readers of clinical trials need to nominate the smallest worthwhile effect of intervention, either by anticipating what most patients would consider to be worthwhile, or by negotiating with individual patients. Now we consider how research might be able to tell us what constitutes the smallest worthwhile effect of intervention. What sorts of research methods can be used to estimate the smallest worthwhile effects of intervention?

Many studies have attempted to estimate the smallest worthwhile effects of intervention, although most do not refer explicitly to the 'smallest worthwhile effect'. Instead they use a range of terms such as 'the minimally important clinical difference' or 'minimal clinically important change' or the 'smallest important difference' or 'patient preferences'. Although we are reluctant to introduce yet another term, we prefer to refer to the 'smallest worthwhile effect' because this makes it clear that we are talking about the smallest effect of intervention that makes the intervention worth its risks, costs and inconveniences.

Many methods have been used to determine the smallest worthwhile effect of intervention. These have been critically reviewed by Barrett et al (2005a) and Ferreira & Herbert (2008). In our opinion, any valid measure of the smallest worthwhile effect of intervention must satisfy three conditions (Ferreira & Herbert 2008):

1. The judgement of whether the effect of intervention is large enough to make the costs, risks and inconveniences of intervention worthwhile must involve recipients of care (patients). Patients can choose whether they will receive physiotherapy intervention or not. Ultimately that choice must be based on patients' decisions about whether the effects of intervention are large enough to be worthwhile. Consequently the smallest worthwhile effect must reflect the values of patients, not of their physiotherapists or doctors.
2. The judgement must take into account the costs, risk and inconveniences of intervention. Some interventions incur greater costs, risks and inconveniences than others. (Compare spinal surgery with provision of an information booklet

for treatment of chronic low back pain.) So different interventions may have very different smallest worthwhile effects. (The smallest worthwhile effect of spinal surgery will be much larger than the smallest worthwhile effect of providing an information booklet, because the costs, risks and inconveniences of spinal surgery are much greater than those of an information booklet.) This means that the smallest worthwhile effect must be intervention-specific, not just outcome-specific.

3. The effect must be defined in terms of the difference in outcomes with and without intervention. As we shall see in Chapter 6, this is the only rigorous way to define the effect of intervention. Thus we need to know how much better a patient's outcome would need to be, compared with the outcome he or she would have experienced had he or she not been given the intervention, to consider that intervention was worthwhile.[16]

Most of the studies that have attempted to determine the smallest worthwhile effect of physiotherapy interventions do not satisfy these criteria.[17] However, a small number of studies have used appropriate methods. In fact, several groups of researchers have independently developed what is essentially the same method. Barrett and colleagues (2005b) call this method the 'benefit–harm trade-off method', and health economists might call it a form of 'contingent valuation'. The method involves describing to patients the expected effect of an intervention and then asking them whether, after considering the risks, costs and inconveniences associated with intervention, they would choose to have the intervention. If the patients say they would have the intervention, they are then asked to imagine that the effect of intervention was smaller and are again asked whether they would choose to have the intervention. The process is repeated, varying the imagined effect of intervention up and down as necessary, until it is possible to establish the smallest worthwhile effect of intervention.

The benefit–harm trade-off method has been used to determine the smallest worthwhile effects of a range of health interventions including chemotherapy for cancer (e.g. Blinman et al 2010, Duric & Stockler 2001, Simes & Coates 2001), pharmacological treatments for the common cold (Barrett et al 2005b, 2007) and, of particular interest here, for physiotherapy interventions for low back pain (Ferreira et al 2009, Yelland & Schluter 2006). A common finding emerges from these studies on remarkably diverse populations and interventions and outcomes: there is a huge amount of variation between patients in what they perceive to be the smallest worthwhile effect for any particular intervention. Some patients are intervention averse (they would consider intervention to have been worthwhile only if it conferred very large beneficial effects), whereas other patients are intervention hungry (they like to have intervention even though the effects are very small). This introduces a difficulty for clinicians who want to use clinical trials to determine whether the effects of an intervention are large enough to warrant offering to their patients. It suggests that it may be difficult to know whether any particular patient would consider the effects of a particular intervention large enough to be worthwhile, and that therefore decisions about the acceptability of an intervention need to be negotiated with each individual patient. Each patient needs to be told of the expected effect of intervention and asked whether they feel that effect is large enough that they would choose to have the intervention.

Estimating uncertainty

Even when clinical trials are well designed and conducted, their findings are associated with uncertainty. This is because the difference between group means observed in the study is only an estimate of the true effect of intervention derived from the sample of participants in the clinical trial. (Our estimate of the effects of compression therapy has uncertainty associated with it because the estimate was obtained from the 80 participants employed in the study by Dini et al (1998), not from all patients in the population we want to make inferences about.) The outcomes in this sample, as in any sample, approximate but do not exactly equal the average outcomes in the populations that the sample represents. Thus the

---

[16]The process of nominating the smallest worthwhile effect is most straightforward in pragmatic trials that compare outcomes with two clinically sensible courses of action. (See Box 5.2 for a discussion of the distinction between pragmatic and explanatory trials.) It is also possible to nominate the smallest worthwhile effect in explanatory trials that compare outcomes with intervention and sham intervention, but in that case the patient must consider how much better the outcome would have to be with intervention compared with sham intervention to be worthwhile. That might be difficult.

[17]The commonly used 'distribution-based' and 'anchor-based' methods for assessing the smallest worthwhile effect of physiotherapy interventions almost always rely on decisions made by the researcher about what is clinically important; they are never intervention-specific, and they typically define 'effects' in terms of changes over time, rather than in terms of differences in outcomes of treated and untreated patients.

average effect of intervention reported in the study approximates but does not equal the true average effect of intervention. Rational interpretation of the clinical trial requires consideration of how good an approximation the study provides. That is,

> to interpret a study's findings properly it is necessary to know how much uncertainty is associated with its results.

The degree of uncertainty associated with an estimate of the effect of an intervention can be described with a confidence interval (Gardner & Altman 1989). Most often the 95% confidence interval is used. Roughly speaking, the 95% confidence interval is the range within which we can be 95% certain that the true average effect of intervention actually lies.[18] (Note that the confidence interval describes the degree of uncertainty about the average effect on the population, not the degree of uncertainty of the effect on individuals.) The 95% confidence interval for the difference between means in the trial by Dini et al (1998) extends from approximately -3 to +3 cm (methods used to calculate confidence intervals are presented in Box 6.1). This suggests that we can suppose that the true average effect of pressure therapy lies somewhere between a reduction in oedema of 3 cm and an increase in oedema of 3 cm. All of the values encompassed by the 95% confidence interval are smaller than what we nominated as the smallest worthwhile effect. (We had nominated a smallest worthwhile effect of 40%; as the initial oedema was 14 cm, this corresponds to a reduction in oedema of 40% of 14 cm, or about 6 cm.) Thus we can conclude that not only is the best estimate of the magnitude of the effect less than the smallest worthwhile effect (0 cm < 6 cm), but also that no value of the effect that is plausibly consistent with the findings of this study (even the most optimistic estimate of 3 cm) exceeds the smallest worthwhile effect. These data strongly suggest that

pressure therapy does not produce clinically worthwhile reductions in lymphoedema.

Some readers will find confidence intervals easier to interpret if they sketch the confidence intervals on a 'tree' plot,[19] as in Figure 6.1. The tree plot consists of a line along which effects of intervention could lie. The middle of the line represents no effect (difference between group means of 0). One end of the line represents a very good effect (intervention group mean minus control group mean is a large positive number) and the other end represents a very harmful intervention (intervention group mean minus control group mean is a large negative number). For any trial we can draw three variables on this graph (Figure 6.2A): the smallest worthwhile effect (in our example this is 6 cm), the best estimate of the effect of intervention (the difference between group means from Dini et al's randomized controlled trial, or 0 cm), and the 95% confidence interval about that estimate (−3 cm to +3 cm). The region to the right of the smallest worthwhile effect is the domain of clinically worthwhile effects of intervention. The graph for the Dini trial (Figure 6.2A) clearly shows that there is not a clinically worthwhile effect, because neither the best estimate of the effect of intervention nor any point encompassed by the 95% confidence interval lie in the region of a clinically worthwhile effect.

Living with uncertainty

In the example just used, the effect of intervention was clearly not large enough to be clinically worthwhile. This is a helpful result because it gives us some certainty about the effect (in this case, the lack of any worthwhile effect) of the intervention. In other examples, such as with the trial by O'Sullivan et al (1997) on specific muscle training for people with spondylolysis and spondylolisthesis, we may find clear answers in the other direction (Figure 6.2B). We have already seen that the mean effect of treatment reported in the O'Sullivan trial was 29 mm, substantially more than the value we nominated as the smallest worthwhile effect (20% of 48 mm, or about 10 mm). The 95% confidence interval for this effect is approximately 15 to 43 mm.[20] Consequently,

---

[18]This interpretation is easy to grasp and easy to use but, strictly speaking, incorrect (see footnote 12). One justification for perpetuating the incorrect interpretation is that it may be a reasonable approximation; 95% confidence intervals for differences between means correspond closely to 1/32 likelihood intervals (Royall 1997), which means that they correspond to the interval most strongly supported by the trial data. Also, in the presence of 'vague priors' (that is, in the presence of considerable uncertainty about the true effect prior to the conduct of the trial), 95% confidence intervals usually correspond quite closely to Bayesian 95% credible intervals which can more legitimately be interpreted as 'the interval within which the true value probably lies' (Barnett 1982).

[19]We call these tree plots because they resemble one element of a forest plot. (For an example of a forest plot, see Figure 6.6.)

[20]Try to do the calculations yourself using the formula in Box 6.1. The key data are that (a) mean pain intensity was 48 mm in the control group and 19 mm in the exercise group, (b) the standard deviations were 23 mm in the control group and 21 mm in the exercise group, and (c) both groups contained 21 participants.

Box 6.1

A method for calculating confidence intervals for differences between means

When confidence intervals about differences between group means are not supplied explicitly in reports of clinical trials, it is usually an easy matter to calculate these from the data reported in trials.

The confidence intervals for the difference between the means for two groups can be calculated from the difference between the two means (*difference*), their standard deviations and the group sizes. An approximate 95% confidence interval is given by first obtaining the average of the two standard deviations (SD_{av}) and the average of the group sizes (n_{av}). Then the 95% confidence interval (95% CI) for the difference between the two means is calculated from:

$$95\% \text{ CI} \approx difference \pm (3 \times SD_{av})/\sqrt{n_{av}}$$

(Herbert 2000a).[21] (The '$\approx$' symbol means 'is approximately equal to'.) In other words, the confidence interval spans an interval from $(3 \times SD)/\sqrt{n_{av}}$ below the difference in group means to $(3 \times SD)/\sqrt{n_{av}}$ above the difference in group means.

This equation is an approximation to the more complex equation that should be used when trialists analyse their data, but it is an adequate approximation for readers of clinical trials to use for clinical decision-making.[22] It has the advantage that it is simple enough to be calculated routinely whenever a clinical trial does not report the confidence interval for the difference between group means.[23]

In the trial by Dini et al (1998) on 80 participants (average group size 40), the authors reported mean measures of oedema for both intervention and control groups (14 cm for both groups), and the standard deviations about those means (6.0 cm for both groups), but they did not report the 95% confidence interval for the difference between means. The 95% confidence interval can be calculated from this data and is:

$$95\% \text{ CI} \approx (14 - 14) \pm (3 \times 6)/\sqrt{40}$$

$$95\% \text{ CI} \approx 0 \pm 3$$

$$95\% \text{ CI} \approx -3 \text{ to} + 3 \text{ cm}$$

Often papers will report standard errors of the means (*SEs*), rather than standard deviations. In that case the calculation is even simpler:[24,25]

$$95\% \text{ CI} \approx difference \pm 3 \times SE_{av}$$

Many trials have more than two groups (as there may be more than one intervention group, or more than one control). The reader must then decide which between-group comparison is (or are) of most interest, and then the 95% confidence intervals for differences between these groups can be calculated in the same way as above. Similarly, most trials report several, and sometimes many, outcomes. It is tedious to calculate 95% confidence intervals for all outcomes, and usually the best approach is to decide which few outcomes are of greatest interest, and then calculate 95% confidence interval for those outcomes only.

Sometimes a degree of detective work is required to find the standard deviations or standard errors. If the standard deviations or standard errors are not given explicitly, they may sometimes be obtained from the error bars in figures. In other trial reports there may be inadequate reporting of trial outcomes and it will not be possible to calculate 95% confidence intervals. Such trials are difficult to interpret. Some trials report medians and interquartile ranges, or sometimes ranges, instead of means and standard deviations, which makes it more difficult to estimate confidence intervals for these trials.[26]

---

[21]The derivation is as follows. If we assume equal group sizes (n) and equal standard deviations (SD) in the two groups, the standard error of the difference in means (SE_{diff}) is $SD/\sqrt{(2/n)}$. For reasonably large samples, the 95% CI is $\approx difference \pm 1.96\ SE_{diff}$ or $difference \pm 1.96\ SD/\sqrt{(2/n)}$, which is $\approx difference \pm 3\ SD/\sqrt{n}$. A simple estimate of the SD is given by SD_{av}, and we can substitute n_{av} for n. Hence the 95% CI is approximated by the $difference \pm 3\ SD_{av}/\sqrt{n_{av}}$.

[22]The procedures described above for calculating the confidence interval of the difference between two means will tend to produce overly conservative confidence intervals (confidence intervals that are too broad) in some circumstances. In particular, this procedure will tend to produce confidence intervals that are too broad when the study is a cross-over study, a study in which participants are matched before randomization, or a study in which statistical procedures (such as ANCOVA) are used to partition out explainable sources of variance. Less often, if the sample size is small and the group sizes are very unequal, or in cluster-randomized trials, the confidence interval may be too narrow. In such studies it is highly desirable that the authors report confidence intervals for the differences between groups.

[23]In fact, if you are prepared to do the calculations roughly, they are easy enough to do without a calculator. Rough calculations can be justified because small differences in the width of confidence intervals are unlikely to make any difference to the clinical decision. The hard part of the equation is in taking the square root of the

sample size. But you can take advantage of the fact that square roots are insensitive to approximation. You will probably make the same clinical decision if you calculate that the square root of 40 is 6.3246, or if you just say it is 'about 6'.

[24]Some readers will wonder why the 95% CI is $\pm 3\ SE_{av}$, and not $\pm 2\ SE_{av}$ (or $\pm 1.96\ SE_{av}$). The explanation is that the 95% CI for the difference between two means is equal to the difference $\pm 1.96\ SE_{diff}$, not the difference $\pm 1.96\ SE_{av}$. When sample sizes and SDs of both groups are equal, $SE_{diff} = \sqrt{2}\ SE_{av}$.

[25]Occasionally papers will report the 95% CI for *each* group's mean. This is unhelpful, because we really want to know the 95% CI for the *difference* between the two means. It is possible, albeit tedious, to convert the 95% CIs for the two group means into a CI for the difference between the two means. To do so we take advantage of the fact that the 95% CI for a group mean is $\approx 4\ SE$ wide.

Here's what to do:

Take the 95% CI for the control group's mean and determine its width by subtracting the lower limit of the confidence interval from the upper limit. Then divide the width of the confidence interval by 4 to get the standard error for the control group mean. Repeat the procedure to calculate the standard error for the intervention group. Then take the average of the two SEs to get the SE_{av}. Then you can calculate the 95% CI for the difference between groups as the $difference \pm 3\ SE_{av}$.

[26]As a rough approximation you can use the equation presented above by treating medians like means and approximating the SD as three-quarters of the interquartile range or one-quarter of the range.

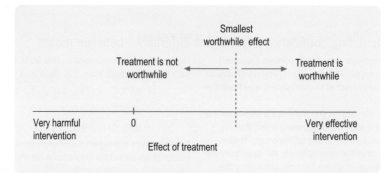

Figure 6.1 • 'Tree plot' of effect size. The tree plot consists of a horizontal line representing the effect of intervention. At the extremes are very harmful and very effective interventions. The smallest worthwhile effect is represented as a vertical dotted line. This divides the tree plot into two regions: the region to the left of this line represents effects of intervention that are too small to be worthwhile, whereas the region to the right of this line represents interventions whose effects are worthwhile.

the entire confidence interval falls in the region that is greater than the smallest worthwhile effect. Again this is helpful because it tells us with some certainty that the intervention produces clinically worthwhile effects.

Unfortunately, when we go through this process with other trials the results will often be less clear. Ambiguity arises when the confidence interval spans the smallest worthwhile effect, because then it is plausible both that the intervention does and does not have a clinically worthwhile effect. Part of the confidence interval is less than the smallest worthwhile effect and part of the confidence interval is greater than the smallest worthwhile effect; either result could be the "true" one. For example, Sand et al (1995) showed that 15 weeks of pelvic floor electrical stimulation for women with genuine stress incontinence produced large reductions in urine leakage (average of 32 ml or 70% reduction) compared with sham stimulation. This result is shown on a tree plot in Figure 6.2C. The mean difference suggests a large and worthwhile effect of intervention, but the 95% confidence interval spanned from a 7% to a 100% reduction. There is, therefore, a high degree of uncertainty about how big the effect actually is, and because the lower end of the confidence interval includes trivially small reductions in urine loss it is not certain, on the basis of this trial alone, that the intervention is worthwhile.

This situation, when the confidence interval spans the smallest worthwhile effect, arises commonly for two reasons. First, the designers of clinical trials conventionally use sample sizes that are sufficient only to rule out no effect of intervention if there truly is a clinically worthwhile effect, but such samples

may be too small to prevent their confidence intervals spanning the smallest worthwhile effect. Second, many interventions have modest effects (their true effects are close to the smallest worthwhile effect), so their confidence intervals must be very narrow if they are not to span the smallest worthwhile effect. Consequently few studies provide unambiguous evidence of an effect, or lack of effect, of intervention.

There are two ways to respond to the uncertainty that is often provided by single trials. First, we can accept uncertainty and proceed on the basis of the best available evidence. In this approach, clinical decisions are based on the difference between group means. When the difference exceeds the smallest worthwhile effect the intervention is thought to be worthwhile, and when the difference between group means is less than the smallest worthwhile effect the intervention is thought to be insufficiently effective. With this approach the role of confidence intervals is to provide an indicator of the degree of self-doubt that should be applied, but they do not otherwise affect clinical decisions. An alternative is to seek more certainty by determining whether the findings of individual studies are replicated in other, similar studies. This is one of the reasons why systematic reviews of randomized controlled trials are potentially a very useful source of information about the effects of intervention. As we saw earlier in this chapter, systematic reviews can combine the results of individual trials in a meta-analysis, effectively providing a single result from many studies. The combined result is derived from a relatively large sample size, so it usually provides a more precise estimate of effects of intervention (its confidence intervals are relatively narrow),

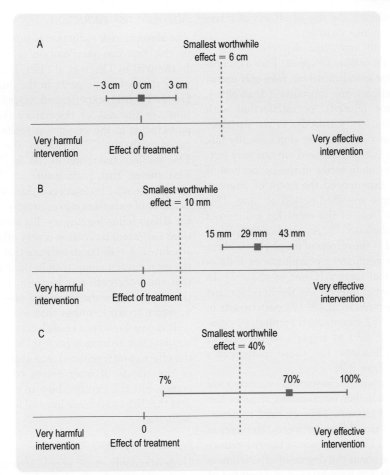

Figure 6.2 • (A) Data from Dini et al (1998) on effects of pressure therapy on post-mastectomy oedema. The smallest worthwhile effect has been nominated as a reduction of oedema of 6 cm (40% of initial oedema levels). The best estimate of the size of the treatment effect (no effect at all) has been illustrated as a small square, and the 95% confidence interval about this estimate (−3 to +3 cm) is shown as a horizontal line. The effect of intervention is clearly smaller than the smallest worthwhile effect. (B) Data from O'Sullivan et al (1997) on effects of specific exercise on pain intensity in people with spondylolisthesis and spondylolysis. The mean effect is a reduction in pain of 29 mm on a 100-mm visual analogue scale (VAS) (95% confidence interval 15 to 43 mm). This is clearly more than the smallest worthwhile effect, which we nominated as a 10-mm reduction (or approximately 20% of the initial pain levels of 48 mm). (C) Data from Sand et al (1995) on effects of a programme of electrical stimulation on urine leakage in women with stress urinary incontinence. The smallest worthwhile effect has been nominated as 40%. The best estimate of the size of the treatment effect (a 70% reduction in leakage) is very worthwhile (much more than a 40% reduction in leakage). However, the 95% confidence interval for this estimate is very wide (7% to 100%). (In this particular case the confidence intervals are not symmetrical because it is not possible to reduce leakage by more than 100%.) The confidence intervals include effects of intervention that are both smaller than the smallest worthwhile effect and greater than the worthwhile effect. Thus, while the best estimate of the treatment effect is that it is clinically worthwhile, this conclusion is subject to a high degree of uncertainty.

and it is more likely to provide unambiguous information about the effect of intervention (narrow confidence intervals are less likely to span the smallest worthwhile effect). We shall consider the role of meta-analysis further later in this chapter.

Dichotomous outcomes

The examples in the preceding section were of clinical trials in which outcomes were measured as continuous variables. Other outcomes are measured as 'dichotomous' variables. This section considers how we might estimate the size of effects of intervention on dichotomous variables.

Dichotomous outcomes are discrete events – things that either do or do not happen. Thus a dichotomous outcome for an individual can take only one of two values. Examples are mortality (dead/alive), injury (injured/not injured), or satisfaction with treatment (satisfied/not satisfied). When variables can take on one of two values we don't usually talk about their mean values.[27] Instead we quantify outcomes of intervention in terms of the proportion of participants that experienced the event of interest, usually within some specified period of time. This tells us about the 'risk' of the event for individuals from that population.[28,29] A good example is provided by a trial of the effects of prophylactic chest physiotherapy on respiratory complications following major abdominal surgery (Olsen et al 1997). In this study the event of interest was the development of a respiratory complication. Of 192 participants in the control group, 52 experienced respiratory complications within 6 days of surgery, so the risk of respiratory complications for these participants was $52/192 = 0.27$, or 27%.

In clinical trials with dichotomous outcomes we are interested in whether intervention reduces the risk of the event of interest. Thus we need to determine whether the risk differs between intervention and control groups. The magnitude of the risk reduction, which tells us about the degree of effectiveness of the intervention, can be expressed in a number of different ways (Guyatt et al 1994, Sackett et al 2000). Three common measures are the *absolute risk reduction* (ARR), *number needed to treat* (NNT) and *relative risk reduction* (RRR).

---

[27]It would be unconventional, but not necessarily inappropriate, to talk about the mean value of a dichotomous outcome. If the alternative events are assigned values of 0 and 1, then their mean is the risk of the alternative assigned a value of 1.

[28]We refer to the risk of an event when the event is undesirable, but we don't usually talk of the risk of a desirable event. (For example, it seems natural to talk of the risk of getting injured, but not of the risk of not getting injured.) There are two ways to deal with this. Given the 'risk' of a desirable event, we can always estimate the risk of the undesirable alternative. The risk (in %) of undesirable event $= 100 - $ the risk (in %) of desirable event. Thus if the risk of not getting injured is 80%, the risk of getting injured is 20%. Alternatively, we could replace the word 'risk' with 'probability' and talk instead about the probability of not getting injured.

[29]Rothman & Greenland (1998: 37) point out that the word 'risk' has several meanings. They call the proportion of participants experiencing the event of interest the 'average risk' or, less ambiguously, the 'incidence proportion'.

Absolute risk reduction

The absolute risk reduction is simply the difference in risk between intervention and control groups. In the trial by Olsen et al (1997), a relatively small proportion of participants in the intervention group $(10/172 = 6\%)$ experienced respiratory complications, so the risk of respiratory complications for participants in the group was relatively small compared with the 27% risk in the control group. The absolute reduction in risk is $27\% - 6\% = 21\%$. This means that participants in the intervention group were at a 21% lower risk than control group participants of experiencing respiratory complications in the 6 days following surgery. Big absolute risk reductions indicate intervention is very effective. Negative absolute risk reductions indicate that risk is greater in the intervention group than in the control group and that the intervention is harmful. (An exception to this rule is when the event is a positive event, such as return to work, rather than a negative event.)

It is possible to put confidence intervals about the absolute risk reduction (as it is about any measure of the effect of intervention), just as we did for estimate of the effects of intervention on continuous outcomes. Box 6.2 explains how to calculate and interpret the 95% confidence interval for the absolute risk reduction.

Number needed to treat

Understandably many people have difficulty appreciating the magnitude of absolute risk reductions. A consequence is that it is often difficult to specify the smallest worthwhile effect in terms of absolute risk reduction, especially when the risk in control participants is low. How big is a 21% reduction in absolute risk? Is a 21% absolute risk reduction clinically worthwhile? A second measure of risk reduction, the number needed to treat, makes the magnitude of an absolute risk reduction more explicit. The number needed to treat is obtained by taking the inverse of the absolute risk reduction. In our example, the absolute risk reduction is 21%, so the number needed to treat is $1/21\%$, or ≈ 5.[30,31] This is the number of people that would need to be treated, on average, to prevent the event of interest happening to one person. In our example, one respiratory complication is prevented for every 5 people given the intervention.

---

[30]Remember that a percentage is a fraction, so $1/21\%$ is the same as $1/0.21$, not $1/21$.

[31]Usual practice is to round NNTs to the nearest whole number.

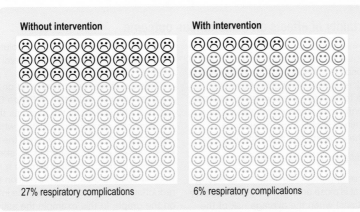

Without intervention

27% respiratory complications

With intervention

6% respiratory complications

Figure 6.3 • A diagram (Cates' plot) illustrating the relationship between the absolute risk reduction and the number needed to treat. The diagram is based on a figure from Cates (2003) and it uses as an example data from the trial by Olsen et al (1997). Each face represents 1% of the population. Sad faces represent people who experienced respiratory complications. Smiley faces represent people who did not experience respiratory complications. The left panel shows outcomes in a population that did not receive the intervention and the right panel shows outcomes in a population that did receive the intervention. The first 6 people (6% of the population) experienced a complication with or without intervention (i.e. in the left and right panels), so intervention made no difference to these participants. The next 21 people, drawn in a brighter blue in the diagram, experienced respiratory complications without intervention but not with intervention. These participants benefited from intervention. The remaining 73 people did not experience respiratory complications with or without intervention, so intervention made no difference to these people. Thus, overall, 21 of 100 people benefited from intervention; we say the absolute risk reduction was 21%. Another way of saying this is that about 1 in every 5 treated patients (21 of 100 people) benefited from treatment, so the number to treat was 5.

For the other 4 of every 5 patients the intervention made no difference: some would not have developed a respiratory complication anyhow, and the others developed a respiratory complication despite intervention. A small number needed to treat (such as 5) is better than a large number needed to treat (such as 100) because it indicates that a relatively small number of patients need to be treated before the intervention makes a difference to one of them.

Figure 6.3 illustrates why it is that a reduction in risk from 27% to 6% corresponds to a number needed to treat of 5 (Cates 2003). This figure illustrates the outcomes of 100 typical patients who did not receive the intervention and another 100 typical patients who did receive the intervention. Twenty-seven of the 100 control group patients experienced a respiratory complication, whereas only 6 of the 100 intervention group patients experienced a respiratory complication (6% of 20 is about 1). That is, for every 100 people who received the intervention, 21 fewer experienced a respiratory complication. Twenty-one of 100 people (or about 1 in 5) benefit from this

intervention.[32] That is why we say the number needed to treat is 5. Conversely, 79 of the 100 people who received the intervention did not benefit from intervention (73 were not going to have a respiratory complication even if they did not receive the intervention, and 6 experienced a respiratory complication despite intervention). In other words, 4 of every 5 patients do not benefit from this intervention.

The number needed to treat is very useful because it makes it relatively easy to nominate what the

---

[32]Strictly speaking, that need not be true. The 21% absolute risk reduction means that the *net* (or *average*) effect was to prevent a complication in 21% of patients. It could also be correctly interpreted as meaning that the intervention prevented respiratory complications in *at least* 21% of patients. Here is why: theoretically an absolute risk reduction of 21% could mean that the intervention *prevented* a respiratory complication in, say, 30% of patients, but *also caused* a respiratory complication in a further 9% of patients. If the intervention prevented a respiratory complication in 30% of patients and caused a respiratory complication in 9% of patients, the absolute risk reduction would still be 21%.

Box 6.2

Estimating uncertainty of effects on dichotomous outcome

As with trials that measure continuous outcomes, many trials with dichotomous outcomes do not report confidence intervals about the absolute risk reduction, number needed to treat or relative risk reduction. Almost all, however, supply sufficient data to calculate the confidence interval. A very rough 95% confidence interval for the absolute risk reduction can be obtained simply from the average sample size (n_{av}) of the experimental and control groups:

$$95\% \text{ CI} \approx difference \text{ } in \text{ } risk \pm 1/\sqrt{n_{av}}$$

(Herbert 2000b).[33] This approximation works well enough (it gives an answer that is close enough to that provided by more complex equations) when the average risk of the events of interest in treated and control groups is greater than $\approx$10% and less than $\approx$90%.

To illustrate the calculation of confidence intervals for dichotomous data, recall that in the study by Olsen et al (1997) the risk to control participants was 27%, the risk to experimental participants was 6%, and the average size of each group was 182, so:

$$95\% \text{ CI} \approx (27\% - 6\%) \pm 1/\sqrt{182}$$

$$95\% \text{ CI} \approx 21\% \pm 0.07$$

$$95\% \text{ CI} \approx 21\% \pm 7\%$$

Thus the best estimate of the absolute risk reduction is 21% and its 95% confidence interval extends from 14% to 28%.

This result has been illustrated on a tree plot of the absolute risk reduction in Figure 6.4. The logic of this tree plot is exactly the same as that used for the tree plot of a continuous variable, which was presented earlier.[34] Again, we plot the smallest worthwhile effect (which we nominated as an absolute risk reduction of 5%, corresponding to a number needed to treat of 20), the effect of intervention (absolute risk reduction of 21% and its confidence interval (14% to 28%) on the graph. In this example the estimated absolute risk reduction and its confidence interval are clearly greater than the smallest worthwhile effect, so we can confidently conclude that this intervention is clinically worthwhile.

In the example just used, we calculated absolute risk reduction and the 95% confidence intervals for the absolute risk reduction. We could, if we wished, have calculated the number needed to treat and the 95% confidence interval for the number needed to treat. As we have already seen, it is a simple matter to calculate the number needed to treat (NNT) from the absolute risk reduction (ARR) – we just invert the absolute risk reduction to obtain the number needed

Figure 6.4 • A 'tree plot' of the size of the treatment effect reported by Olsen et al (1997). The tree plot consists of a horizontal line representing treatment effect. At the extremes of the horizontal axis are very harmful and very effective treatments. The smallest worthwhile effect is represented as a vertical dotted line. This example shows the effect (expressed as an absolute risk reduction, ARR) of chest physiotherapy on risk of respiratory complications following upper abdominal surgery. The smallest worthwhile effect has been nominated as an absolute reduction in risk of 5%. The best estimate of the size of the treatment effect (21%) and all of the 95% confidence interval about this estimate (14% to 28%) fall to the right of the line of the smallest worthwhile effect. Thus the treatment effect is clearly greater than the smallest worthwhile effect.

[33]The 'proof is as follows. If we assume that the sample sizes of the two groups are equal, the normal approximation for the 95% CI for the ARR reduces to the $ARR \pm 1.96 \times \sqrt{[(R_c \,(1 - R_c) + R_t \,(1 - R_t)]/\sqrt{n}}$, where R_c and R_t are the risks in the control and treated groups and n is the number of participants in each group. To a very rough approximation, the term $1.96 \times \sqrt{[(R_c \,(1 - R_c) + R_t \,(1 - R_t)]} = 1$, provided $0.1 < R < 0.9$. Thus, to a very rough approximation, the 95% CI for the ARR $\approx ARR \pm 1/\sqrt{n}$. We can substitute n_{av} for n, so the 95% CI for the ARR $\approx ARR \pm 1/\sqrt{n_{av}}$.

[34]You will often see forest plots of the effects of intervention on dichotomous outcomes arranged so that beneficial treatment effects are to the left and harmful effects to the right. One of the reasons for this is that most forest plots are of the relative risk or odds ratio, and, by convention, smaller relative risks or odds ratios correspond to more beneficial effects of intervention. Here we have described the effect of intervention in terms of the absolute risk reduction. Larger absolute risk reductions correspond to more beneficial effects, so the natural convention is to plot beneficial effects of intervention to the right.

Box 6.2

Estimating uncertainty of effects on dichotomous outcome—cont'd

to treat.[35] The same applies to the ends of the confidence intervals (the 'confidence limits'). Once we have calculated the confidence limits for the absolute risk reduction we can obtain the 95% confidence interval for the number needed to treat by inverting the confidence limits of the absolute risk reduction. There is, however, a complication with the interpretation of confidence intervals for the number needed to treat (Altman 1998). When the confidence interval for the absolute risk reduction includes zero, confidence intervals for the number needed to treat don't appear to make sense. The problem and explanation are best illustrated with an example.

Pope et al (2000) investigated the effects of stretching before sport on all-injury risk in army recruits undergoing a 12-week training programme. Subjects were randomly allocated to groups that stretched or did not stretch prior to activity. Of the 803 participants in the control group, 175 were injured (risk of 21.8%) and 158 of the 735 participants in the stretch group were injured (risk of 21.5%).

Thus the effect of stretching was an absolute risk reduction of 0.3%, with an approximate 95% confidence interval from −3% to +4%. If we re-cast these estimates in terms of numbers needed to treat, we get a number needed to treat of 333 and an approximate 95% confidence interval for the number needed to treat of −33 to 25. The interpretation of the number needed to treat of 333 is quite straightforward. It means that 333 people would need to stretch before activity for 12 weeks to

Figure 6.5 • Explanation of confidence intervals for numbers needed to treat (NNTs). The data of Pope et al (2000) suggest that stretching before exercise reduces injury risk (absolute risk reduction, ARR) by 0% (95% confidence interval −3% to 4%) in army recruits undergoing a 12-week training programme (tree plot shown in top panel). When, as in this example, the confidence interval for the ARR includes zero, the confidence interval for the NNT looks a little strange. In this example the estimated NNT is infinity and the 95% confidence interval extends from -33 to 25. Bizarrely, the estimated effect (infinity) does not seem to lie within its confidence intervals (-33 to 25). The explanation is that the tree plot for the NNT has a strange number line. A tree plot for the NNT is drawn in the lower panel; it has been scaled and aligned so that it corresponds exactly to the tree plot for the ARR shown in the upper panel. The NNT of infinity lies in the middle of the tree plot (no effect of intervention). Smaller numbers lie at the tails of the number line. On this bizarre number line the estimated NNT always lies within its confidence interval.

Continued

---

[35]The same operation is used to convert a NNT into an ARR: the ARR = 1/NNT.

Box 6.2

Estimating uncertainty of effects on dichotomous outcome—cont'd

prevent one injury.[36],[37] But the confidence limits are, at first, a little perplexing, because the estimate of 333 does not appear to lie within the confidence interval (−33 to 25).

The explanation is that numbers needed to treat lie on an unusual number scale (Figure 6.5; Altman 1998). In fact it is easiest to visualize the number scale as the inverse of the normal number scale that we use for the absolute risk reduction. Instead of being centred on zero, like the

number scale for the absolute risk reduction, the number scale for the number needed to treat is centred on 1/0, or infinity. This number scale is big in the middle and little at the edges! If we refer back to our example, you can see that, on this strange number scale, the best estimate of the number needed to treat (333) really does lie within the 95% confidence interval of −33 to 25!

---

smallest worthwhile effect might be. With the number needed to treat, we can more easily weigh up the benefits of preventing the event in one participant against the costs and risks of giving the intervention. (Note that the benefit is received by a few, but costs are shared by all.) In our example, most would agree that a number needed to treat of 10 would be worthwhile, because preventing one respiratory complication is a very desirable thing, and the risks and costs of this simple intervention are minimal, so little is lost from ineffectively treating 9 of every 10 patients. Most would agree, however, that a number needed to treat of 100 would be too small to make the intervention worthwhile. There may be little risk associated with this intervention, but it probably incurs too great a cost (too much discomfort caused to patients, for example) for us to justify treating 99 people ineffectively to prevent one respiratory complication.

What, then, is the largest number needed to treat for prophylactic chest physiotherapy we would accept as being clinically worthwhile (what is the smallest worthwhile effect)? When we polled some experienced cardiopulmonary therapists they indicated that they would not be prepared to instigate this therapy if they had to treat more than about 20 patients to prevent one respiratory complication. That is, they nominated a number needed to treat of 20 as the smallest worthwhile effect. This corresponds to an absolute risk reduction of 5%. It would be interesting to survey patients facing major abdominal surgery to determine what they considered to be

the smallest worthwhile effect. The effect of intervention demonstrated in the trial by Olsen et al (number needed to treat = 5) is greater than most therapists would consider to be minimally clinically worthwhile (number needed to treat ≈20; remember that a small number needed to treat indicates a large effect of intervention).

Clearly there is no one value for the number needed to treat that can be deemed to be the smallest worthwhile effect. The size of the smallest worthwhile effect will depend on the seriousness of the event and the costs and risks of intervention. Thus the smallest worthwhile effect of a 3-month exercise programme may be as little as 2 or 3 if the event being prevented is not a very serious problem (such as infrequent giving way of the knee), whereas the smallest worthwhile effect for the use of incentive spirometry in the immediate postoperative period after chest surgery may be a number needed to treat of many hundreds if the event being prevented is death from respiratory complications.[38] When intervention is ongoing, the number needed to treat, like the absolute risk reduction, should be related to the period of intervention. A number needed to treat of 10 for a 3-month course of therapy aimed at reducing respiratory complications in children with cystic fibrosis is similar in the size of its effect to another therapy that has a number needed to treat of 5 for a 6-month course of therapy.

---

[36]Following the same approach as in footnote 35, this is a bit like saying that, on average, a person would need to stretch before activity for 333 × 12 weeks, or 77 years, to prevent an injury.

[37]This analysis differs slightly from the analysis reported in the trial by Pope et al (2000) because the authors of the original trial report used more sophisticated methods to analyse the data than are used here.

[38]A simple way of weighing up benefit and harm is to assign (very subjectively) a number to describe the benefit of intervention. The benefit of intervention is described in terms of how much worse the event being prevented is than the harm of the intervention. In the example of prevention of respiratory complications with prophylactic chest physiotherapy, we might judge that respiratory complications are 10 times as bad (unpleasant, expensive, etc.) as the intervention of prophylactic physiotherapy. If the benefit is greater than the number needed to treat, the benefit of therapy outweighs its harm. In our example, respiratory complications are 10 times as bad as prophylactic physiotherapy, and the NNT is 5, so the therapy produces more benefit than harm.

Relative risk reduction

A more commonly reported but less immediately helpful way of expressing the reduction in risk is as a proportion of the risk in control group patients. This is termed the relative risk reduction. The relative risk reduction is obtained by dividing the absolute risk reduction by the risk in the control group. Thus the relative risk reduction produced by prophylactic chest physiotherapy is 21%/27%, which is 78%. In other words, prophylactic chest physiotherapy reduced the risk of respiratory complications by 78% *of the risk in untreated patients*. You can see that the relative risk reduction (78%) looks much larger than the absolute risk reduction (21%), even though they are describing exactly the same effect.[39] Which, then, is the best measure of the magnitude of an intervention's effects? Should we use the absolute risk reduction, its inverse (the number needed to treat), or the relative risk reduction?

The relative risk reduction has some properties that make it useful for comparing the findings of different studies, but it can be deceptive when used for clinical decision-making. This might best be illustrated with an example. Lauritzen et al (1993) showed that the provision of hip protector pads to residents of nursing homes produced relative reductions in risk of hip fracture of 56%. This might sound as if the intervention has a big effect, and it may be tempting to conclude on the basis of this statistic that the hip protectors are clinically worthwhile. However, the incidence of hip fractures in the study sample was about 5% per year (Lauritzen et al 1993), so the absolute reduction of hip fracture risk with hip protectors in this population is 56% *of* 5%, or just less than 3%. By converting this to a number needed to treat, we can see that 36 people would need to wear hip protectors for 1 year to prevent one fracture.[40] When the risk reduction is expressed as an absolute risk reduction or, better still as a number needed to treat, the effects appear much smaller than when presented as a relative

risk reduction. (Nonetheless, because hip fractures are serious events, a 1-year number needed to treat of 36 may still be worthwhile.) This example illustrates that it is probably better to make decisions about the effects of interventions in terms of absolute risk reductions or numbers needed to treat than relative risk reductions.

The importance of baseline risk

In general, even the best interventions (those with large relative risk reductions) will produce small absolute risk reductions only when the risk of the event in control group patients (the 'baseline risk') is low. Perhaps this is intuitively obvious-if few people are likely to experience the event, it is not possible to prevent it very often. There are two very practical implications. First, even the best interventions are unlikely to produce clinically worthwhile effects if the event that is to be prevented is unlikely. The converse of this is that an intervention is more likely to be clinically worthwhile when it reduces risk of a high-risk event. (For a particularly clear discussion of this issue see Glasziou & Irwig 1995.) Second, as the magnitude of the effect of intervention is likely to depend very much on the risk to which untreated participants are exposed, care is needed when applying the results of a clinical trial to a particular patient if the risk to patients in the trial differs markedly from the risk in the patient for whom the intervention is being considered. If the risk in control participants in the trial is much higher than in the patient in question, the effect of intervention will tend to be overestimated (that is, the absolute risk reduction calculated from trial data will be too high, and the number needed to treat will be too low).[41]

There is a simple work-around that makes it possible to apply the results of a clinical trial to patients with higher or lower levels of risk. The approach described here is based on the method used by Straus & Sackett (1999; see also McAlister et al 2000). The absolute risk reduction or number needed to treat is calculated as described above, directly from the results of the trial, but is then adjusted by a factor, let's call it f, which describes how much more risk participants are at than the untreated (control) participants in the trial. A value of f of greater than 1 is used when the patients to whom the result is to be applied are at

---

[39]In fact the relative risk reduction always looks larger than the absolute risk reduction because it is obtained by dividing the absolute risk reduction by the probability of the event in untreated patients, and the probability of the event in untreated patients is always less than 1.

[40]Some people find NNTs per year hard to conceptualize. If a 1-year NNT for wearing hip protectors of 36 means nothing to you, try looking at it in another way. If 36 people need to wear hip protectors for 1 year to prevent one fracture, that is a bit like (though not exactly the same as) having to wear a hip protector for 36 years to prevent a hip fracture. Then the decision becomes easier still: would you wear a hip protector for 36 years if you thought it would prevent a hip fracture?

[41]The underlying assumption here is that measures of relative effects of treatment are constant regardless of baseline risk. This has been investigated by a number of authors, notably Furukawa et al (2002), Deeks & Altman (2001) and Schmid et al (1998). McAlister et al (2000) provides an excellent commentary on this literature.

a greater risk than control participants in the trial, and a value of *f* of less than 1 is used when patients to whom the result is to be applied are at a lower risk than untreated participants in the trial. The absolute risk reduction is adjusted by multiplying by *f*, and the number needed to treat is adjusted by dividing by *f*.

The following example illustrates how this approach might be used. A physiotherapist treating a morbidly obese patient undergoing major abdominal surgery might estimate that the patient was at twice the risk of respiratory complications as participants in the trial of Olsen et al (1997). To obtain a reasonable estimate of the effects of intervention (that is, to take into account the greater baseline risk in this participant than in participants in the trial), the number needed to treat (which we previously calculated as 5) could be divided by 2. This gives a number needed to treat of 2.5 (which rounds to 3) for morbidly obese participants. Thus we can anticipate an even larger effect of prophylactic physiotherapy among high-risk patients.[42] This approach can be used to adjust estimates of the likely effects of intervention for any individual patient up or down on the basis of therapists' perceptions of their patients' risks.

See Box 6.3 for a summary of this section.

Box 6.3

Is the evidence relevant to me and my patient/s?

Are the participants in the study similar to the patients I wish to apply the study's findings to?

Look at the inclusion and exclusion criteria used to determine eligibility for participation in the trial or systematic review.

Were interventions applied appropriately?

Look at how the intervention was applied.

Are the outcomes useful?

Determine whether the outcomes matter to patients.

Does the therapy do more good than harm?

Obtain an estimate of the size of the effect of treatment. Assess whether the effect of therapy is likely to be large enough to make it worth applying.

What does this systematic review of effects of intervention mean for my practice?

In the preceding section we considered how to assess whether a particular clinical trial provides us with relevant evidence, and what that evidence means for clinical practice. Now we turn our attention to interpreting systematic reviews of the effects of intervention.

Is the evidence relevant to me and my patient/s?

Making decisions about the relevance of a systematic review is very much like making decisions about the relevance of a clinical trial. (See 'Is the evidence relevant to me and my patient/s?' at the beginning of this chapter.) All of the same considerations apply. Just as with individual trials, we need to decide whether the review is able to provide information about the participants, interventions and outcomes we are interested in.

With systematic reviews, decisions about relevance of participants, interventions and outcomes can be made at either of two levels. The simpler approach is to look at the question addressed by the review and the criteria used to include and exclude studies in the review. In most systematic reviews there are explicit statements about the review question and the criteria used to determine what trials were eligible for the review. For example, a Cochrane systematic review by the Outpatient Service Trialists (2004) stipulated that the objective of the review was to 'assess the effects of therapy-based rehabilitation services targeted towards stroke patients resident in the community within 1 year of stroke onset/discharge from hospital following stroke'. The review was explicitly concerned with the effects of therapist-based rehabilitation services (defined at considerable length in the review) on death, dependency or performance in activities of daily living of patients who had experienced a stroke, were resident in a community setting, and had been randomized to treatment within 1 year of the index stroke. This clear statement of the scope of the review is typical of Cochrane systematic reviews.

To some readers, particularly those with a specific interest in the field of the review, this level of detail may be insufficient. These readers may be

---

[42]To see whether you've got the hang of this, try using the data from our earlier example to calculate the number needed to treat with hip protectors to prevent a hip fracture in a high risk population with a 1-year risk of hip fracture of 20%.

interested in the precise characteristics of participants included in each trial, or the precise nature of the intervention, or the precise method used to measure outcomes. It may be possible to obtain this level of information if the review separately reports details of each trial considered in the review. This information is often presented in the form of a table. Typically the table describes the participants, interventions and outcomes measured in each trial. When systematic reviewers provide this degree of detail the reader can decide for himself or herself which trials study relevant participants, interventions and outcomes. It may be that a particular trial has investigated the precise combinations of participants, interventions and outcomes that are of greatest interest.

By way of example, if you were interested in the potential effects of weight-supported walking training for a particular patient who recently had a stroke, you might consult the Cochrane review by Moseley et al (2005). This review assessed the effects of treadmill training or body weight support in the training of walking after stroke, so it included all trials with participants who had suffered a stroke and exhibited an abnormal gait pattern. Some trials were conducted on ambulatory patients and others on patients who were non-ambulatory. The authors described, in the text of their review, that eight of the 15 trials in the review[43] were conducted on ambulatory patients, and they provided detailed information about the participants, interventions and outcomes of these trials. When systematic reviews provide the details of each of the reviewed studies, as in this review, readers can base their conclusions on the particular trials that are most relevant to their own clinical questions.

What does the evidence say?

Good systematic reviews provide us with a wealth of information about the effects of interventions. They usually provide a detailed description of each of the individual trials included in the review and may, in addition, provide summary statements or conclusions that indicate the reviewers' interpretation of what the trials collectively say. Either or both may be helpful to the reader. In the following section we consider how to interpret the data presented in systematic reviews.

We begin by considering how systematic reviews can draw together the evidence from individual clinical trials into summary statements about the effects of intervention. As readers of systematic reviews, we want these summary statements to tell us both about the strength of the evidence and, if the evidence is strong enough to draw some conclusions, about the size of the effect of the intervention.

There are several distinctly different approaches that reviewers use to generate summary statements. Unfortunately, not all generate summary statements that are entirely satisfactory. As we shall see, a common problem is that the effect of the intervention is given in simplistic terms: the intervention is said to be either 'effective' or 'ineffective'.

> Statements about the effects of intervention that are not accompanied by estimates of the magnitudes of those effects are of little use for clinical decision-making.

Readers should be wary of systematic reviews with summary statements that claim the intervention is or is not effective when that claim is not supported with a statement of the estimated magnitude of the effect.

The simplest method used to generate summary statements about the effects of intervention is called *vote counting*. Vote counting is used in many narrative reviews and some systematic reviews. In the vote counting approach, the reviewer assigns one 'vote' to each trial, and then counts up the number of studies that do and do not find evidence for an effect of intervention. Some reviewers apply a simple rule: the conclusion with the most votes wins! Other reviewers are more conservative: they stipulate that a certain (high) percentage of trials must conclude there is a significant effect of intervention before there is collective evidence of an effect. Sometimes the vote counting threshold is not made explicit. In that case the reviewer informally assesses the proportion of significant trials and decides whether 'most' trials are significant or not, without explicitly stating the threshold that defines 'most'. But regardless of what threshold is used, vote counting generates one of two conclusions: either there is evidence of an effect, or there is not.

An example of the use of vote counting comes from a systematic review of preventive interventions for back and neck problems (Linton & van Tulder 2001). This review reports that 'Six of the nine randomised controlled trials did not find any significant differences on any of the outcome variables

---

[43]The review will be updated in late 2010 and it is expected that new trials will be added to the review at that time.

compared between the back school intervention and usual care or no intervention or between different types of back or neck schools ... Thus, there is consistent evidence from randomized controlled trials that back and neck schools are not effective interventions in preventing back pain' (pp 789 & 783). In this review, there were more non-significant than significant trials of back and neck schools, so the authors concluded back and neck schools are not an effective intervention.

The shortcomings of vote counting have been understood since the very early days of systematic reviews. Hedges & Olkin (1980, 1985) showed that vote counting is toothless; it lacks statistical power. That is, even when an intervention has clinically important effects the vote counting approach is likely to conclude that there is no evidence of an effect of intervention. The power of the vote counting procedure is determined by the threshold required to satisfy the reviewer that there is an effect (for example, 50% of trials or 66% of trials), the number of trials, and the statistical power of the individual trials. (The statistical power of an individual trial refers to the probability that the trial will detect a clinically meaningful effect if such an effect truly exists. Many trials have low statistical power because they are too small; that is, many trials have too few participants to enable them to detect clinically meaningful effects of intervention if such effects exist.) Typically, the power of the vote counting approach is low.[44] For this reason, systematic reviews that use vote counting and conclude there is no evidence of an effect of intervention should be treated with suspicion.

There is a second serious problem with vote counting. Vote counting provides a dichotomous answer: it concludes that there is or is not evidence that the intervention is effective. Earlier in this chapter it was argued that there is little value in learning if the intervention is effective. What we need to know, instead, is how effective the intervention is. The 'answer' provided by vote counting methods is not clinically useful.

An alternative to vote counting is the *levels of evidence approach*. This approach differs from vote counting in that it attempts to combine information about both the quality of the evidence and the effects

Box 6.4

Levels of evidence criteria of van Poppel et al (1997)

Level 1 (strong evidence): multiple relevant, high-quality randomized clinical trials (RCTs) with consistent results.

Level 2 (moderate evidence): one relevant, high-quality RCT and one or more relevant low-quality RCTs or non-randomized controlled clinical trials (CCTs) (high or low quality). Consistent outcomes of the studies.

Level 3 (limited evidence): only one high-quality RCT or multiple low-quality RCTs and non-randomized CCTs (high or low quality). Consistent outcomes of the studies.

Level 4 (no evidence): only one low-quality RCT or one non-randomized CCT (high or low quality); no relevant studies or contradictory outcomes of the studies.

Results were considered contradictory if less than 75% of studies reported the same results; otherwise outcomes were considered to be consistent.

of the intervention. In some versions of this approach, the reviewer defines 'strong evidence', 'moderate evidence', 'weak evidence' (or 'limited evidence') and 'little or no evidence'. Usually the definitions are based on the quantity, quality and consistency of evidence. A typical example is given in Box 6.4.

As an example, the same systematic review that used vote counting to examine effects of back and neck schools also used levels of evidence criteria to examine the effects of exercise for preventing neck and back pain (Linton & van Tulder 2001). Strong ('Level A') evidence was defined as 'generally consistent findings from multiple randomized controlled trials'. It was concluded that 'there is consistent evidence that exercise may be effective in preventing neck and back pain (Level A)'.

One of the problems with the levels of evidence approach is that different authors use slightly different criteria to define levels of evidence. Indeed, some authors use different criteria in different reviews. For example, van Poppel et al (1997: 842) define limited evidence as 'only one high quality randomized controlled trial or multiple low quality randomized controlled trials and non-randomized controlled clinical trials (high or low quality). Consistent outcome of the studies', whereas Berghmans et al (1998: 183) define limited evidence as 'one relevant randomized controlled trial of sufficient methodologic quality or multiple low quality randomized controlled trials.' These small differences in wording are not just untidy; they can profoundly affect the conclusions

---

[44]Another, remarkably bad, property of the vote counting approach is that the power of vote counting may actually decrease with an increasing number of trials (Hedges & Olkin 1985). Consequently, the probability of detecting an effect of intervention may decrease as evidence accrues.

that are drawn. Even apparently small differences in definitions of levels of evidence can lead to surprisingly different conclusions. Ferreira and colleagues (2002) applied four different sets of levels of evidence criteria to six Cochrane systematic reviews and found only 'fair' agreement (kappa = 0.33) between the conclusions reached with the different criteria. Application of the different criteria to one particular review, of the effects of back school programme for low back pain, lead to the conclusion that there was 'strong evidence that back school was effective' or 'weak evidence' or 'limited evidence' or 'no evidence', depending on which criteria were used. As the conclusions of systematic reviews can be very sensitive to the criteria used to define levels of evidence, readers of systematic reviews should be reluctant to accept the conclusions of systematic reviews which use the levels of evidence approach.

Another significant problem with the levels of evidence approach is that it, too, is likely to lack statistical power. This is because most levels of evidence criteria are based on vote counting. For example, the definition of 'strong evidence' used by van Poppel et al (1997: 842) ('multiple relevant, high quality randomized clinical trials with consistent outcomes') is based on vote counting because it requires that there be 'consistent' findings of the trials. In fact the levels of evidence approach is likely to be even less powerful than vote counting because it usually invokes additional criteria relating to trial quality. That is, to meet the definition of strong evidence there must be at least a certain proportion of significant trials (vote counting) *and* the trials must be of a certain quality. Thus, in general, the levels of evidence approach will have even less power than vote counting.

A quick inspection of the systematic reviews in physiotherapy that use vote counting or levels of evidence approaches shows that only a small proportion conclude there is strong evidence of an effect of intervention. This low percentage may indicate that there is not yet strong evidence of the effects of many interventions, but an equally plausible explanation is that true effects of intervention have been missed because the levels of evidence approach lacks the statistical power required to detect such effects.

Recent efforts have focused on developing qualitative methods of summarizing evidence that do not have the shortcomings of vote counting and levels of evidence approaches. One promising initiative is the Grading of Recommendations Assessment, Development and Evaluation (GRADE) project, which seeks to summarize several dimensions of the quality of evidence (GRADE Working Group 2004). GRADE assesses dimensions of study design, study quality, consistency (the similarity of estimates of effect across studies) and directness (the extent to which people, interventions and outcome measures are similar to those of interest). It uses the following definitions of the quality of evidence:

- *High-quality evidence.* Further research is very unlikely to change our confidence in the estimate of effect.
- *Moderate-quality evidence.* Further research is likely to have an important impact on our confidence in the estimate of effect and may change the estimate.
- *Low-quality evidence.* Further research is very likely to have an important impact on our confidence in the estimate of effect and may change the estimate.
- *Very low-quality evidence.* Any estimate of effect is very uncertain.

The focus on robustness of estimates of magnitude of the effect makes GRADE attractive. The Cochrane Collaboration now encourages authors of Cochrane systematic reviews to use GRADE, and as a consequence a substantial proportion of Cochrane reviews now scale the quality of evidence using GRADE.

An alternative to vote counting and the levels of evidence approach is *meta-analysis*. Meta-analysis is a statistical tool for summarizing effects of interventions. Usually the process of meta-analysis does not involve consideration of the quality of evidence.[45] It involves extracting estimates of the size of the effect of intervention from each trial and then statistically combining ('pooling') the data to obtain a single estimate based on all the trials.

An example of meta-analysis is provided in a systematic review of effects of pre- and post-exercise stretching on muscle soreness, risk of injury and athletic performance (Herbert & Gabriel 2002). This systematic review identified five studies that reported useful data on the effects of stretching on muscle soreness. The results of the five studies were pooled in a meta-analysis to produce a pooled estimate of the effects of stretching on subsequent muscle soreness.

To conduct a meta-analysis the researcher must first describe the magnitude of the effect of intervention reported in each trial. This can be done with any of a number of statistics. In trials that report continuous outcomes, the statistic most used to

---

[45]It is possible to include measures of trial quality as weights in meta-analysis, However, this practice lacks a strong theoretical justification. It is not common practice.

describe the size of effects of intervention is the mean difference between groups. This is the same statistic we used to describe the size of effects of interventions when appraising individual trials earlier in this chapter, and it has the same interpretation. Alternatively, some reviews will report the standardized mean difference between groups (usually calculated as the difference between group means divided by a pooled estimate of the within-group standard deviation).[46] The advantage of dividing the difference between means by the standard deviation is that this makes it possible to pool the findings of studies that report findings on different scales. However, when the size of the effect of intervention is reported on a standardized scale it can be very difficult to interpret, because it is difficult to know how big a particular standardized effect size must be to be clinically worthwhile.

When outcomes are reported on a dichotomous scale, different statistics are used to describe the effects of intervention. Unfortunately, the statistics we preferred to use earlier in this chapter to describe the effects of intervention on dichotomous outcomes in individual trials (the absolute risk reduction and number needed to treat) are not well suited to meta-analysis. Instead, in meta-analyses, the effect of intervention on dichotomous outcomes is most often reported as a relative risk or an odds ratio.[47]

The relative risk is simply the ratio of risks in intervention and control groups. Thus, if the risk in the intervention group is 6% and the risk in the control group is 27% (as in the trial by Olsen et al (1997) that we examined earlier in this chapter), the relative risk is 6/27 or 0.22. A relative risk of less than 1.0 indicates that risk in the intervention group was lower than that in the control group, and a risk of greater than 1.0 indicates that the risk in the intervention group was higher than that in the control group. A relative risk of 1.0 indicates that both groups had the same risk, and implies there was no effect of the intervention. The further the relative risk departs from 1.0, the bigger the effect of the intervention.

The odds ratio is similar to relative risk except that it is a ratio of odds, instead of a ratio of risks

(or probabilities). Odds are just another way of describing probabilities,[48] so the odds ratio behaves in some ways very like the relative risk. In fact, when the risk in the control group is low, the odds ratio is nearly the same as the relative risk. When the risk in the control group is high (say, more than 15%), the odds ratio diverges from the relative risk. The odds ratio is always more extreme (that is, it is further from 1.0) than the relative risk.

Usually the summary statistic for each trial is presented in either a table or a forest plot, such as the one reproduced in Figure 6.6. This is a particularly useful feature of systematic reviews. They provide, at a glance, a summary of the effects of intervention from each trial.

Regardless of what summary statistic is used to describe the effect of intervention observed in each trial, meta-analysis proceeds in the same way. The summary statistics from each trial are combined to produce a pooled estimate of the effect of intervention. The pooled estimate is really just an average of the summary statistics provided by each trial. But the average is not a simple average because some trials are given more 'weight' than others. The weight is determined by the standard error of the summary statistic, which is nearly the same as saying that the weight is determined by sample size: bigger studies (those with lots of participants) provide more precise estimates of the effects of intervention, so they are given more influence on the final pooled (weighted average) estimate of the effect of intervention.

The allure of meta-analysis is that it can provide more precise estimates of the effects of intervention than individual trials. This is illustrated in the meta-analysis of effects of stretching before or after exercise on muscle soreness, mentioned earlier (Herbert & Gabriel 2002). None of the five studies included in the meta-analysis found a statistically significant effect of stretching on muscle soreness, and all found the effects of stretching on muscle soreness was near zero. However, most of the individual studies were small and had fairly wide confidence intervals, meaning that individually they could not rule out small but marginally worthwhile effects. Pooling estimates of the effects of stretching

---

[46]There are several minor variations of this statistic.

[47]The relative risk (RR) is closely related to the relative risk reduction (RRR) that we considered earlier in this chapter. In fact the RR is just 1 − RRR. Thus if the RRR = 10%, the RR = 90%. The RR is the ratio of risks in the treated and control groups. So ratios of 1 (or 100%) indicate that the two groups have the same risk (indicating that the intervention has no effect) and ratios that depart from 1 are indicative of an effect of intervention. A number of other measures, notably the hazard ratio and incidence rate ratio, are also used, though rarely.

[48]The odds is the ratio of the risk of the event happening to the 'risk' of the event not happening. So if the risk is 33%, the ratio of risks is 33/67 or 0.5. If the risk is 80%, the odds are 80/20, or 4, and so on. You can convert risks (probabilities, R) to odds (O) with the equation $O = R/(1 − R)$. And you can convert back from odds to risks with $R = O/(1 + O)$.

Figure 6.6 • An example of a forest plot. Forest plots summarize the findings of several randomized trials of intervention, in this case the effects of stretching on post-exercise muscle soreness. Each row corresponds to one randomized trial; the names of the trial authors are given at the left. For each trial, the estimate of effect of intervention is shown as a diamond. (In this case the effect of intervention is expressed as the average reduction in muscle soreness, given in millimetres on a 100-mm soreness visual analogues scale, VAS.) The horizontal lines indicate the extent of the 95% confidence intervals, which can be loosely interpreted as the range within which the true average effect of stretching probably lies. The big symbol at the bottom is the pooled estimate of the effect of intervention, obtained by statistically combining the findings of all of the individual studies. Note that the confidence intervals of the pooled estimate are narrower than the confidence intervals of individual studies. Data are from Herbert & Gabriel (2002).

from all five trials in a meta-analysis provided a more precise estimate of the effects of stretching (see Figure 6.6). The authors concluded that 'the pooled estimate of reduction in muscle soreness 24 hours after exercising was only 0.9 mm on a 100-mm scale (95% confidence interval −2.6 mm to 4.4 mm) ... most athletes will consider effects of this magnitude too small to make stretching to prevent later muscle soreness worthwhile.' The meta-analysis was able to provide a very precise estimate of the average effect of stretching (between − 2.6 and 4.4 mm on a 100-mm scale), which permitted a clear conclusion to be drawn about the ineffectiveness of stretching in preventing muscle soreness.[49]

> The important difference between meta-analysis and both the vote counting and the levels of evidence approaches is that meta-analysis focuses on estimates of the *size* of the effect of the intervention, rather than on whether the effect of intervention was statistically significant or not.

[49]At least the meta-analysis permitted a clear conclusion about the effects of the stretching protocols used in the trials that were reviewed, on the types of people who participated in the trials that were reviewed. A limitation of the trials was that they examined the effects of a very small number of sessions of stretching and participants may not have been representative of the majority of people who stretch before or after exercise. These limitations were addressed in a recent randomized trial by Jamtvedt et al (2010).

This is important for two reasons. First, as we have already seen, information about the size of the effects of intervention is critically important for clinical decision-making. Rational clinical decision-making requires information about how much benefit intervention gives, not just information about whether intervention is 'effective' or not. Second, by using estimates of the magnitude of effects of interventions, meta-analysis accrues more information about the effects of intervention than vote counting or the levels of evidence approach. Consequently meta-analysis is much more powerful than either vote counting or the levels of evidence approach. Under some conditions, meta-analysis is statistically optimal. That is, meta-analysis can provide the maximum possible information about the effects of an intervention, so it is less likely than vote counting or the levels of evidence approach to conclude that there is 'not enough evidence' of the effects of intervention if there really is a worthwhile effect of the intervention. For this reason meta-analysis is the strongly preferred method of synthesizing findings of trials in a systematic review.

Why is meta-analysis not used in all systematic reviews? The main reason is that the pooled estimates of effects of intervention provided by meta-analysis are interpretable only when each of the trials is trying to estimate something similar. Meta-analysis is interpretable only when the estimates to be pooled are from trials that measure similar outcomes and apply similar sorts of intervention to similar types of patient. (That is, the trials need to be 'homogeneous' with respect to outcomes, interventions and patients.) The trials need not be identical-they just need to be sufficiently similar for the pooled estimate to be interpretable. However, the practical reality is that when several trials investigate the effects of an intervention they typically recruit participants from quite different sorts of populations, apply interventions in quite different sorts of ways, and use quite different outcome measures (that is, they are typically 'heterogeneous'). Thus, in their systematic review, Ferreira et al (2002) reported that only 11 of 34 trials could be included in meta-analyses 'due primarily to heterogeneity of outcome measures and comparison groups'. In these circumstances it is often difficult for the reader to decide whether it was appropriate or inappropriate statistically to pool the findings of the trials in a meta-analysis. In fact this issue of when it is and is not appropriate to pool estimates of effects of intervention in a meta-analysis is one of the most difficult methodological issues in systematic reviews. Readers of meta-analyses must carefully examine the details of the individual trials to decide whether the pooled estimate is interpretable. The reader needs to ask: 'Is it reasonable to combine estimates of the effect of interventions from these studies?'

One way to deal with heterogeneity is to divide the pool of studies available for meta-analysis into subgroups of trials with common characteristics and analyse each subgroup separately. (The subgroups are usually referred to as 'strata', and this approach is usually called a 'stratified analysis'.) A more sophisticated approach uses specialized regression techniques (collectively known as meta-regression techniques) to model explicitly the sources of heterogeneity. These approaches potentially enable reviewers to provide stratum-specific estimates of the effect of intervention, and they make it possible to examine the effect of various study characteristics (such as the specific way in which the intervention was administered) on the effect of intervention.

An example of a stratified analysis is given in the review of interventions for disabled workers by Tompa et al (2008). This review included trials of a diverse range of interventions, so the analysis was stratified by category of intervention (ergonomics and other education, physiotherapy, behavioural therapy and work/vocational rehabilitation) as well as by features of the interventions (early contact with

worker by the workplace, work accommodation offer, contact between health care provider and workplace, ergonomic work site visits, supernumerary replacements, and return to work coordination). The effects of intervention were reported separately for each stratum.

An example of the use of meta-regression to explore sources of heterogeneity is provided by a review conducted by Sherrington et al (2008). The authors used meta-regression to explore characteristics of falls prevention programmes associated with the effects of the falls risk programmes on the rate or risk of falls. The analysis suggested that the most effective programmes employed a high dose of exercise and challenging balance exercises, but did not include a walking programme. The estimated effect of a programme with all three of these characteristics was that it would reduce the risk of falling (relative risk reduction) by 42% of the risk in people who did not undertake a falls risk programme (95% confidence interval 31% to 52%). Risk reductions of this magnitude might be considered worthwhile by many potential participants in falls risk programmes.

We caution, however, that stratified analyses and meta-regression approaches to modelling heterogeneity are potentially misleading. This is because such analyses share all of the potential problems of subgroup analyses of individual randomized trials (discussed on page 95 and in footnote 1 of this chapter; Herbert & Bø 2005).[50] Thus stratified analyses and meta-regressions, like subgroup analyses of individual randomized trials, are prone to report spurious subgroup effects. Few such analyses are conducted in a way that would minimize the risk of spurious effects. We recommend caution when

---

[50]There are other problems with stratified analyses and meta-regression modeling of heterogeneity. Most meta-regressions produce estimates of the effects of study-level characteristics (for example they may produce estimates of the effect of administering the intervention in a particular way), but these estimates are based on between-study comparisons rather than within-study comparisons. That is, the analysis of these effects involves comparisons of the findings of trials that do and do not administer intervention in a particular way. But such comparisons are of non-randomized alternatives, so, unlike randomized comparisons, they are potentially exposed to serious confounding. It would be far better to estimate the effects of administering intervention in a particular way using randomized trials or meta-analysis of randomized trials in which individual patients are randomized to receive the intervention administered in one way or the other. A related limitation of these analyses is that the characteristic of interest is usually a study-level characteristic yet inference is usually made at the level of individual patients. This may lead to an inferential fallacy known as the 'ecological fallacy' or 'Simpson's paradox' (Robinson 1950).

interpreting findings of systematic reviews that involve stratified analyses or use meta-regression to examine heterogeneity. Ideally such findings are subsequently subject to confirmation in randomized trials designed specifically for that purpose.

These impediments to meta-analysis (insufficient data for meta-analysis, and heterogeneity of participants, interventions or outcomes) may be thought to provide a justification for using vote counting or the levels of evidence approach. But, as we have seen, vote counting and the levels of evidence approach lack statistical power and, at any rate, do not provide useful summaries of the effects of intervention because they do not estimate the size of effects of intervention. And the levels of evidence approach has the additional problem that it is sensitive to the precise definitions of each of the levels of evidence, which are somewhat arbitrary. That is not to say that reviews that employ vote counting or the levels of evidence approach are not useful. Such reviews may still provide the reader with results of a comprehensive literature search and an assessment of quality, and perhaps a detailed description of the trials and their findings. But their conclusions should be regarded with caution.

When meta-analysis is not possible, vote counting and levels of evidence are not a good alternative. So what is? The best information we can get from a systematic review, if meta-analysis is not appropriate or not possible, is a detailed description of each of the trials included in the review. Fortunately, as we have seen, estimates of effects of intervention provided by each trial are usually given in a table or a forest plot, and this information is often complemented by information about the methodological quality of each trial and the details of the patients, interventions and outcomes in each trial.

> So even if meta-analysis has not been conducted, or if it has been conducted inappropriately, we can still get useful information from systematic reviews. The reviews fulfil the very useful role of locating, summarizing and evaluating the quality of relevant trials.

Readers may find the prospect of examining the estimates of individual trials less attractive than being presented with a summary meta-analysis. In effect, the reader is provided with many answers ('the effect on a particular outcome of applying intervention in a particular way to a particular population was X, and the effect on another outcome of applying intervention in another way to another population was Y'),

rather than a simple summary ('the intervention has effect Z'). Also, because the findings of individual studies are not pooled, conclusions must be based on the (usually imprecise, and possibly less credible) estimates of the effects of intervention provided by individual trials. Nonetheless, this is the only truly satisfactory alternative to meta-analysis when meta-analysis is not appropriate or not possible because, unlike vote counting and the levels of evidence approach, the description of estimates of effects of intervention provided by individual trials provides clinically interpretable information.

Typical physiotherapy interventions, such as exercises, are multifaceted; they contain numerous components. Consequently they are sometimes referred to as complex health interventions. The interpretation and implementation of results from systematic reviews of complex interventions presents particular issues. First, there is a problem that interventions are often not sufficiently well described, in reports of trials of complex interventions, to enable the interventions to be replicated in clinical practice. Glasziou and colleagues (2008) assessed the extent of this problem by assessing 80 consecutive studies (55 randomized trials and 25 systematic reviews) selected for abstraction in the journal *Evidence-Based Medicine*. Forty-four of the 80 studies were of drug treatments. Descriptions of elements of the intervention were missing in 41 of 80 of the published reports. Not surprisingly, information was better in reports of individual trials than in systematic reviews, and it was also better for drug treatments than for non-drug treatments. The missing element was most often a description of the content or method of delivery of the intervention. Several initiatives have now been taken to improve the description of interventions in reports of clinical trials and systematic reviews (e.g. Glasziou et al 2010). A recent extension to the CONsolidated Standards of Reporting Trials (CONSORT) statement (available at http://www.consort-statement.org/extensions) recommends that authors of reports of randomized trials provide detailed descriptions of non-pharmacological treatments.

A second problem relates to the fact that the quality of interventions in individual trials is often not considered when results are summarized in systematic reviews. Herbert & Bø (2005) provide an example of how the quality of intervention in individual trials can affect the results (i.e. the pooled estimate of effect) in a systematic review. Four randomized trials of the effects of pelvic floor training to prevent urinary incontinence during pregnancy were identified, of which three presented enough data to permit meta-analysis. The studies were heterogeneous with respect to intervention. Two showed clinically important effects of antenatal training, whereas one study reported clinically trivial effects. In the two trials with positive effects, training was supervised regularly by a physiotherapist, whereas in the study with negative effects women saw the physiotherapist only once. The pooled estimate of effect obtained from a meta-analysis of all three trials did not show a convincing effect of pelvic floor training (odds ratio 0.67, 95% confidence interval 0.39 to 1.16). However, when the large trial of a low-intensity intervention was excluded from the meta-analysis, a clinically worthwhile effect of antenatal training (odds ratio 0.50, 0.34 to 0.75) was found. The largest trial may have reported a smaller effect because of its size. Resource limitations often mean that large trials provide less intensive interventions, and in large trials it may be logistically difficult to provide well-supervised interventions. Yet large trials are most heavily weighted in meta-analyses. If large studies with less intense interventions show smaller effects, they will tend to dilute the effects of smaller studies that show larger effects. Thus, an uncritical synthesis of the data could suggest that the intervention is ineffective, but a more accurate interpretation might be that the intervention is effective only if administered intensively.

To summarize this section, systematic reviews that use vote counting or the levels of evidence approach do not generate useful conclusions about effects of intervention. Moreover, reviews that use these methods may conclude there is insufficient evidence of effects of intervention even when the data say otherwise. Systematic reviews that employ meta-analysis potentially provide better evidence of effects of intervention because meta-analysis involves explicit quantification of effects of interventions, and is statistically optimal. However, meta-analysis is not always possible and, even when meta-analysis is possible, may not be appropriate. When a meta-analysis has been conducted, readers must examine whether the trials pooled in the meta-analysis were sampled from sufficiently similar populations, used sufficiently similar interventions, and measured outcomes in sufficiently similar ways. Where meta-analysis is not appropriate or possible, or has not been done, the best approach is to inspect details of individual trials. In any case, readers should consider how well the intervention was administered in the individual trials.

What does this study of experiences mean for my practice?

It has been said that the strength of the quantitative approach lies in its *reliability* (repeatability), by which is meant that replication of quantitative studies should yield the same results time after time, whereas the strength of qualitative research lies in *validity* (closeness to the truth). That is, good qualitative research can touch what is really going on rather than just skimming the surface (Greenhalgh 2001). Specifically, high-quality interpretive research offers an understanding of roles and relationships. This implies that qualitative research can help physiotherapists better understand the context of their practice and their relationships with patients and their families. But this requires that the research findings be presented clearly, and that the findings are transferable to other settings.

Was there a clear statement of findings?

Are the findings explicit? Is it clear how the researchers arrived at their conclusion?

What do findings from qualitative research look like? The product of a qualitative study is a narrative that tries to represent faithfully and accurately the social world or phenomena being studied (Giacomini et al 2002). The findings may be presented as descriptions or theoretical insights or theories.

The interpretation of findings is closely related to the analytical path. This was discussed in Chapter 5, but we revisit these ideas here. The findings should be presented explicitly and clearly and it should be clear how the researchers arrived at their conclusion. Interpretation is an integral part of qualitative inquiry, and there is an emerging nature of qualitative research in the way that the research alters as the data are collected. In qualitative research, unlike quantitative research, the results cannot be distinguished from the data, so it is not reasonable to expect separation of what the researchers found from what they think it means (Greenhalgh 2001). Consequently, in qualitative research, the results and the discussion are sometimes presented together. If so, it is still important that the data and the interpretation are linked in a logical way. As described in Chapter 5, the analytical path should be clearly described so that readers can follow the way the authors arrived at their conclusions. Triangulation can improve the credibility of the study and strengthen the findings.

The findings of qualitative studies are often grouped into themes, patterns or categories, and may involve the development of hypothesis and theories. This process is carried out from within a theoretical framework. The theoretical framework can be likened to reading glasses that are worn by the researcher when she or he asks questions about the materials (Malterud 2001); the framework influences how the researcher sees the data. A frequent shortcoming of reports of qualitative research is omission of information about the theoretical framework. It may not be clear whether the themes or patterns or categories identified in a qualitative study represent empirical findings or whether they were identified in advance. It is not sufficient for a researcher simply to say that the materials were coded in a way that identified patterns of responses. The reader needs to know the principles and choices underlying pattern recognition and category foundation (Malterud 2001). Hjort and colleagues (1999) describe a two-step process that they used to identify categories of patients with rheumatoid arthritis. The aim of their study was to describe and analyse patients' ideas and perceptions about home exercise and physical activity. Five categories emerged from the first step of open coding and categorization, ending up with three idealized types of people: the action-oriented, the compliant and the resigned. By integrating results such as these into practice, physiotherapists are more likely to be able to identify and understand individual needs, and may be better equipped to collaborate with patients.

The findings of qualitative studies are often supported with quotations. Quotations and stories can be used to illustrate insights gained from the data analysis. One important function of quotations is to demonstrate that the findings are based on data (Greenhalgh 2001). Statements such as 'The participants became aware of their breathing' would be more credible if one or two verbatim quotes from the interviews were reproduced to illustrate them. For example:

> Breathing – it always comes back to breathing. I stop, become aware of how I breathe, and discover again and again that when I start to breathe deeply, my body relaxes. I do this several times a day, especially at work.
>
> (Steen & Haugli 2001)

Quotes and examples should be indexed by the researcher so that they can be traced back to an identifiable participant or setting (Greenhalgh 2001).

It is a challenge to present complex material from qualitative research in a clear, transparent and meaningful way without overloading the reader with details and theories that do not relate directly to the phenomenon that is studied. Still, readers should look for whether the results of a qualitative research report address the way the findings relate to other theories in the field. An empirically developed theory need not agree with existing beliefs (Giacomini et al 2002). But, regardless of whether a new theory agrees with existing beliefs or not, the authors should describe the relationship between the new theory and prevailing theories and beliefs in a critical manner (Giacomini et al 2002).

How valuable is the research?

Does the study contribute to existing knowledge or understanding? Have avenues for further research been identified? Can the findings be transferred to other populations or settings?

The aim of most research, and almost all useful research, is to produce information that can be shared and applied beyond the study setting. No study, irrespective of the method used, can provide findings that are universally transferable. Nonetheless, studies whose findings cannot be generalized to other contexts in some way can have little direct influence on clinical decision-making. Thus, readers should ask whether a study's findings are generalizable. One criterion for the generalizability of a qualitative study is whether it provides a useful 'road map' for the reader to navigate similar social settings.

A common criticism of qualitative research is that the findings of qualitative studies pertain only to the limited setting in which they were obtained. Indeed, it has been argued that issues of generalizability in qualitative research have been paid little attention, at least until quite recently (Schofield 2002). A major factor contributing to disregard of issues of generalizability (or 'external validity'[51]) appears to be a widely shared view that external validity is unimportant, unachievable or both (Schofield 2002). However, several trends, including the growing use of qualitative studies in evaluation and policy-oriented research, have led to an increased awareness of the importance of structuring qualitative research in a way that enhances understanding of other situations. Generalizability can be enhanced by studying the

---

[51] 'External validity' is another term for 'generalizability' or 'applicability' (Campbell & Stanley 1966).

typical, the common and the ordinary, by conducting multisite studies, and by designing studies to fit with future trends (Schofield 2002).

Still, the generalizability of qualitative research is likely to be conceptual rather than numerical. Interpretive research offers clinicians an understanding of roles and relationships, not effect sizes or rates or other quantifiable phenomena. Many studies of interest to clinicians focus on communication among patients, therapists, families and caregivers. Other studies describe behaviours of these groups, either in isolation or during interactions with others (Giacomini et al 2002). A study that explored views held by health professionals and patients about the role of guided self-management plans in asthma care suggested that attempts to introduce such plans in primary care were unlikely to be successful because neither patients nor professionals were enthusiastic about guided self-management plans (Jones et al 2000). Neither health professionals nor patients felt positive towards guided self-management plans, and most patients felt that the plans were largely irrelevant to them. A fundamental mismatch was apparent between the views of professionals and patients on the characteristics of a 'responsible' asthma patient, and on what patients should be doing to control their symptoms. Studies like this provide findings that could, for example, help clinicians to understand why patients with asthma might not 'comply' with treatment plans. This might suggest (but would not prove the effectiveness of) modifications to care processes, and it suggests ways that practice could be made more patient-centred.

What does this study of prognosis mean for my practice?

This section considers how we can interpret good-quality evidence of the prognosis of particular conditions. That evidence may be in the form of a cohort study or a clinical trial, or even a systematic review of prognosis.

Is the study relevant to me and my patient/s?

The first step in interpreting evidence of prognosis is much the same as for studies of the effects of therapy. We need to consider whether the patients in the

study are similar to the patients that we wish to make inferences about, and whether the outcomes are those that are of interest to patients. These issues are very similar to those discussed at length with randomized trials or systematic reviews of the effects of therapy, so we will not elaborate further on them here. Instead we focus on some issues that pertain particularly to interpretation of evidence of prognosis.

When we ask questions about prognosis we could be interested in the natural course of the condition (what happens to people who are untreated) or, instead, we might be interested in the clinical course of the condition (what happens to people treated in the usual way). We can learn about the natural course of the condition from studies that follow untreated cohorts, and we learn about the clinical course of the condition from studies that follow treated cohorts.[52] What clinical value can this information have? How is this information relevant to clinical practice?

Perhaps the most important role of prognostic information is that it can be used to inform patients of what the likely outcome of having a particular condition is likely to be. For some conditions, particularly relatively minor ailments, one of the main reasons that patients seek out professionals is to obtain a clear prognosis. People are naturally curious about what their futures are likely to be, and they often ask about their prognoses. They may seek reassurance that their conditions are not serious, or that the conditions will resolve without intervention. In responding, physiotherapists are required to be fortune tellers. It is best, where possible, that they be evidence-based fortune tellers! We need to be provisioned with good-quality evidence about prognosis for the conditions we often see. Of course, we should not divulge prognoses just because we know what they are. Some patients do not want to know their prognosis, particularly if the prognosis is bleak. It may take a great deal of wisdom to know if, when and how to inform patients of poor prognoses.

Information about the natural history of a condition also tells us whether we should be alarmed about prognosis, and whether we should look for some way to manage the condition. For example, the parents of a young child with talipes valgus (also called pes calcaneovalgus or pes abductus or pes valgus) might be interested in the natural history of the condition

---

[52]Some controlled trials may be able to tell us about both the natural course of the condition (using data from an untreated control group) and the clinical course of the condition (using data from the intervention group).

124

because they want to know whether it is likely to become a persistent problem, or whether it is something that will resolve with time. If the natural course was one of ongoing disability, we might consider investigating interventions that might improve outcomes. But if, as is the case for talipes valgus in very young children, the long-term prognosis is favourable (Widhe et al 1988), then we will probably not consider intervention, and we would probably choose simply to monitor development of the child's foot.

We can extend this idea further. Information about the natural course of a condition sets an upper limit for the benefit that can be provided by intervention. For example, we may learn that the prognosis for a 42-year-old man with primary shoulder dislocation is good: the risk of subsequent re-dislocation is around 6% within 4 years (te Slaa et al 2004). Theoretically, then, the best possible intervention is one that reduces the risk of dislocation by around 6% over 4 years. The implication is that there is little point in considering interventions (such as a long-term exercise programme) to prevent re-subluxation, because, even if the intervention prevented all dislocations (an unrealistically optimistic scenario), the number needed to treat for 10 years would be 11. That is, even in this unrealistically optimistic scenario, the intervention would prevent only 1 subluxation for every 11 patients who exercised for 10 years. Most patients would consider this benefit (an average of 110 years of exercise to prevent one subluxation) insufficient to make the intervention worthwhile. This example illustrates how information about a good prognosis might discourage consideration of intervention.

In a similar vein, prognostic information can be used to supplement decisions about therapy. Early in this chapter we considered whether the effects of particular interventions were big enough to be clinically worthwhile and we used the example of a clinical trial that showed that, in the general population of patients undergoing upper abdominal surgery, prophylactic chest physiotherapy produced substantial reductions in risk of respiratory complications (number needed to treat = 5). Then we noted that the effects would be twice as big (number needed to treat of 2 or 3) in a morbidly obese population at twice the risk of respiratory complications. The information required for these calculations, about the prognosis (risk of respiratory complications) in morbidly obese patients, can be obtained from studies of prognosis. That is, prognostic studies

can be used to scale estimates of the effects of therapy to particular populations.

A particular consideration in studies of prognosis concerns whether the follow-up was sufficiently prolonged to be useful. For some conditions (such as acute respiratory complications of surgery) most of the interest focuses on a short follow-up period (days or weeks), whereas for other conditions (such as cystic fibrosis or Parkinson's disease) the long-term prognosis (prognosis over years or even decades) is of more interest. Readers should ascertain whether follow-up was sufficiently prolonged to capture important prognoses.

What does the evidence say?

What does prognosis look like? Essentially prognoses come in two styles. Prognoses about events (dichotomous outcomes) are expressed in terms of the risk of the event. And prognoses about continuous outcomes are expressed in terms of the expected value of the outcome (usually the mean outcome, but sometimes the median outcome). Usually prognoses have to be associated with a time frame to be useful. Thus we say 'in patients who have undergone ACL [anterior cruciate ligament] reconstruction, the 5 year risk of injury of the contralateral ACL is approximately 11%' (Deehan et al 2000; this is a prognosis about a dichotomous variable) or 'In the 3 months following hemiparetic stroke, hand function recovers, on average, by approximately 2 points on the 6 point Hand Movement Scale' (Katrak et al 1998) this is a prognosis about a continuous variable).

This means that calculating prognosis is straightforward. For dichotomous outcomes we need determine only the proportion of people (that is, the risk of) experiencing the event of interest. And for continuous outcomes we need determine only the mean (or median) outcome. But, although the calculations are straightforward, finding the data can be difficult. Often the prognostic information is contained in studies that were not explicitly designed to measure prognosis. It can require a degree of detective work to snoop out key data that appear incidentally perhaps in among statistical summaries or in the headings to tables.

Sometimes outcome data are presented in the form of survival curves, such as the one illustrated in Figure 6.7. Survival curves are particularly informative because they indicate how the risk of

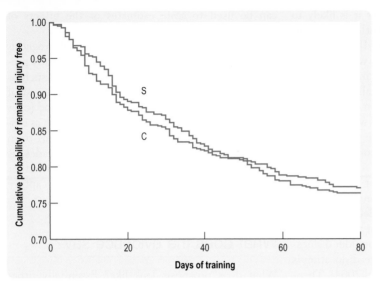

Figure 6.7 • An example of survival curves from a randomized trial of the effects of pre-exercise stretching on risk of injury. The survival curves show the cumulative probability of army recruits in stretch (S) and control groups (C) remaining injury free over the course of a 12-week training programme. Redrawn from Pope et al (2000).

experiencing an event changes with time.[53] The risk for any particular prognostic time frame can be obtained from this curve. Figure 6.7 gives an example of a survival curve that shows the risk of lower-limb musculoskeletal injury in army recruits undergoing military training. As the study was a randomized trial, there are two survival curves: one for each group. However the curves are very similar, so either curve could be used to generate information about risk of injury in army recruits undergoing training. The curves show that risk of injury in the first fortnight is 6% or 8%, and risk of injury in the first 10 weeks is 22% or 23%.

Estimates of prognosis, like estimates of the effects of intervention, are at best only approximations, because they are obtained from finite samples of patients. Earlier in this chapter we considered how to quantify the uncertainty associated with estimates of effects of intervention using confidence intervals. We saw that large studies were associated with relatively narrow confidence intervals. The same applies for estimates of prognosis: large studies provide more certainty about the prognosis.

It may be useful to determine the degree of uncertainty to attach to an estimate of prognosis. This is best done by inspecting the confidence intervals associated with the prognosis. If we are lucky the paper will report confidence intervals for estimates of prognosis, but if not it is a relatively easy matter to calculate the confidence ourselves, at least approximately. Again, there are some simple equations that we can use to obtain approximate confidence intervals for estimates of prognosis. These are given in Box 6.5.

Up to now we have considered how to obtain global prognoses for broadly defined groups. But prognosis often varies hugely from person to person. Some people have characteristics that are likely to make their prognosis much better or much worse than average. For example, the prognosis of return to work in young head-injured adults probably varies enormously with degree of physical and psychological impairment, age, level of education and social support. Ideally, we would use information about prognostic variables such as these to refine the prognosis for any individual.

Many studies aim to identify prognostic variables, and to quantify how prognosis differs across people with and without (or with varying degrees of) the prognostic variables. The simplest approach involves separately reporting prognosis for participants with and without a prognostic factor (or, for continuous variables, for people with low and high levels of the prognostic factor). An example comes from

---

[53] The survival curve is not just the proportion of survivors at any one point in time, because if the probability of surviving were calculated in this way it would be biased by loss to follow-up. Instead, the survival curve is calculated by estimating the survival probability over each successive increment of time, and then obtaining the product of the successive probabilities of surviving each successive time interval.

Box 6.5

Confidence intervals for prognosis

These equations are similar to those we used to generate confidence intervals for estimates of effects of intervention.[54] When outcomes are measured on continuous scales we can calculate the approximate 95% confidence interval for the mean outcome at some point in time:

$$95\% \, CI \approx mean \pm 3 \times SD/\sqrt{2N}$$

where N is the number of participants in the group of interest.

When the outcome is measured on a dichotomous scale we can calculate an approximate 95% confidence interval for the risk of an event within some time period:

$$95\% \, CI \approx risk \pm 1/\sqrt{2N}$$

To illustrate the use of these formulae, consider the study of long-term prognosis of whiplash-associated disorder conducted by Bunketorp et al (2005). These authors followed up patients who had presented to hospital emergency departments with a whiplash injury 17 years earlier.

At 17 years, the mean total score on the 100-point Neck Disability Index was 22 (SD 22, N = 99). This is the expected level of disability in a patient in this population 17 years after injury. The mean score of 22 indicates that on average patients had fairly mild disability. We can calculate an approximate 95% confidence interval for this prognosis:

$$95\% \, CI \approx mean \pm 3 \times SD/\sqrt{2N}$$
$$95\% \, CI \approx 22 \pm (3 \times 22)/\sqrt{2 \times 99}$$
$$95\% \, CI \approx 22 \pm 5$$
$$95\% \, CI \approx 17 \text{ to } 27$$

Thus we expect an average level of disability in this population of between 17 and 27 points on the Neck Disability Index 17 years after whiplash injury.

Fifty-five of 108 participants reported persistent pain related to the initial injury. That is, in this cohort the risk of persistent pain after 17 years was 55/108 or 51%. The 95% confidence interval for this prognosis is:

$$95\% \, CI \approx risk \pm 1/\sqrt{2N}$$
$$95\% \, CI \approx 51\% \pm 1/\sqrt{2 \times 108}$$
$$95\% \, CI \approx 51\% \pm 7\%$$
$$95\% \, CI \approx 44 \text{ to } 58\%$$

We could say that we anticipate a risk of persistent pain of between 44% and 58% at 17 years.

---

the prospective cohort study by Albert et al (2001) of the prognosis of pregnant women with pelvic pain that we examined in Chapter 5. These authors separately reported prognoses for women with each of four syndromes of pelvic pain.

More recent studies tend to use a different and more complex approach. These studies develop multivariate predictive models to ascertain the degree to which prognosis is independently associated with each of a number of prognostic factors. The results are often reported in a table describing the importance and strength of the independent associations with each prognostic factor. Interpretation of the independent associations of prognostic factors is beyond the scope of this book.[55] Suffice it to say that information about the independent associations of prognostic factors with prognosis is potentially important for two reasons. First, this can tell us how much the presence of a particular prognostic factor modifies prognosis. Second, we can potentially generate more precise estimates of prognosis if we take into account the prognostic factor when making the prognosis.

What does this study of the accuracy of a diagnostic test mean for my practice?

In the final section of this chapter we consider the interpretation of high-quality studies of the accuracy of diagnostic tests.

---

[54]The only difference is that, for prognosis of continuous variables, we now need to estimate a confidence interval for the mean of a single group (rather than for the difference in the means of control and experimental groups, as we did for effects of therapy). Likewise for prognosis of dichotomous variables, we now need to estimate a confidence interval for the risk of a single group (rather than for the absolute risk reduction, which is the difference in the risks of control and experimental groups, as we did for effects of therapy). The width of the confidence intervals for estimates of prognosis differ from those used to estimate the size of effects of intervention only in that we use 2N (twice the number of participants in the group of interest) rather than n_{av} (the average number of participants in each group) in the denominator.

[55]Grobbee & Hoes (2009) provide an excellent introduction to the field. A more advanced text is Harrell (2001).

Is the evidence relevant to me and my patient/s?

The interpretation of the relevance of evidence about the accuracy of diagnostic tests is very similar to the interpretation of studies of the effects of therapy and prognosis. Most importantly we need to consider whether the patients in the study are similar to the patients about which we wish to make inferences.

An additional consideration is the skill of the tester. Many of the diagnostic tests used by physiotherapists require manual skill to implement and clinical experience to interpret. When reading studies of diagnostic tests that require skill and experience it is good practice to look for an indication that the test was conducted by people with appropriate levels of training and expertise. This is particularly critical when the test performs poorly; you then want to be satisfied that it was the test, rather than the tester, that was incapable of generating an accurate diagnosis.

Another issue concerns the setting in which the tests were conducted. Tests may perform well in one setting (say, a private practice that sees a broad spectrum of cases) and poorly in other settings (say, a specialist clinic). We will revisit this issue towards the end of this chapter. For now we simply allude to the idea that readers will obtain the best estimates of the accuracy of diagnostic tests from studies conducted in clinical settings similar to their own.

What does the evidence say?[56]

We say that a test is positive when its findings are indicative of the presence of the condition, and we say the test is negative when its findings are indicative of the absence of the condition. However, most tests are imperfect. Thus, even good clinical tests will sometimes be negative when the condition being tested for is present (false negative), or positive when the condition being tested for is absent (false positive). The process of applying and interpreting diagnostic tests is probabilistic – the findings of a test often increase or decrease suspicion of a particular diagnosis but, because most tests are imperfect, it is rare that a single test clearly rules in or rules out a diagnosis. Good diagnostic tests have sufficient accuracy that positive findings greatly increase

suspicion of the diagnosis and negative tests greatly reduce suspicion of the diagnosis.

The most common way of describing the accuracy of diagnostic tests (the concordance of the findings of the test and the reference standard) is in terms of sensitivity and specificity. Sensitivity is the probability that people who truly have the condition, as determined by testing with the reference standard, will test positive. So it is the proportion (or percentage) of people who truly have the condition that test positive. Specificity is the probability that people who do not have the condition (again, as determined by testing with the reference standard) will test negative. So it is the proportion (or percentage) of people who truly do not have the condition that test negative. Clearly, it is desirable that sensitivity and specificity are as high as possible – that is, it is desirable that sensitivity and specificity are close to 100%.

Though widely used, there is a major limitation to the use of sensitivity and specificity as indexes of the accuracy of diagnostic tests (Anonymous 1981). Fundamentally, sensitivity and specificity are quantities that we do not need to know about. Sensitivity tells us the probability that a person who has the condition will test positive. Yet, when we test patients in the course of clinical practice we *know* whether the test was positive or negative so we don't need to know the probability of a positive test occurring. Moreover, we *don't know*, when we apply the test in clinical practice, whether the person actually has the condition. If we did, there would be no point in carrying out the test. There is no practical value in knowing the probability that the test is positive when the condition is present. Instead, we need to know the probability of the person having the condition if the test is positive. There is a similar problem with specificities – we don't need to know the probability of a person testing negative when he or she does not have the condition, but we do need to know the probability of the person having the condition when he or she tests negative.

Likelihood ratios

Likelihood ratios provide an alternative way of describing the accuracy of diagnostic tests (Sackett et al 1985). Importantly likelihood ratios can be used to determine what we really need to know about. With a little numerical jiggery-pokery,

---

[56]This next section has been reproduced with only minor changes from Herbert (2005). We are grateful to the publisher for permission to reproduce this material.

likelihood ratios can be used to determine the probability that a person with a particular test finding has the diagnosis that is being tested for.

The likelihood ratio tells us how much more likely a particular test result is in people who have the condition than it is in people who don't have the condition. As most tests have two outcomes (positive or negative), this means we can talk about two likelihood ratios – one for positive test outcomes (we call this the positive likelihood ratio) and one for negative test outcomes (we call this the negative likelihood ratio).

The positive likelihood ratio tells us how much more likely a positive test finding is in people who have the condition than it is in those who don't. Obviously it is desirable for tests to be positive more often in people who have the condition than in those who don't, so consequently it is desirable to have positive likelihood ratios with values greater than 1. In practice, positive likelihood ratios with values greater than about 3 may be useful, and positive likelihood ratios with values greater than 10 are typically very useful.

The negative likelihood ratio tells us how much more likely a negative test finding is in people who have the condition than those who don't. This means that it is desirable for tests to have negative likelihood ratios of less than 1. The smallest value negative likelihood ratios can have is zero. In practice, tests with negative likelihood ratios with values less than about one-third (0.33) may be useful, and tests with negative likelihood ratios of less than about one-tenth (0.10) are typically very useful.

Many studies of diagnostic tests report only the sensitivity or the specificity of the tests, but not likelihood ratios. Fortunately it is an easy matter to calculate likelihood ratios from sensitivity and specificity:

$$LR+ = sensitivity/(100 - specificity)$$
$$LR- = (100 - sensitivity)/specificity$$

where $LR+$ is the positive likelihood ratio and $LR-$ is the negative likelihood ratio, and sensitivity and specificity are given as percentages.[57,58] Therefore, if sensitivity is 90% and specificity is 80%, the positive likelihood ratio is $90/(100 - 80) = 4.5$ and the negative likelihood ratio is $(100 - 90)/80 = 0.125$.

Likelihood ratios provide more relevant information than sensitivities and specificities. So it is a worthwhile practice, when reading papers of the accuracy of diagnostic tests, routinely to calculate likelihood ratios (even if only roughly, in your head) and to note

them in the margins. The likelihood ratios are what you should try to remember because they provide the most useful summary of a test's accuracy.[59]

Using likelihood ratios to calculate the probability that a person has a particular diagnosis

From the moment a person presents for a physiotherapy consultation most physiotherapists will begin to make guesses about the probable diagnosis. For example, a young adult male may attend physiotherapy and begin to describe an injury incurred the previous weekend. Even before he describes the injury, his physiotherapist may have arrived at a provisional diagnosis. It may be obvious from the way in which the patient walks into the room that he has an injury of the ankle. Most commonly, injuries to the ankle are ankle sprains or ankle fractures. But it is rare that someone can walk soon after an ankle fracture, so the physiotherapist's suspicion is naturally directed towards an ankle sprain. And most ankle sprains are sprains of the lateral ligaments. So the physiotherapist may guess, even before talking to the patient, that the injury is a lateral ankle sprain. This simple scenario provides an important insight into the process of diagnosis: physiotherapists usually develop hypotheses about the likely diagnosis very early in the examination. Thereafter, most of the examination is directed towards confirming or refuting those diagnoses. Additional pieces of information are accrued with the aim of proving or disproving the diagnosis. Thus we can think of the examination as a process of progressive refinement of the probability of a diagnosis.

> The real value of likelihood ratios is that they tell us *how much* to change our estimates of the probability of a diagnosis on the basis of a particular test's finding.[60]

If we want to use likelihood ratios to refine our estimates of the probability of a diagnosis, we need first to be able to quantify probabilities. Probabilities can lie on a scale from 0 (no possibility) to 1 (definite) or, more conveniently, on a scale of 0% to 100%. Consider the following case scenarios:

---

[57]Alternatively, if sensitivity and specificity are calculated as proportions, you can insert 1 instead of 100 in the equations.

[58]The use of likelihood ratios extends easily to tests that have more than two categories of outcome. (A common example is tests whose outcomes are given as positive, uncertain or negative.) In that case there is a likelihood ratio for each possible test outcome.

[59]If you find it too hard to remember the numerical value of likelihood ratios, try to commit to memory a qualitative impression of the accuracy of the test: are the likelihood ratios such that the test is weakly discriminative, or moderately discriminative, or highly discriminative?

[60]More generally, likelihood ratios tell us about *strength of evidence*, or the degree to which the evidence favours one hypothesis over another. This is the basis of the likelihood approach to statistical inference (Royall 1997).

Case 1: A 23-year-old man reports that 3 weeks ago he twisted his knee during an awkward tackle while playing football. Although he experienced only moderate pain at the time, the knee swelled immediately. In the 3 weeks since the injury, the swelling has only partly subsided. The knee feels unstable and there have been several occasions of giving way.

Given this meagre history, what probability would you assign to the diagnosis of a torn anterior cruciate ligament? Most physiotherapists would assign a high probability, perhaps between 70% and 90%, implying that most patients presenting like this are subsequently found to have a tear of the anterior cruciate ligament. For now, let us assign a probability of 80%. Because we have not yet formally tested the hypothesis that this patient has a torn anterior cruciate ligament, we will call this the *pre-test* probability (Sox et al 1988). That is, we estimate that the pre-test probability this patient has a torn anterior cruciate ligament is 80%.

It appears likely that this patient has a torn anterior cruciate ligament, but the diagnosis is not yet sufficiently likely that we can act as though that diagnosis is certain. The usual course of action would be to test this diagnostic hypothesis, probably with an anterior drawer test, or Lachman's test, or the pivot shift test (Magee 2002). Clearly, if these tests are positive we should be more inclined to believe the diagnosis of anterior cruciate ligament tear, and if the tests are negative we should be less inclined to believe that diagnosis. The question is, if the test is positive *how much* more inclined should we be to believe the diagnosis? And if the test is negative *how much* less inclined should we be to believe the diagnosis? Likelihood ratios provide a measure of how much more or how much less we should believe a particular diagnosis on the basis of particular test findings (Go 1998).

A recent systematic review of diagnostic tests for injuries of the knee (Solomon et al 2001) concluded that the positive likelihood ratio for the anterior drawer test was 3.8 (this is higher than 1, which is necessary for the test to be of any use at all, and high enough to make it marginally diagnostically useful). The negative likelihood ratio was 0.3 (this is less than 1, which is necessary for the test to be of any use, and low enough to be marginally useful).

Now we need to combine three pieces of information: our estimate of the pre-test probability; our test finding (whether or not the test was positive); and information about the diagnostic accuracy of the test (the positive or negative likelihood ratio, depending upon whether the test was positive). The easiest way to combine these three pieces of

Figure 6.8 • Example of a likelihood ratio nomogram. Reproduced with permission from Davidson (2002), after Fagan (1975).

information is with a likelihood ratio nomogram, such as that in Figure 6.8, reproduced from Davidson (2002), after Fagan (1975). The nomogram contains three columns. Reading from left to right, the first is the pre-test probability, the second is the likelihood ratio for the test, and the third is what we want to know: the probability that the person has the diagnosis (the 'post-test probability'). All we need do is draw a line from the point on the first column that is our estimate of the pre-test probability. The line should pass through the second column at the likelihood ratio for the test (we use the positive likelihood ratio if the test was positive and the negative likelihood ratio if the test was negative). When we extrapolate the line to the right-most column, it intersects that column at the post-test probability. What we have done is to estimate the probability that the person has the condition on the basis of our estimate of the pre-test probability the test result (positive or negative), and what we know about the properties of the test (expressed in terms of its likelihood ratios). By using the nomogram we have used mathematical rules to combine these three pieces of information.[61]

Returning to our example, we find that the young man with the suspected anterior cruciate ligament tear tests positive with the anterior drawer test. Using the nomogram we can estimate a revised (post-test) probability of anterior cruciate ligament lesion given the positive test finding. The post-test probability is 94%. (Try using the nomogram yourself and see whether you get approximately this answer.) If the test had been negative, we would have used the negative likelihood ratio in the nomogram and would have concluded that this man's post-test probability of having an anterior cruciate ligament tear was 55%.

This illustrates a central concept in diagnosis:

> The proper interpretation of a diagnostic test can be made only after consideration of pre-test probabilities.

Theoretically, these pre-test probabilities could be 'evidence based'.[62] However, good evidence of pre-test probabilities is rarely available. More often pre-test probabilities are based on clinical intuition and experience – the physiotherapist estimates the pre-test probability based on the proportion of people with such a presentation who, in his or her experience, have subsequently been found to have this diagnosis. Thus *rational* diagnosis is inherently *subjective* and *experience based*.

Some physiotherapists feel suspicious about the inherent subjectivity of this approach to diagnosis. Subjectivity, where it produces variation in practice, is probably undesirable. However, the alternatives (such as ignoring what intuition says about pre-test probabilities and making uniform assumptions about pre-test probabilities such as 'all pre-test probabilities are 50%') are likely to produce much less accurate diagnoses. So, for the foreseeable future, it

seems sensible to retain the subjective elements of rational diagnosis; the process of diagnosis will remain as much an art as a science.

Viewed in this way, the process of diagnosis is one in which intuition-based estimates of the probability of a diagnosis are replaced with progressively more objective estimates based on test findings. Indeed, if, after conducting a test, the diagnosis remains uncertain (that is, if the post-test probability is still neither very high nor very low), the post-test probability can be used as a refined estimate of the next pre-test probability. Sequential testing can proceed in this way, the post-test probability of one test becoming the pre-test probability of the next test, until the post-test probability becomes very high or very low and the diagnosis is confirmed or rejected. The diagnosis is confirmed once the post-test probability has become very high. Alternatively, the diagnosis is rejected once the post-test probability has become very low.

A consequence is that a given test finding should be interpreted quite differently when applied to different people, because different people will present with different pre-test probabilities. To illustrate this point, consider a second case.

> Case 2: A 32-year-old netball player reports that she twisted her knee in a game 3 weeks ago. At the time her knee locked and she was unable to straighten it fully. She does not recall significant swelling, and reports no instability. However, in the 3 weeks since her injury there have been several occasions when the knee locked again. Between locking episodes the knee appears to have functioned near normally.

This is not a classical presentation of an anterior cruciate ligament lesion. A more likely explanation of this woman's knee symptoms is that she has a meniscal tear. We might estimate the pre-test probability of an anterior cruciate ligament lesion for this woman to be 15%. If she tests positive to the anterior drawer test, we would obtain a post-test probability of 40%. (Try it and see whether you get the same answer.) In other words, after conducting the anterior drawer test we would conclude there is a 60% probability (100% − 40%) that she does *not* have an anterior cruciate ligament lesion, even though she tested positive to the anterior drawer test. This illustrates that a positive anterior drawer test should be considered to be much less indicative of an anterior cruciate ligament lesion when the pre-test probability is low. Perhaps that is not clever statistics, just common sense!

---

[61]The nomogram allows us to bypass some maths. But the maths is pretty easy: the post-test odds of the diagnosis is simply the pre-test odds multiplied by the likelihood ratio. An important assumption underlying this approach (the use of both the nomogram and the equation) is that likelihood ratios remain constant across pre-test probabilities.

[62]For example, pre-test probabilities could be based on epidemiological data about the prevalence of the condition being tested for in the population to whom the test is applied. The prevalence, or the proportion of people in this population who have the condition, provides us with an empirical estimate of the pre-test probability of having the condition.

If we had used a more accurate test (of which Lachman's test may be an example – one study estimated that its positive likelihood ratio was 42; Solomon et al 2001), we should have expected further to modify our estimates of the probability of the diagnosis. With a positive likelihood ratio of 42 and pre-test probability of 15%, a positive Lachman test gives a post-test probability of 88%. This illustrates simply that discriminative tests (those with high positive likelihood ratios or low negative likelihood ratios) should influence the diagnosis more than tests with low discrimination.

References

Ada, L., Foongchomcheay, A., 2002. Efficacy of electrical stimulation in preventing or reducing subluxation of the shoulder after stroke: a meta-analysis. Aust. J. Physiother. 48, 257–267.

Albert, H., Godskesen, M., Westergaard, J., 2001. Prognosis in four syndromes of pregnancy-related pelvic pain. Acta Obstetrica et Gynecologica Scandinavica 80, 505–510.

Altman, D.G., 1998. Confidence intervals for the number needed to treat. BMJ 317, 1309–1312.

Anonymous, 1981. How to read clinical journals: II. To learn about a diagnostic test. Can. Med. Assoc. J. 124, 703–710.

Armitage, P., Berry, G., 1994. Statistical methods in medical research, third ed. Blackwell, Oxford.

Barnett, V., 1982. Comparative statistical inference. Wiley, New York.

Barrett, B., Brown, D., Mundt, M., et al., 2005a. Sufficiently important difference: expanding the framework of clinical significance. Med. Decis. Making 25, 250–261.

Barrett, B., Brown, R., Mundt, M., et al., 2005b. Using benefit harm tradeoffs to estimate sufficiently important difference: the case of the common cold. Med. Decis. Making 25, 47–55.

Barrett, B., Harahan, B., Brown, D., et al., 2007. Sufficiently Important difference for common cold: Severity reduction. Ann. Fam. Med. 5, 216–223.

Berghmans, L.C., Hendriks, H.J., Bo, K., et al., 1998. Conservative treatment of stress urinary incontinence in women: a systematic review of randomized clinical trials. Br. J. Urol. 82, 181–191.

Blinman, P., Duric, V., Nowak, A.K., et al., 2010. Adjuvant chemotherapy for early colon cancer: what survival benefits make it worthwhile? Eur. J. Cancer 46, 1800–1807.

Brookes, S.T., Whitely, E., Egger, M., et al., 2004. Subgroup analyses in randomized trials: risks of subgroup-specific analyses; power and sample size for the interaction test. J. Clin. Epidemiol. 57, 229–236.

Bunketorp, L., Stener-Victorin, E., Carlsson, J., 2005. Neck pain and disability following motor vehicle accidents – a cohort study. Eur. Spine J. 14, 84–89.

Cambach, W., Chadwick-Straver, R.V., Wagenaar, R.C., et al., 1997. The effects of a community-based pulmonary rehabilitation programme on exercise tolerance and quality of life: a randomized controlled trial. Eur. Respir. J. 10, 104–113.

Campbell, D.T., Stanley, J.C., 1966. Experimental and quasi-experimental designs for research. Rand McNally, Chicago.

Cates, C., 2003. Dr Chris Cates' EBM web site. Visual Rx, version 1.7 (software). Online. Available: http://www.nntonline.net 8 Nov 2010.

Cohen, J., 1988. Statistical power analysis for the behavioral sciences. Erlbaum, Hillsdale, NJ.

Counsell, C.E., Clarke, M.J., Slattery, J., et al., 1994. The miracle of DICE therapy for acute stroke: fact or fictional product of subgroup analysis? BMJ 309, 1677–1681.

Davidson, M., 2002. The interpretation of diagnostic tests: a primer for physiotherapists. Aust. J. Physiother. 48, 227–233.

Deehan, D.J., Salmon, L.J., Webb, V.J., et al., 2000. Endoscopic reconstruction of the anterior cruciate ligament with an ipsilateral patellar tendon autograft. A prospective longitudinal five-year study. J. Bone Joint Surg. Br. 82, 984–991.

Deeks, J.J., Altman, D.G., 2001. Effect measures for meta-analysis of trials with binary outcomes. In: Egger, M., Davey Smith, G., Altman, D.G.

(Eds.), Systematic reviews in health care: meta-analysis in context. BMJ Books, London, pp. 313–335.

de Gruttola, V.G., Clax, P., DeMets, D.L., et al., 2001. Considerations in the evaluation of surrogate endpoints in clinical trials: summary of a National Institutes of Health workshop. Control. Clin. Trials 22, 485–502.

Dini, D., Del Mastro, L., Gozza, A., et al., 1998. The role of pneumatic compression in the treatment of postmastectomy lymphedema. A randomized phase III study. Ann. Oncol. 9, 187–190.

Duric, V., Stockler, M., 2001. Patients' preferences for adjuvant chemotherapy in early breast cancer: a review of what makes it worthwhile. Lancet Oncol. 2, 691–697.

Echt, D.S., Liebson, P.R., Mitchell, L.B., et al., 1991. Mortality and morbidity in patients receiving encainide, flecainide, or placebo. The Cardiac Arrhythmia Suppression Trial. N. Engl. J. Med. 324, 781–788.

Efron, B., Tibshirani, R.J., 1993. An introduction to the bootstrap. Chapman & Hall, New York.

Fagan, T.J., 1975. Nomogram for Bayes theorem. N. Engl. J. Med. 293, 257.

Ferreira, M.L., Herbert, R.D., 2008. What does 'clinically important' really mean? Aust. J. Physiother. 54, 229–230.

Ferreira, P.H., Ferreira, M.L., Maher, C.G., et al., 2002. Effect of applying different "levels of evidence" criteria on conclusions of Cochrane reviews of interventions for low back pain. J. Clin. Epidemiol. 55, 1126–1129.

Ferreira, M.L., Ferreira, P.H., Herbert, R.D., et al., 2009. People with low back pain typically need to feel 'much better' to consider intervention worthwhile: an observational study. Aust. J. Physiother. 55, 123–127.

Flynn, T., Fritz, J., Whitman, J., et al., 2002. A clinical prediction rule for classifying patients with low back pain who demonstrate short-term improvement with spinal manipulation. Spine 27, 2835–2843.

Furukawa, T.A., Guyatt, G.H., Griffith, L.E., 2002. Can we individualize the 'number needed to treat'? An empirical study of summary effect measures in meta-analyses. Int. J. Epidemiol. 31, 72–76.

Gardner, M.J., Altman, D.G., 1989. Statistics with confidence. Confidence intervals and statistical guidelines. BMJ Books, London.

Giacomini, M., Cook, D., Guyatt, G., 2002. Qualitative research. In: Guyatt, G., Rennie, D., the Evidence-based Medicine Working Group, (Eds.), Users' guide to the medical literature. A manual for evidence-based clinical practice. American Medical Association, Chicago.

Gigerenzer, G., Swijtink, Z., Porter, T., et al., 1989. The empire of chance: how probability changed science and everyday life. Cambridge University Press, New York.

Glasziou, P.P., Irwig, L.M., 1995. An evidence based approach to individualising treatment. BMJ 311, 1356–1359.

Glasziou, P., Meats, E., Heneghan, C., et al., 2008. What is missing from descriptions of treatment in trials and reviews? BMJ 336, 1472–1474.

Glasziou, P., Chalmers, I., Altman, D., et al., 2010. Taking healthcare interventions from trial to practice. BMJ 341, c3852.

Go, A.S., 1998. Refining probability: an introduction to the use of diagnostic tests. In: Friedland, D.J., Go, A.S., Davoren, J.B., et al. (Eds.), Evidence-based medicine. A framework for clinical practice. Lange/McGraw-Hill, New York, pp. 11–33.

GRADE Working Group, 2004. Grading the quality of evidence and the strength of recommendations. BMJ 328, 1490.

Greenhalgh, T., 2001. How to read a paper. BMJ Books, London.

Grobbee, D.E., Hoes, A.W., 2009. Clinical epidemiology: principles, methods, and applications for clinical research. Jones & Bartlett, Sudbury.

Guyatt, G.H., Berman, L.B., Townsend, M., et al., 1987. A measure of quality of life for clinical trials in chronic lung disease. Thorax 42, 773–778.

Guyatt, G.H., Feeny, D.H., Patrick, D.L., 1993. Measuring health-related quality of life. Ann. Intern. Med. 118, 622–629.

Guyatt, G.H., Sackett, D.L., Cook, D.J., 1994. Users' guides to the medical literature. II. How to use an article about therapy or prevention. B. What were the results and will they help me in caring for my patients? JAMA 271, 59–63.

Hancock, M., Herbert, R.D., Maher, C., 2009. A guide to interpretation of studies investigating subgroups of responders to physical therapy interventions. Phys. Ther. 89, 698–704.

Harrell, F.E., 2001. Regression modeling strategies: with applications to linear models, logistic regression, and survival analysis. Springer, New York.

Hedges, L.V., Olkin, I., 1980. Vote-counting methods in research synthesis. Psychol. Bull. 88, 359–369.

Hedges, L.V., Olkin, I., 1985. Statistical methods for meta-analysis. Academic Press, Orlando.

Herbert, R.D., 2000a. How to estimate treatment effects from reports of clinical trials. I: Continuous outcomes. Aust. J. Physiother. 46, 229–235.

Herbert, R.D., 2000b. How to estimate treatment effects from reports of clinical trials. II: Dichotomous outcomes. Aust. J. Physiother. 46, 309–313.

Herbert, R.D., 2005. The accuracy of diagnostic tests. In: Gass, E., Refshauge, K. (Eds.), Musculoskeletal physiotherapy: clinical science and evidence-based practice. Butterworth-Heinemann, London, pp. 109–113.

Herbert, R.D., Bø, K., 2005. Analysis of quality of interventions in systematic reviews. BMJ 331, 507–509.

Herbert, R.D., Gabriel, M., 2002. Effects of pre- and post-exercise stretching on muscle soreness, risk of injury and athletic performance: a systematic review. BMJ 325, 468–472.

Hjort, I., Lundberg, E., Ekegård, H., et al., 1999. Motivation for home exercise in patients with rheumatoid arthritis. Nordisk Fysioterapi 3, 31–37.

Jamtvedt, G., Herbert, R.D., Flottorp, S., et al., 2010. A pragmatic randomised trial of stretching before and after physical activity to prevent injury and soreness. Br. J. Sports Med. 44, 1002–1009.

Jones, A., Pill, R., Adams, S., 2000. Qualitative study of views of health professionals and patients on guided self management plans for asthma. BMJ 321, 1507–1510.

Jull, G., 2002. Use of high and low velocity cervical manipulative therapy procedures by Australian manipulative physiotherapists. Aust. J. Physiother. 48, 189–193.

Katrak, P., Bowring, G., Conroy, P., et al., 1998. Predicting upper limb recovery after stroke: the place of early shoulder and hand movement. Arch. Phys. Med. Rehabil. 79, 758–761.

Laakso, E.L., Robertson, V.J., Chipchase, L.S., 2002. The place of electrophysical agents in Australian and New Zealand entry-level curricula: is there evidence for their inclusion? Aust. J. Physiother. 48, 251–254.

Lauritzen, J.B., Petersen, M.M., Lund, B., 1993. Effect of external hip protectors on hip fractures. Lancet 341, 11–13.

Lilford, R., Royston, G., 1998. Decision analysis in the selection, design and application of clinical and health services research. J. Health Serv. Res. Policy 3, 159–166.

Linton, S.J., van Tulder, M.W., 2001. Preventive interventions for back and neck pain problems: what is the evidence? Spine 26, 778–787.

Lotters, F., van Tol, B., Kwakkel, G., et al., 2002. Effects of controlled inspiratory muscle training in patients with COPD: a meta-analysis. Eur. Respir. J. 20, 570–576.

McAlister, F.A., Straus, S.E., Guyatt, G.H., et al., 2000. Users' guides to the medical literature: XX. Integrating research evidence with the care of the individual patient. JAMA 283, 2829–2836.

McDonagh, M.J.N., Davies, C.T.M., 1984. Adaptive response to mammalian skeletal muscle to exercise with high loads. Eur. J. Appl. Physiol. 52, 139–155.

McIlwaine, P.M., Wong, L.T., Peacock, D., et al., 2001. Long-term comparative trial of positive expiratory pressure versus oscillating positive expiratory pressure (flutter) physiotherapy in the treatment of cystic fibrosis. J. Pediatr. 138, 845–850.

Magee, D., 2002. Orthopedic physical assessment. Saunders, Philadelphia.

Malterud, K., 2001. Qualitative research: standards, challenges, and guidelines. Lancet 358, 483–489.

Meyer, K., Steiner, R., Lastayo, P., et al., 2003. Eccentric exercise in coronary patients: central hemodynamic and metabolic responses. Med. Sci. Sports Exerc. 35, 1076–1082.

Moseley, A.M., Stark, A., Cameron, I.D., et al., 2005. Treadmill training and body weight support for walking after stroke. In: The Cochrane Library, Issue 4. Wiley, Chichester.

Moyé, L.A., 2000. Statistical reasoning in medicine: the intuitive p-value primer. Springer, New York.

Nickerson, R.S., 2000. Null hypothesis significance testing: a review of an old and continuing controversy. Psychol. Methods 5, 241–301.

Olsen, M.F., Hahn, I., Nordgren, S., et al., 1997. Randomized controlled trial of prophylactic chest physiotherapy in major abdominal surgery. Br. J. Surg. 84, 1535–1538.

O'Sullivan, P.B., Twomey, L.T., Allison, G.T., 1997. Evaluation of specific stabilizing exercise in the treatment of chronic low back pain with radiologic diagnosis of spondylolysis or spondylolisthesis. Spine 22, 2959–2967.

Outpatient Service Trialists, 2004. Therapy-based rehabilitation services for stroke patients at home. In: The Cochrane Library, Issue 3. Wiley, Chichester.

Pope, R., Herbert, R.D., Kirwan, J., 2000. Effects of pre-exercise stretching on risk of injury in army recruits: a randomized trial. Med. Sci. Sports Exerc. 32, 271–277.

Robinson, W.S., 1950. Ecological correlations and the behaviour of individuals. Am. Sociol. Rev. 15, 351–357.

Rothman, K.J., Greenland, S., 1998. Modern epidemiology. Williams & Wilkins, Philadelphia.

Royall, R.M., 1997. Statistical evidence: a likelihood paradigm. Chapman & Hall, New York.

Sackett, D.L., Haynes, R.B., Tugwell, P., 1985. Clinical epidemiology: a basic science for clinical medicine. Little, Brown, Boston.

Sackett, D.L., Straus, S.E., Richardson, W.S., et al., 2000. Evidence-based medicine. How to practice and teach EBM, second ed. Churchill Livingstone, Edinburgh.

Sand, P.K., Richardson, D.A., Staskin, D.R., et al., 1995. Pelvic floor electrical stimulation in the treatment of genuine stress incontinence: a multicenter, placebo-controlled trial. Am. J. Obstet. Gynecol. 173, 72–79.

Schmid, C.H., Lau, J., McIntosh, M.W., 1998. An empirical study of the effect of control rate as a predictor of treatment efficacy in meta-analysis of clinical trials. Stat. Med. 17, 1923–1942.

Schofield, J.W., 2002. Increasing the generalisability of qualitative research. In: Huberman, A.M., Miles, M.B. (Eds.), The qualitative researcher's companion. Sage, Thousand Oaks, CA.

Second International Study of Infarct Survival Collaborative Group, 1988. Randomised trial of intravenous streptokinase, oral aspirin, both, or neither among 17187 cases of suspected acute myocardial infarction: ISIS-2. Lancet 2, 349–360.

Sherrington, C., Lord, S.R., Herbert, R.D., 2004. A randomized controlled trial of weight-bearing versus non-weight-bearing exercise for improving physical ability after hip fracture and completion of usual care. Arch. Phys. Med. Rehabil. 85, 710–716.

Sherrington, C., Whitney, J.C., Lord, S.R., et al., 2008. Effective exercise for the prevention of falls – a systematic review and meta-analysis. J. Am. Geriatr. Soc. 56, 2234–2243.

Simes, R.J., Coates, A.S., 2001. Patient preferences for adjuvant chemotherapy of early breast cancer: how much benefit is needed? J. Natl. Cancer Inst. Monogr. 30, 146–152.

Solomon, D.H., Simel, D.L., Bates, D.W., et al., 2001. Does this patient have a torn meniscus or ligament of the knee? Value of the physical examination. JAMA 286, 1610–1620.

Sox, H.C., Blatt, M.A., Higgins, M.C., et al., 1988. Medical decision making, second ed. Butterworths, Stoneham, MA.

Steen, E., Haugli, L., 2001. From pain to self-awareness: a qualitative analysis of the significance of group participation for persons with chronic musculoskeletal pain. Patient Educ. Couns. 42, 35–46.

Straus, S.E., Sackett, D.L., 1999. Applying evidence to the individual patient. Ann. Oncol. 10, 29–32.

te Slaa, R.L., Wijffels, M.P., Brand, R., et al., 2004. The prognosis following acute primary glenohumeral dislocation. J. Bone Joint Surg. Br. 86, 58–64.

Tijhuis, G.J., de Jong, Z., Zwinderman, A.H., et al., 2001. The validity of the Rheumatoid Arthritis Quality of Life (RAQoL) questionnaire. Rheumatology 40, 1112–1119.

Tompa, E., de Oliveira, C., Dolinschi, R., Irvin, E., 2008. A systematic review of disability management interventions with economic evaluations. J. Occup. Rehabil. 18, 16–26.

van der Windt, D.A.W.M., van der Heijden, G.J.M.G., van den Berg, S.G.M., et al., 2004. Ultrasound therapy for acute ankle sprains. In: The Cochrane Library, Issue 3. Wiley, Chichester.

van Poppel, M.N., Koes, B.W., Smid, T., et al., 1997. A systematic review of controlled clinical trials on the prevention of back pain in industry. Occup. Environ. Med. 54, 841–847.

Widhe, T., Aaro, S., Elmstedt, E., 1988. Foot deformities in the newborn: incidence and prognosis. Acta Orthop. Scand. 59, 176–179.

Yelland, M.J., Schluter, P.J., 2006. Defining worthwhile and desired responses to treatment of chronic low back pain. Pain Med. 7, 38–45.

Yusuf, S., Wittes, J., Probstfield, J., et al., 1991. Analysis and interpretation of treatment effects in subgroups of patients in randomised clinical trials. JAMA 266, 93–98.

Clinical guidelines as a resource for evidence-based physiotherapy

7

CHAPTER CONTENTS

Overview 135
What are clinical guidelines? 135
History of clinical guidelines and why
they are important 136
Where can I find clinical guidelines? 137
How do I know if I can trust the
recommendations in a clinical guideline? . . 138
Who developed the guideline? 138
How were the recommendations
developed? 140
References 141

OVERVIEW

This chapter describes what clinical guidelines are and why they are important in current health care. The chapter identifies databases where clinical guidelines can be found and discusses how to assess the quality and trustworthiness of a clinical guideline. It highlights the importance of patient involvement in guideline development and introduces the concepts of quality of evidence and strength of recommendations.

What are clinical guidelines?

Many clinical problems are complex and require the synthesis of findings from several kinds of research. Management of a particular patient's condition may require information about diagnosis, prognosis, effects of therapy and attitudes. It is time-consuming to explore the evidence relating to each aspect of the management of each clinical problem separately.

Clinical guidelines provide an efficient alternative. They provide a single source of information about the management of clinical conditions. Evidence-based clinical guidelines integrate high-quality clinical research with contributions from clinical experts and patients, in order to formulate reliable recommendations for practice. Where there are practice issues relevant to the guideline topic for which there is little or no evidence, a rigorous and systematic process is used to reach consensus about best practice.

> The purpose of a clinical guideline is to provide a ready-made resource of high-quality information for both practitioner and patient, so they can discuss together the different options for treatment and the different degrees of benefit or risk that interventions may have for that patient. A shared and informed decision can then be made about how to proceed with treatment.

Field and Lohr's description of clinical guidelines (Institute of Medicine 1992) has stood the test of time. It is now an internationally accepted definition (p 27):

> Clinical guidelines are systematically developed statements to assist practitioner and patient decisions about appropriate health care for specific circumstances.

In Chapter 3 we saw that systematic reviews provide a way of synthesizing evidence. There are some similarities between systematic reviews and clinical guidelines. At the heart of both is a comprehensive, rigorous review of high-quality clinical research. However, there are also a number of differences. A summary of these is presented in Table 7.1.

Table 7.1 Differences between systematic reviews and clinical guidelines

Systematic review	Clinical guideline
Focus is likely to be on a single clinical question, or a limited aspect of patient care	Usually covers the whole process of disease management, with many clinical questions, so may require a number of systematic reviews
Likely to be developed by a small group of researchers	Developed by a wide range of stakeholders: patients, clinical experts, researchers, professional groups
Conclusions of the review are based on results from high-quality clinical research alone	Conclusions (recommendations) are based on a complex synthesis of high-quality clinical research, but also expert opinion, patient experience and consensus views
Patients have a limited role or no role in production of the review. Rarely, patients may be involved in framing review question(s) and helping with the assessment and interpretation of evidence	Patients have a key role in production of the guidelines. They may participate in framing of questions, interpretation of evidence and, with the rest of the guideline development group, making judgements about information from patients and health care practitioners
Validity of conclusions depends on methodological rigour	Validity of conclusions (recommendations) depends on methodological rigour and judgements made by guideline development group
Can be developed relatively quickly (evidence can be very current)	Takes a longer time to develop (risk of evidence being out of date at time of publication)
Typically published as a technical report for health professionals	Patient versions often produced, in addition to a publication for health professionals

Some people are concerned that clinical guidelines, because they include recommendations for practice, become recipes for health care that take away the individual practitioner's autonomy to make his or her own decisions about treatment. But clinical guidelines are not there to be implemented slavishly without thought being given to the implications of the recommendations for individual patients. It may be that the patient has a co-morbidity or a social situation that means that the recommendations are not applicable *in those circumstances*, or that, even though the patient is aware of the evidence described in the guideline, his or her preference is for a different approach or specific treatment. It is a patient's right to make such decisions, and it is the physiotherapist's responsibility to facilitate those decisions by providing relevant, accurate and accessible information. However, if a recommendation in a guideline is based on high-quality evidence, it may reasonably be expected that the recommendations should be implemented unless there is a patient-related reason not to do so. So, although the implementation of clinical guidelines is not mandatory, a decision not to implement guideline recommendations ought to be justified.

History of clinical guidelines and why they are important

Since the early 1990s, more and more has been written about what clinical guidelines are, and how they should be developed. There are a number of reasons why they have become popular. The introduction of the notion of 'evidence-based' clinical guidelines links closely to the development of evidence-based medicine and evidence-based practice, described in Chapter 1. This led to a greater awareness of the importance of utilizing the results of high-quality clinical research in practice. Also, the exponential increase in the volume of published literature means that it is increasingly difficult to keep up to date with new research. Clinical guidelines, which provide summaries of high-quality clinical research, patient views and clinical expertise, provide a more manageable resource for busy practitioners.

In some countries, such as the UK, there have been calls from the government and from the general public for more consistency in the provision of health care for any particular condition or clinical problem. The goal is to ensure that people can expect the same (excellent) health care, regardless of where they live, and to reduce variation in practice. This can be achieved only if what constitutes best practice is known. Recommendations for practice need to be developed in a systematic, reliable and credible way if they are to be applied across a whole population. Lastly, but of equal importance, patients increasingly request information about what treatments will work best for them, what options they may have, and the basis for the information health care professionals give them.

Physiotherapists have always wanted to know that they are doing the best for their patients, and many look to their peers for guidance on what is expected 'best practice'. This could be a personal network of one or more colleagues of perceived similar or greater expertise, or local colleagues working in the same service, or an organized regional, national or international group of specialists.

But how reliable is such guidance? On what is it based? Is it based on opinion and experience, or is it based on high quality clinical research? Many 'guidelines' are based on informal consensus, which in turn is based on a combination of opinion and shared experience. Is this reliable enough? How do we know whether the recommendations really reflect effective practice that will lead to health benefits for patients? How can we discern what is effective practice without looking *systematically* at the available evidence and considering its implications for practice?

Before the early 1990s, most clinical guidelines in health care were developed informally, often by groups from a single health care profession, who produced, by informal consensus, statements of 'best practice'. But over the following few years a literature developed that described a more systematic and evidence-based approach to developing guidelines.

There was a common view about the key processes required in the development of a good guideline (Grimshaw & Russell 1993, Grimshaw et al 1995):

- The scientific evidence is assembled in a systematic fashion.
- The panel that develops the guideline includes representatives of most, if not all, relevant disciplines.
- The recommendations are explicitly linked to the evidence from which they are derived.

There was an acknowledgement (Grimshaw & Russell 1993) that guidelines that were not supported by a literature review may be biased towards reinforcing *current* practice, rather than promoting *evidence-based* practice. And there were concerns that guidelines developed using non-systematic literature reviews may suffer from bias and provide 'false reassurance'.

The literature on clinical guideline development suggests that, from 2000 onwards, a more systematic approach to guideline development methodology has become accepted in many countries (Burgers et al 2003). Developments in methods have, more recently, tended to focus on the difficult problem of formulating recommendations where there is limited research evidence – a situation that most guideline developers find themselves in. Methodological initiatives have focused on the impact of people on guideline development, as opposed to the research literature focus of the 1990s. One such initiative is the Grading of Recommendations Assessment, Development and Evaluation (GRADE) Working Group. Information about the GRADE initiative and relevant publications can be found at http://www.gradeworkinggroup.org.

Where can I find clinical guidelines?

Only a minority of clinical guidelines are published in journals, so the major databases such as MEDLINE, Embase and CINAHL provide a poor way of locating practice guidelines. The most complete database of evidence-based practice guidelines relevant to physiotherapy is PEDro (http://www.pedro.org.au). PEDro was described in some detail in Chapter 4.

PEDro archives only *evidence-based* practice guidelines. Evidence-based practice guidelines are defined by the makers of PEDro as guidelines in which:

1. a systematic review was performed during the guideline development *or* the guidelines were based on a systematic review published in the 4 years preceding publication of the guideline, and
2. at least one randomized controlled trial related to physiotherapy management is included in the review of existing scientific evidence, and
3. the clinical practice guideline must contain systematically developed statements that include recommendations, strategies or information that assist physiotherapists or patients to make decisions about appropriate health care for specific clinical circumstances.

At the time of writing there are 725 evidence-based clinical guidelines on the database.

To find clinical practice guidelines on PEDro, use the *Advanced Search* option, and choose *Clinical Guidelines* in the drop-down menu of the *'Methods'* field. You can add additional search terms and combine them with AND or OR to refine your search.

A National Guidelines Clearing House can be found at http://www.guideline.gov/. This contains mostly guidelines developed in North America. Criteria for inclusion in the database include the presence of a systematic literature review based on published, peer-reviewed evidence and systematically developed statements that include recommendations to assist health care decision-making.

Some countries have national clinical guideline programmes that produce multiprofessional clinical guidelines. Many of these include reference to physiotherapy management. Sites of national clinical guideline programmes and information include:

- (in England) http://www.nice.org.uk
- (in Australia) http://www.nhmrc.gov.au/guidelines/health_guidelines.htm
- (in New Zealand) http://www.nzgg.org.nz
- (in the USA) http://www.guideline.gov

There are also several international societies that have developed guidelines for the management of specific diseases. One example is the Osteoarthritis Research Society International (http://www.oarsi.org).

The Guidelines International Network (G-I-N) is an international association of organizations involved in clinical guidelines. Its aims include facilitating the sharing of information and knowledge and working between guideline programmes, and improving and harmonizing methodologies for guideline development. You can find more information about G-I-N at http://www.g-i-n.net/

How do I know if I can trust the recommendations in a clinical guideline?

With the growing number of clinical guidelines being developed by many different international, national and local organizations, it is important for physiotherapists to be able to distinguish between high- and low-quality clinical guidelines.

In 1999, Cluzeau et al argued for the development of criteria for the critical appraisal of guidelines,

> **Box 7.1**
>
> **Domains of the AGREE instrument**
> Scope and purpose
> Stakeholder involvement
> Rigour of development
> Clarity and presentation
> Applicability
> Editorial independence

following the same principles as work that was already becoming established to assess the quality of a randomized controlled trial or systematic review. A checklist was developed containing 37 items (Cluzeau & Littlejohns 1999, Cluzeau et al 1999) addressing different aspects of guideline development. Later, this instrument was further developed and validated by an international group of researchers from 13 countries, known as the Appraisal of Guidelines, REsearch and Evaluation (AGREE) Collaboration (The AGREE Collaboration 2003). The instrument is divided into six theoretical quality domains (Box 7.1) where

> the 'quality' of guidelines is defined as 'the confidence that the biases linked to the rigour of development, presentation, and applicability of a clinical practice guideline have been minimized and that each step of the development process is clearly reported' (p 18).

The AGREE instrument was revised in 2010. Box 7.2 provides an overview of the original AGREE items and the changed implemented in the 2010 version. The tool can be found at www.agreetrust.org.

In the next sections we consider how to assess some elements of a clinical guideline, by focusing on two important questions: 'Who developed the guideline?' and 'How were recommendations developed?'

Who developed the guideline?

The guideline should describe all those who have been involved at some stage of the development process. Some will have been part of the guideline development group, which carries out the guideline development process. Others will have been involved at particular consultation stages of the development process, or as an expert adviser at a particular point in the development process. Guideline developers should describe the process that they used to identify

Box 7.2

Comparison between the AGREE Instrument and the AGREE II

Domain	Original AGREE item	AGREE II item
Scope and purpose	1 The overall objective(s) of the guideline is (are) specifically described	No change
	2 The clinical question(s) covered by the guideline is (are) specifically described	The health question(s) covered by the guideline is (are) specifically described
	3 The patients to whom the guideline is meant to apply are specifically described	The population (patients, public, etc.) to whom the guideline is meant to apply is specifically described
Stakeholder involvement	4 The guideline development group includes individuals from all the relevant professional groups	No change
	5 The patients' views and preferences have been sought	The views and preferences of the target population (patients, public, etc.) have been sought
	6 The target users of the guideline are clearly defined	No change
	7 The guideline has been piloted among end users	Delete item. Incorporated into user guide description of item 19
Rigour of development	8 Systematic methods were used to search for evidence	No change in item. Renumber to 7
	9 The criteria for selecting the evidence are clearly described	No change in item. Renumber to 8
		NEW Item 9. The strengths and limitations of the body of evidence are described
	10 The methods for formulating the recommendations are clearly described	No change
	11 The health benefits, side-effects and risks have been considered in formulating the recommendations	No change
	12 There is an explicit link between the recommendations and the supporting evidence	No change
	13 The guideline has been externally reviewed by experts prior to its publication	No change
	14 A procedure for updating the guideline is provided	No change
Clarity of presentation	15 The recommendations are specific and unambiguous	No change
	16 The different options for management of the condition are clearly presented	The different options for management of the condition or health issue are clearly presented
	17 Key recommendations are easily identifiable	No change
Applicability	18 The guideline is supported with tools for application	The guideline provides advice and/or tools on how the recommendations can be put into practice AND Change in domain (from Clarity of Presentation) AND renumber to 19
	19 The potential organizational barriers in applying the recommendations have been discussed	The guideline describes facilitators and barriers to its application AND change in order – renumber to 18
	20 The potential cost implications of applying the recommendations have been considered	The potential resource implications of applying the recommendations have been considered
	21 The guideline presents key review criteria for monitoring and/or audit purposes	The guideline presents monitoring and/or auditing criteria
Editorial independence	22 The guideline is editorially independent from the funding body	The views of the funding body have not influenced the content of the guideline
	23 Conflicts of interest of guideline development members have been recorded	Competing interests of guideline development members have been recorded and addressed

key stakeholders. Stakeholders include any groups of health professionals involved with the care of patients for the topic being considered, patients themselves, people with technical skills that will support the rigour of the guideline development process, and those who have responsibility for the successful implementation of the guideline.

A number of authors describe the importance of having representatives from a range of different backgrounds in a guideline development group. This is thought to be critical to ensure potential biases are balanced (Shekelle et al 1999). A group with diverse values, perspectives and interests is less likely to skew judgements, particularly during the stage of formulating recommendations, than if the group consists solely of like-minded people (Murphy et al 1998).

Patients provide a particularly valuable source of evidence about what constitutes clinically effective health care (Duff et al 1996), and in clinical guideline development the involvement of patients is an increasingly established part of the process. A number of studies have been conducted to evaluate the ways in which patients and users can contribute most effectively to the guideline development process; however, we do not know the effect of different methods to involve users in guideline development (Nilsen et al 2006).

How were the recommendations developed?

High-quality clinical guidelines are based on up-to-date and high-quality systematic reviews. Appraisal of systematic reviews has already been discussed in Chapters 5 and 6. The principles discussed in those chapters can be used to appraise the systematic reviews upon which clinical guidelines are based.

Clinical guidelines should explicitly report 'quality of evidence' or 'levels of evidence' upon which recommendations are based. Almost all of the systems used to describe quality or levels of evidence presume that there is a 'hierarchy' of evidence. High-quality systematic reviews of randomized controlled trials are placed at the top of the evidence hierarchy. This is usually followed by individual randomized controlled trials, then cohort studies and other types of observational study. Consensus and the views of expert groups are placed at the bottom of the hierarchy, as they are considered to provide the least reliable evidence. This type of hierarchy can be useful, but is sometimes used inappropriately. Sometimes these hierarchies are used in a way that fails to recognize that different clinical questions lend themselves to different research designs. For example, evidence about diagnostic tests may draw on cross-sectional studies, yet such studies are not represented in the typical hierarchy. Similarly evidence about patients' experiences may be discerned by qualitative research, but qualitative methods are typically unrepresented in the information hierarchy. Readers should appreciate that the hierarchies used to categorize levels of evidence in clinical guidelines are usually applicable only to evidence about intervention; typically these hierarchies refer to the strength of evidence concerning the effects of interventions.

From quality (level) of evidence to strength of recommendations

Guidelines must go one step further than systematic reviews: rather than just summarizing evidence, guidelines must also make recommendations for practice. This makes development of guidelines difficult, but it is also what makes them important.

As a consequence, readers of clinical practice guidelines must be concerned not just with the quality of evidence, but also with the strength of the recommendations that can be made on the basis of the evidence. Generating recommendations for practice involves not only consideration of the research evidence, but also consideration of the trade-off between benefit and harm. Making that trade-off inevitably involves placing, implicitly or explicitly, a relative value on each outcome. It requires that judgements be made about what the evidence really means for patients. The results of such judgements must then be translated into meaningful recommendations for practice. Finally, users of guidelines need to know how much trust they should place in a recommendation, so each recommendation needs to be accompanied by an indication of the strength of the recommendation.

The GRADE Working Group (2004) suggests that recommendations should consider four main factors:

- the balance between benefits and harms, taking into account the estimated size of the effect for the main outcomes, the confidence limits around those estimates, and the relative value placed on each outcome
- the quality of evidence
- translation of the evidence into practice in a specific setting
- uncertainty about baseline risk for the population.

Based on these four criteria, the following categories for recommendations are suggested:

- 'Do it' or 'Don't do it', indicating 'a judgement that most well-informed people would make'.
- 'Probably do it' or 'Probably don't do it', indicating 'a judgement that a majority of well-informed people would make, but a substantial minority would not'.

Other clinical guidelines include systems for grading the strength of recommendations. For example, some guidelines define a 'Grade A' recommendation as one that is based on at least one randomized controlled trial, whereas a 'Grade C' recommendation is based on expert opinion or clinical experience. However, more and more organizations and institutions, such as the National Institute for Health and Clinical Excellence, now use GRADE to rate the strength of recommendations.

For guideline developers, formulation of recommendations is difficult for two reasons. First, there is unlikely to be sufficient high-quality clinical research on which to base clear recommendations for the whole range of interventions or care processes described in the guideline scope, so other methods have to be used to gather information that can be used as a reliable resource. Second, formulating recommendations for practice from the available information, whether high-quality clinical research or consensus or expert views, requires a degree of judgement and interpretation by the guideline development group that is potentially open to the biases of the guideline development group participants and the group process.

The guideline should explicitly consider the health benefits, side-effects and risks of the recommendations. This allows patients and physiotherapists to understand the relative benefits and risks of different options for intervention, so that shared decisions can be made.

There are also other important issues that should be considered when assessing whether you can trust a clinical guideline. These relate to clarity, applicability and editorial independence (see Box 7.2). There should also be a clear and detailed description of the clinical questions covered by the guideline, as well as a clear description of the population to whom the guideline recommendations apply. Readers of guidelines must be satisfied that the process of formulating recommendations described in the guideline is transparent and free of bias.

To conclude, high-quality clinical guidelines provide a valuable resource for practice in the form of recommendations for practice based on a systematic evidence review integrated with information from a consensus process and expert judgement. However, clinical guidelines are expensive and time-consuming to develop. A real challenge for the years ahead will be to set up international collaborations between organizations that will trust each others' work sufficiently to avoid the current duplication of guidelines across countries. A second challenge will be to determine with more clarity whether clinical guidelines actually lead to health benefits for patients. Finally, optimal mechanisms for facilitation and implementation of guidelines need to be found and used.

Chapter 9 will describe what is currently known about strategies for the successful implementation of clinical guidelines.

References

Burgers, J., Grol, R., Klazinger, N., et al., 2003. Towards evidence-based clinical practice: an international survey of 18 clinical guidelines programs. Int. J. Qual. Health Care 15 (1), 31–45.

Cluzeau, F.A., Littlejohns, P., 1999. Appraising clinical practice guidelines in England and Wales: the development of a methodological framework and its application to policy. Jt. Comm. J. Qual. Improv. 25 (10), 514–521.

Cluzeau, F.A., Littlejohns, P., Grimshaw, J.M., et al., 1999. Development and

application of a generic methodology to assess the quality of clinical guidelines. Int. J. Qual. Health Care 11 (1), 21–28.

Duff, L.A., Kelson, M., Marriott, S., et al., 1996. Clinical guidelines: involving patients and users of services. Journal of Clinical Effectiveness 1 (3), 104–112.

GRADE Working Group, 2004. Grading quality of evidence and strength of recommendations. BMJ 328, 1490–1497.

Grimshaw, J., Russell, I., 1993. Achieving health gain through clinical

guidelines I: developing scientifically valid guidelines. Qual. Health Care 2, 243–248.

Grimshaw, J., Eccles, M., Russell, I., 1995. Developing clinically valid practice guidelines. J. Eval. Clin. Pract. 1 (1), 37–48.

Institute of Medicine, 1992. Field, M.J., Lohr, K.N. (Eds.), Guidelines for clinical practice: from development to use. National Academy Press, Washington, DC.

Murphy, M.K., Black, N.A., Lamping, D.L., et al., 1998. Consensus development methods, and their use in clinical guideline development. Health Technol. Assess. 2 (3), 1–88.

Nilsen, E.S., Myrhaug, H.T., Johansen, M., et al., 2006. Methods of consumer involvement in developing healthcare policy and research, clinical practice guidelines and patient information material. Cochrane Database Syst Rev (3), CD004563.

Shekelle, P.G., Woolf, S.H., Eccles, M., et al., 1999. Developing guidelines. BMJ 318, 593–596.

The AGREE Collaboration, 2003. Development and validation of an international appraisals instrument for assessing the quality of clinical practice guidelines: the AGREE project. Qual. Saf. Health Care 12, 18–23.

When and how should new therapies be introduced into clinical practice?[1]

8

CHAPTER CONTENTS

Overview 143
The life cycle of a medical innovation 143
A case study 145
Proposal for a protocol for introduction
of new therapies 145
Anticipation of some objections 146
References 147

OVERVIEW

The process by which new therapies enter clinical practice is frequently suboptimal. Often ideas for new therapies are generated by clinical observations or laboratory studies; therapies based on those ideas may enter clinical practice without any further scrutiny. As a consequence, some ineffective practices become widespread. We propose a six-stage protocol for the implementation of new therapies. Hypotheses about therapy based on pre-clinical research should be subject to clinical exploration and pilot studies prior to rigorous assessment with randomized clinical trials. If randomized clinical trials suggest that the intervention produces clinically important effects, further randomized studies can be conducted to refine the intervention. New interventions should not be recommended, or included in teaching curricula, or taught in continuing education courses, until their effectiveness has been demonstrated in high-quality randomized clinical trials.

---

[1]This section is reproduced, with only minor changes, from Bø & Herbert (2009). We are grateful to Professor Kari Bø and the publishers of the journal *Physiotherapy* for granting permission to reproduce this material.

As has been mentioned earlier in this book, physiotherapy has undergone a remarkable transformation in the last two decades. Whereas practice was once based almost exclusively on clinical experience and theory, today practice is increasingly based on the findings of high-quality randomized clinical trials. This transformation has been built on a rapid proliferation of research evidence (Moseley et al 2002).

That does not mean that physiotherapy practice is now dominated by high-quality research evidence, or that current clinical practice is primarily evidence based. Several recent studies suggest that physiotherapy practice often departs from that recommended in evidence-based clinical practice guidelines (Bekkering et al 2005, Rebbeck et al 2006, Swinkels et al 2005).

In this chapter we consider how innovations in therapy become incorporated into clinical practice. We argue that the current state is far from optimal because innovative therapies still become accepted practice on the basis of laboratory research alone. We conclude by making recommendations about how and when new therapies should be incorporated into routine clinical practice.

The life cycle of a medical innovation

In 1981, John McKinlay, a distinguished epidemiologist, described seven stages in the 'career' of medical innovations. The description was offered in a slightly humorous vein, but it illustrates a not-unfamiliar phenomenon. The seven stages, slightly modified for the current context, are as follows.

Stage 1. The Promising Report: A new approach to therapy or a new therapeutic procedure is presented at a conference or in professional journals. Occasionally the new therapy may be based on a clinical observation. (An example is McKenzie's famous observation of a remarkable reduction in low back pain that a patient experienced when lying prone; McKenzie 1981.) More often the therapy is developed by a clinician or clinician–researcher who has read and thought about the implications of pre-clinical (laboratory) research. Claims about the effectiveness of the new therapy are usually based on the presumed mechanisms of action, but may also be supplemented with case reports or descriptions of case series.

Stage 2. Professional adoption: Soon the most innovative clinicians begin to practise the new therapy. The therapy may be enthusiastically endorsed, in which case it permeates into wider clinical practice.

Stage 3. Public acceptance: Professional enthusiasm spawns enthusiasm from consumers. The public comes to expect that the new therapy should be available to those who want it.

Stage 4. Standard practice: Eventually the new therapy becomes standard practice. It is described in textbooks. Clinicians who do not provide the therapy are considered to be behind the times.

Stage 5. Randomized clinical trials: High-quality randomized clinical trials are conducted that show the therapy is much less effective than first assumed. Some trials suggest that the effects of the therapy are too small to be worthwhile, or even that the therapy is harmful.

Stage 6. Professional denunciation: The profession defends the therapy against the findings of the randomized clinical trials. The defence often focuses on limitations to the external validity (generalizability) of the trial findings.

Stage 7. Extinction: Damning evidence accumulates. The profession becomes used to negative findings, and individual clinicians start to look for alternative interventions. Eventually all but the truest believers abandon the intervention for a more recent innovation. Textbooks continue to recommend the practice decades later.

Every clinician who has practised for more than 10 years has observed parts of this life cycle of new therapies. As one therapy slips quietly into obscurity, others spring up, competing for the attention of clinicians. Sometimes new therapies adapt to protect themselves from the negative findings of randomized clinical trials. Nowadays randomized clinical trials increasingly determine which therapies survive, which change, and which disappear from practice (Bekkering et al 2005, Hagen et al 2004, Rebbeck et al 2006). A particularly clear example is the practice of recommending bed rest for people with low back pain or sciatica; this practice has rapidly declined in popularity since the publication of a landmark systematic review of randomized trials that showed the practice had little effect or was even harmful (Hagen et al 2004).

Not all interventions go through this cycle. Some therapies are adopted widely only after the publication of high-quality randomized clinical trials, but this is the exception rather than the rule. Other new therapies are too implausible, or too difficult to implement, or lack a charismatic advocate; such therapies might never be widely adopted, or they might be practised only at the margins of the professions. When randomized clinical trials or systematic reviews of randomized clinical trials provide evidence of a lack of effect, the evidence is rarely definitive and therapists are understandably reluctant to abandon the practice. (In physiotherapy, there are few therapies that were practised in the 1950s that are not still practised by some therapists, and of those that have been more or less discontinued (such as the use of infra-red radiation) few have been discontinued because of the findings of randomized clinical trials.) Of course, many therapies survive scrutiny; these are found to be effective in well-designed randomized clinical trials (Herbert et al 2001) and provide a solid core of contemporary professional practice.

McKinlay's observations of the life cycle of a medical innovation were published in 1981, but in many respects the model is still valid today. Indeed, in 2000 Imrie & Ramey reviewed literature which indicated that, although much of medical practice was based on some sort of evidence, only a relatively modest proportion of medical interventions (typically somewhere between one- and two-thirds) was supported by randomized clinical trials.

Of course these observations do not apply only to medicine. They apply equally well to all the health professions, including physiotherapy. In our opinion the most damning observation made by McKinley is not that randomized clinical trials often disprove the effectiveness of therapies, or that the findings of randomized clinical trials are often disputed by clinicians. The more problematic observation is that many therapies become widely practised prior to demonstration of their effectiveness with randomized clinical trials.

A case study

A case in point is the recent adoption of the practice of training abdominal muscles to treat stress urinary incontinence. Stress urinary incontinence can be prevented and treated with pelvic floor muscle training, as demonstrated by over 50 randomized clinical trials and several systematic reviews (Bø et al 2007). Sapsford (2001, 2004) has advocated a new approach to pelvic floor muscle training. She argues that exercise for stress urinary incontinence should involve training of the abdominal muscles, especially the transversus abdominis, claiming that voluntary activity in the abdominal muscles results in increased pelvic floor muscle activity and that abdominal muscle training to rehabilitate the pelvic floor muscles may be useful in treating dysfunction of the pelvic floor. According to Sapsford, 'pelvic floor muscle rehabilitation does not reach its optimum level until the muscles of the abdominal wall are rehabilitated as well' (Sapsford 2004: 627). Sapsford's recommendations have been enthusiastically received, and there are now many physiotherapists routinely training the abdominal muscles of women with stress urinary incontinence.

This is an example of a therapy that has entered clinical practice on the basis of a promising report. It appears that the first proposal to train the abdominal muscles for stress urinary incontinence was presented by Sapsford & Hodges in 2001. That proposal was based on the findings of a small laboratory study on healthy women (women without stress urinary incontinence) showing that contraction of the transversus abdominis muscle was associated with co-contraction of the pelvic floor muscles. The theory and recommendations for this training model were published first in *Physiotherapy*, which has a circulation of about 50000, and later in *Manual Therapy*, which currently has the highest impact factor of all therapy journals. Soon thereafter, many physiotherapists had begun to incorporate abdominal training into programmes designed to prevent and treat stress urinary incontinence. Now, only few years after the first laboratory experiments showing that transversus abdominis contractions are associated with pelvic floor muscle contractions,

the intervention is endorsed in textbooks (Godel-Purrer 2006, Jones 2008).

In 2004 Dumoulin and colleagues published a randomized clinical trial comparing the addition of deep abdominal muscle training to pelvic floor muscle training. The deep abdominal muscle training was carried out in accordance with recommendations made by Sapsford (2001). Little additional beneficial effect was observed from adding abdominal muscle training to pelvic floor muscle training. The absolute difference in the proportion of women whose incontinence was cured was 4% (95% confidence interval −3% to 22%). (Positive values favour the group that received abdominal training.) These data are not absolutely definitive because the confidence intervals are too wide to rule out, with certainty, clinical benefits of abdominal training, and because the trial has not yet been replicated. Nonetheless these data, the best currently available, suggest that addition of deep abdominal muscle training does not substantially improve the outcome of pelvic floor rehabilitation beyond the effect provided by specific pelvic floor muscle training.

The early indications are that the innovation of abdominal training to treat stress urinary incontinence is unlikely to be helpful. Unfortunately the innovation has already become routine clinical practice in many clinical settings. It may eventually prove that it would have been better to wait on the findings of randomized clinical trials before advocating abdominal training for stress urinary incontinence.

Proposal for a protocol for introduction of new therapies

We propose a protocol for the introduction of new therapies into clinical practice (Table 8.1).

Table 8.1 A protocol for implementation of new therapies

Stage	Phase
1: Clinical observation or laboratory studies 2: Clinical exploration 3: Pilot studies	Development phase
4: Randomized clinical trials	Testing phase
5: Refinement 6: Active dissemination	Refinement and Dissemination phase

Stage 1. Clinical observation or laboratory studies: In this stage, clinicians develop hypotheses about new therapeutic strategies based on their clinical observations. Alternatively, clinicians who read reports of laboratory research or conduct their own laboratory studies generate and test hypotheses about the causes of dysfunction and responses to interventions. The studies may be conducted on animals or on humans, with or without disease. The result is an unconfirmed hypothesis about clinical intervention. The hypothesis may suggest how the intervention should be administered (Herbert & Bø 2005).

Stage 2. Clinical exploration: The hypothesis is subject to clinical exploration. Expert clinicians administer a prototype of the intervention to volunteer patients. Trial and error is used to explore different ways of administering the intervention, including different doses of the intervention, and to assess whether predictions of hypotheses concerning the intervention are borne out by clinical observation. The process is explicitly exploratory. Patients are fully informed of the exploratory nature of the intervention.

Stage 3. Pilot studies: If clinical exploration suggests that administration of the intervention is feasible and that the predictions of the hypothesis appear to be supported, pilot studies (typically case series, or small randomized studies) are conducted to document, in a more systematic and objective way, the feasibility and outcomes of the intervention. These data are used to determine whether to proceed to a randomized clinical trial. The data are not used to support claims about the effectiveness of the intervention.

Stage 4. Randomized clinical trials and systematic reviews: If pilot studies are sufficiently promising, randomized clinical trials are conducted. Usually it is necessary to conduct more than one trial to ensure the robustness and generalizability of the findings. The first trials may be explanatory in orientation, but eventually it is necessary to conduct pragmatic trials, including trials with cost-effectiveness analyses (Herbert 2009). It is only after several high-quality trials have demonstrated consistent findings that claims can be made of the effectiveness of the intervention.

Stage 5. Refinement: If randomized clinical trials suggest that an intervention may have clinically important effects, additional studies are conducted to test further the usefulness of the intervention and to maximize its effectiveness. These could involve randomized head-to-head comparisons of the intervention with competing interventions, and large randomized studies to evaluate the size of the effects of intervention in different patient subgroups. Note that issues of the differential responses of subgroups can be tested only in large randomized studies; such studies are difficult to do well (Herbert 2007).

Stage 6. Active dissemination: The intervention is recommended in clinical practice guidelines, undergraduate teaching curricula and continuing education courses. There is active dissemination of information about the effectiveness of the intervention to therapists, other health professionals, and consumers of therapy (Bekkering et al 2005, Rebbeck et al 2006).

Stages 1, 2 and 3 can be considered to be the Development phase, Stage 4 is the Testing phase, and Stages 5 and 6 are the Refinement and Dissemination stage. This staged process is broadly similar to the familiar classification of the phases of drug development (Pocock 1983). Importantly (with the possible exception of Stages 5 and 6), the stages should occur in order. There is a case for arguing that the findings of Stages 2 and 3 are best communicated only amongst the clinicians and researchers who are developing the intervention, because positive results may be misinterpreted by the wider professional community as providing substantive evidence of the effectiveness of the intervention. Active promotion of the intervention should not occur until Stage 4 is complete.

Anticipation of some objections

Many clinicians would argue that it is not possible to delay introduction of new therapies until there is strong evidence of the effects of the intervention from randomized clinical trials because it is not possible to conduct randomized clinical trials on all new interventions. In the past that may have been true. Until recent times, the rate of publication of trial reports was low. However, as we saw in Chapter 4, there has been a spectacular increase in the number of reports of randomized clinical trials published in recent years. In our opinion there is plenty of capacity to subject new interventions to randomized clinical trials prior to their widespread implementation.

Substantial resources are required to conduct high-quality randomized trials. It will certainly be expensive to subject every new therapy to a randomized trial prior to introduction of the therapy into clinical practice. In the long run, however, subjecting new therapies to randomized trials is likely to be a cost-effective strategy both because it will reduce the costly introduction of ineffective therapies and because questions about efficacy can be more easily resolved, with fewer trials, in the period before the therapy becomes established clinical practice.

Many clinicians are frustrated by clinical research. They believe that the research process is too slow and unresponsive to the ever-growing body of new knowledge generated by pre-clinical research. They want to see a continuous rapid evolution of clinical practice emerge from a close relationship between skilled physiotherapists and laboratory researchers. This model, in which laboratory studies directly influence clinical practice, has been the dominant model driving practice in physiotherapy for the last 20 years. But in our view it is counter-productive and, in the long-term, damaging to professional progress.

Good decisions about whether to implement new therapies into clinical practice must be informed by high-quality randomized clinical trials. By introducing new therapies prior to the conduct of high-quality trials we risk administering ineffective therapies. History has shown that once new therapies become established in clinical practice it is very difficult to discontinue them if high-quality evidence subsequently shows the therapy to be ineffective.

That does not mean that all innovation in clinical practice needs to be preceded by clinical trials. It is sensible to distinguish between small changes to the way in which interventions of proven interventions are administered (for example, new positions for doing exercises), and new therapies (a new way of intervening based on a new therapeutic hypothesis, or application of a proven intervention to a very different patient group for whom the original hypothesis might not apply). The former is a legitimate part of the day-to-day struggle to administer intervention as well as possible, but the latter, in our view, represents a degree of clinical innovation that requires scrutiny. New therapies need to be subjected to an explicit protocol of development.

References

Bekkering, G.E., van Tulder, M.W., Hendriks, E.J., et al., 2005. Implementation of clinical guidelines on physical therapy for patients with low back pain: randomized trial comparing patient outcomes after a standard and active implementation strategy. Phys. Ther. 85 (6), 544–555.

Bø, K., Herbert, R., 2009. When and how should new therapies become routine clinical practice? Physiotherapy 95, 51–57.

Bø, K., Morkved, S., Berghmans, B., et al., 2007. Evidence-based physical therapy for the pelvic floor – bridging science and clinical practice. Elsevier, Oxford.

Dumoulin, C., Lemieux, M.C., Bourbonnais, D., et al., 2004. Physiotherapy for persistent postnatal stress urinary incontinence: a randomized controlled trial. Obstet. Gynecol. 104 (3), 504–510.

Godel-Purrer, B., 2006. Training and functional exercises for the muscles of the pelvic floor. In: Carriere, B., Feldt, C.M. (Eds.), The pelvic floor. Georg Thieme, New York, pp. 69–142.

Hagen, K.B., Hilde, G., Jamtvedt, G., et al., 2004. Bed rest for acute low-back pain and sciatica. Cochrane Database Syst. Rev. 4, CD001254.

Herbert, R.D., 2007. Dealing with heterogeneity in clinical trials (editorial). Man. Ther. 12, 1–2.

Herbert, R.D., 2009. Explanatory and pragmatic clinical trials. In: Gad, S.C. (Ed.), Clinical trails handbooks. Wiley, Chichester, pp. 1081–1098.

Herbert, R.D., Bø, K., 2005. Analysis of quality of interventions in systematic reviews. BMJ 331, 507–509.

Herbert, R.D., Maher, C.G., Moseley, A.M., et al., 2001. Effective physiotherapy. BMJ 323, 788–790.

Imrie, R., Ramey, D.W., 2000. The evidence for evidence-based medicine. Complement. Ther. Med. 8 (2), 123–126.

Jones, R.C., 2008. Pelvic floor stability and trunk muscle co-activation. In: Laycock, J., Haslam, J. (Eds.), Therapeutic management of incontinence and pelvic pain: pelvic organ disorders, second ed. Springer, London, pp. 99–104.

McKenzie, R., 1981. The lumbar spine: mechanical diagnosis and therapy. Spinal Publications, Waikanae, New Zealand.

McKinlay, J.B., 1981. From 'promising report' to 'standard procedure': Seven stages in the career of a medical innovation. Milbank Mem. Fund Q. Health Soc. 59 (3), 374–411.

Moseley, A.M., Herbert, R.D., Sherrington, C., et al., 2002. Evidence for physiotherapy practice: a survey of the Physiotherapy Evidence Database (PEDro). Aust. J. Physiother. 48 (1), 43–49.

Pocock, S.J., 1983. Clinical trials: a practical approach. Wiley, Chichester.

Rebbeck, T., Maher, C.G., Refshauge, K.M., 2006. Evaluating two implementation strategies for whiplash guidelines in physiotherapy: a cluster randomised trial. Aust. J. Physiother. 52 (3), 165–174.

Sapsford, R., 2001. The pelvic floor. A clinical model for function and rehabilitation. Physiotherapy 87, 620–630.

Sapsford, R., 2004. Rehabilitation of pelvic floor muscles utilizing trunk stabilization. Man. Ther. 9 (1), 3–12.

Sapsford, R.R., Hodges, P.W., 2001. Contraction of the pelvic floor muscles during abdominal maneuvers. Arch. Phys. Med. Rehabil. 82 (8), 1081–1088.

Swinkels, I.C., van den Ende, C.H., van den Bosch, W., et al., 2005. Physiotherapy management of low back pain: does practice match the Dutch guidelines? Aust. J. Physiother. 51 (1), 35–41.

Making it happen

9

CHAPTER CONTENTS

Overview 149
What do we mean by 'making it
happen? 149
   Two approaches 150
Changing is hard 150
   Theories of change 150
   Barriers to change 152
   Barriers to implementing the steps of
   evidence-based practice 152
   Barriers to implementing a change
   in specific practice behaviour 153
Evidence-based implementation 154
   What helps people to change
   practice? 154
   Implementing the steps of
   evidence-based practice 154
   Implementing a change in specific
   practice behaviour 154
   Implementing clinical guidelines 155
Evidence-based physiotherapy in the
context of continuous quality
improvement 159
References 159

OVERVIEW

The availability of high-quality clinical research does not necessarily ensure evidence-based practice. Translation of research into practice is difficult for many reasons. This chapter focuses on the process of implementing evidence-based physiotherapy. Barriers to change for physiotherapists are presented, and some theories of change are discussed. The chapter provides an overview of evidence-based implementation of evidence-based care, with a specific emphasis on guideline implementation. The implementation of evidence-based physiotherapy should be viewed in the context of a range of other organizational and individual quality improvement activities.

What do we mean by 'making it happen'?

The availability of high-quality clinical research does not, on its own, ensure evidence-based practice. There is often a gap between research and practice. Evidence-based practice must be made to happen.

Researchers have sometimes assumed that, if they publish reports of their research in professional journals, clinicians will read those reports and use the findings of the research in clinical practice. This is referred to as passive diffusion. At best, passive diffusion occurs slowly, and it may not occur at all. Sometimes a more active strategy, called dissemination, is employed: dissemination involves targeting the message to defined groups. A third strategy, implementation, is even more active, planned and tailored. 'Implementation involves identifying and assisting in overcoming the barriers to the use of the knowledge ... It ... uses not only the message itself, but also organizational and behavioural tools that are sensitive to constraints and opportunities of [*health professionals*] in identified settings' (Lomas 1993: 227). That is, implementation involves addressing and overcoming barriers to change.

As discussed in Chapter 1, there are a number of reasons why we might wish for practice to be informed by high-quality clinical research. However, in practice, there are barriers to changing practice behaviour. Making evidence-based physiotherapy happen is a challenge to both individuals and organizations, so action is needed from both of these perspectives. Up to now this book has focused on how individual physiotherapists can identify, appraise, interpret and use high-quality clinical research. But bringing about change is a responsibility not just of practising physiotherapists. Often implementation programmes are initiated 'top-down'. For example, there may be a national or local strategy to improve physiotherapy for low back pain or for the management of osteoporosis. This means that someone is responsible at a management level for the implementation of a specific practice change or a guideline. Such management activities are important because, to make evidence-based practice happen, individuals need support, access to resources and a culture that supports change. That is why we have focused on a broader perspective of implementation in this book. The target group for this chapter is, therefore, primarily physiotherapy and health service leaders, managers of health services and policy-makers.

Two approaches

Evidence-based physiotherapy can be made to happen in two main ways. The first is by implementing the five steps of evidence-based practice (described in Chapter 1) as an integral part of everyday practice. This involves physiotherapists formulating questions of relevance for practice, searching, critically appraising research and informing current practice with high-quality clinical research. In the clinical decision-making process this information is combined with practice knowledge and patient preferences. These 'steps' provide the infrastructure for, or foundations of, evidence-based physiotherapy. Application of the steps requires the skills to ask questions, search, appraise and interpret the evidence. It also requires ready access to the internet and journals. Chapter 10 will consider how you can evaluate whether or not you are implementing the steps in your own practice.

A second approach to making evidence-based physiotherapy happen is through the implementation of a personal and/or organizational practice or behaviour change related to a specific condition. This may be necessary because there is current variation in practice, or because that practice needs to be improved or changed in a particular area. A typical

example is the implementation of new strategies for management of low back pain. Organizations have to decide which strategies to use to improve professional performance and quality of care, and on what to base the choice of strategies.

Changing is hard

Change is always difficult, in every area of human life. We guess you will have experienced how hard change can be. Most physiotherapists provide a good service for their patients. Sometimes it is clear why there are large variations in practice among physiotherapists, or gaps between current practice and high-quality clinical research. It may be that the patient or the physiotherapist has strong preferences for, or positive experiences of, a certain treatment, or it may simply be due to a lack of knowledge by the physiotherapist. Sometimes, however, the explanations for gaps between research and practice are less obvious. Clinical behaviour, like other behaviours (for example physical activity, sexual behaviour or smoking habits), is determined by a number of factors, and the link between knowledge and behaviour is often weak. Anyone who has tried to change patient behaviour, or their own behaviour, will recognize how difficult it is. Knowledge alone is often not sufficient for behaviour change. Physiotherapists' behaviours and practice patterns are influenced by a number of factors. Factors related to resources, social support, practice environment, prevailing opinions and personal attitudes might all act as barriers to desired change.

Before moving on to a discussion of barriers that have been identified in physiotherapy, it will be useful to consider some theories of change.

Theories of change

Implementation research has been defined as the scientific study of methods to promote the uptake of research findings for the purpose of improving the quality of care. It includes the study of factors that influence the behaviour of health care professionals and organizations, and the interventions that enable them to use research findings more effectively. Research in this area has followed two related tracks: the transfer or diffusion of knowledge, and behaviour change (Agency for Healthcare Research and Quality 2004).

Theories of change can be used both to understand the behaviour of health professionals and to guide the development and implementation of interventions intended to change behaviour. Numerous theories of behaviour change have developed from a variety of perspectives: psychology, sociology, economics, marketing, education, organizational behaviour and others. The theories relate to changing the behaviours of patients, professionals and organizations. One type of theory is often called the classical, or descriptive, model (Agency for Healthcare Research and Quality 2004) and the most referred to is Rogers' Diffusion of Innovation Theory (Rogers 1995). This is a passive model that describes the naturalistic process of change. The innovation-decision process is derived from Rogers' theory and consists of five stages that potential adopters pass through as they decide to adopt an innovation. Rogers developed the model of adopter types in which he classified people as innovators (the fastest adopter group), early adopters, the early majority, the late majority and laggards (the slowest to change). However, these classical models provide little information about how actually to accelerate and promote change.

Another type of change theory is planned change models (Agency for Healthcare Research and Quality 2004). These models aim to explain how planned change occurs and how to alter ways of doing things in social systems. Most such models are based on social cognitive theories. Three examples of planned change theories are Green's precede–proceed model, the social marketing model and the Ottawa Model of Research Use.

The precede–proceed model outlines steps that should precede an intervention and gives guidance on how to proceed with implementation and subsequent evaluation (Green et al 1980). The 'precede' stage involves identifying the problem and the factors that contribute to it. The factors are categorized as predisposing, enabling or reinforcing. The key 'proceed' stages are implementation and evaluation of the effect the intervention had on behaviour change, and on predisposing, enabling and reinforcing factors.

Social marketing provides a framework for identifying factors that drive change. According to this model, change should be carried out in several stages (Kotler 1983). The first stage is a planning and strategy development stage. The next stage involves selecting the relevant channels and materials for the intervention. At this stage the target group is 'segmented' to create homogeneous subgroups based, for example, on individuals' motivations for change.

Subsequently, materials are developed and piloted with the target audience. Finally, there is implementation, evaluation and feedback, after which the intervention may be refined. Social marketing has focused largely on bringing about health behaviour change at a community level, but it has also been used as the basis for other quality improvement strategies, for example academic detailing or outreach visits, discussed later in this chapter.

The *Ottawa Model of Health Care Research* requires quality improvement facilitators to conduct an assessment of the barriers to implementing evidence-based recommendations. They then identify the potential adopters, and look at the practice environment to determine factors that might hinder or support the uptake of recommendations (Agency for Healthcare Research and Quality 2004). The information is then used to tailor interventions to overcome identified barriers or enhance the supporters. Finally, the impact of the implementation is evaluated and the interactive process begins again.

Motivational theories, including the social cognition model, propose that motivation determines behaviour, and therefore the best predictors of behaviour are factors that predict motivation. This assumption is the basis for *social psychological* theories. *Bandura's social cognitive theory* is one example (Bandura 1997). This theory proposes that behaviour is determined by incentives and expectations. Self-efficacy expectations are beliefs about one's ability to perform the behaviour (for example, 'I can start being physically active') and have been found to be a very important construct and predictor of behaviour change. A refinement of social cognitive theory is *stage models* of behaviour, which describe the factors thought to influence change in different settings. Individuals are thought to go through different stages to achieve a change, and different interventions are needed at different stages. Such theory might be applied to the types of change required for evidence-based practice. One model (Prochaska & Velicer 1997) involves five stages: pre-contemplation, contemplation, preparation, action and maintenance. One can easily understand that a person who is in a pre-contemplation stage (someone for whom no reason for change has been given) would need strategies to raise awareness and acknowledge information needs. In contrast, a person at an action or maintenance stage needs easy access to high-quality clinical research, and reminders to keep up the achieved behaviour. This theory is widely used, as in a study to improve physical activity (Marcus et al 1998).

Nonetheless a recent systematic review found that there was little evidence to support the use of stage model theories for smoking cessation (Riemsma et al 2003).

Most of the theories described above focus on individuals, but organizational factors play an important role in change processes as well. One type of *organizational theory* is *rational system models*, which focus on the internal structure and processes of an organization (Agency for Healthcare Research and Quality 2004). These models describe four stages in the process of organizational change and different perspectives that need to be addressed in each stage. The stages relate to awareness of a problem, identification of actions, implementation and institutionalization of the change. *Institutional models* assume that management has the freedom to implement change and the legitimacy to ask for behaviours to drive the implementation. Institutional models can explain important factors of quality improvement involving *total quality management*, an organizational intervention that is carried out by a range of philosophies and activities. All organizational models emphasize the complexity of organizations and the need to take account of multiple factors that influence the process of change.

Learning theory, derived from educational research, emphasizes the role of intrinsic personal motivation. From these theories have developed activities based on consensus development and problem-based learning. In contrast, *marketing approaches* are widely used to target physician behaviour (for example prescribing) and also to promote health to the general public, as in health promotion campaigns.

As demonstrated here, there are many theories of change. All have shortcomings because implementation is a complex process. The only way to know whether interventions based on these theories are effective is to evaluate the interventions in clinical and practice settings. There is much debate about how such evaluations should be conducted. It has been suggested that, in the future, implementation strategies should have a stronger theoretical basis than is typical of current intervention strategies (Grimshaw et al 2004).

Barriers to change

In the introduction to this chapter we presented two different approaches to 'making it happen'. The first was through implementation of the 'steps' of evidence-based physiotherapy in everyday practice. The second approach was by implementing a desired change in current practice for a particular patient group. The outcome measures for the first approach would be measures of the extent to which physiotherapists formulate questions, search and read papers critically, and use high-quality clinical research to inform their everyday practice. The outcome measure for the second approach would be the extent to which current practice is matched to high-quality clinical research. Both approaches require a change in behaviour, but the barriers to using the steps for evidence-based physiotherapy as part of everyday practice might differ from the barriers to achieving a desired practice for a patient group. The barriers might also differ between patient groups and cultures. There are no universal barriers to or one-size-fits-all solutions for good practice (Oxman & Flottorp 1998). Specific barriers and solutions have to be identified for every implementation project, which might then not be relevant to other settings or circumstances.

The identification of barriers to implementation of evidence-based physiotherapy is often carried out with qualitative research methods, as the aim is to explore attitudes, experiences and meanings. Many of us will have a limited insight into barriers to using evidence in our own practices. Critical reflection is the starting point for identifying determinants for practice.

Barriers to implementing the steps of evidence-based practice

Several studies have tried to identify barriers to evidence-based practice among health professionals (Freeman & Sweeny 2001, Young & Ward 2001). In a survey of Australian general practitioners, 45% stated that the most common barrier was 'patient demand for treatment despite lack of evidence for effectiveness' (Young & Ward 2001: 215). The next three highest-rated barriers were all related to lack of time. This was rated as a 'very important barrier' by significantly more participants than lack of skills.

Humphris and colleagues (2000) used qualitative methods to identify barriers to evidence-based occupational therapy and followed this qualitative study with a survey to evaluate the importance of the identified factors. The three most discouraging factors were workload pressure, time limitations and insufficient staff resources. Another survey, carried out with dieticians, occupational therapists, physiotherapists, and speech and language therapists, identified barriers related to skills, understanding research methodology, and having access to research and time. The relevance of research and institutional barriers seemed to be less of a problem (Metcalfe et al 2001). More specifically, the top three barriers were 'statistical analysis in papers is not understandable', 'literature not compiled in one place' and 'literature reports conflicting results'. More than one-third (38%) of the physiotherapists felt that doctors would not co-operate with implementation, and 30% felt that they did not have enough authority to change practice.

A well-conducted study was carried out in the Wessex area of the UK with the aim of identifying physiotherapists' attitudes and experiences related to evidence-based physiotherapy (Barnard & Wiles 2001). Junior physiotherapists and physiotherapists working in hospital settings felt that they had the skills needed to appraise research findings prior to implementation. Others, particularly senior physiotherapists working in community settings, felt that they did not. Community physiotherapists also felt that they were not able to engage in evidence-based practice due to poor access to library facilities and difficulties in meeting with peers. Some physiotherapists also described problems with the culture working against evidence-based physiotherapy where senior staff were resistant to change. A more recent study by Bridges et al (2007) found that personal characteristics, especially a desire for learning and self-directed learning, were associated with the propensity to adopt evidence-based physiotherapy, whereas characteristics of the social system made a minimal contribution to observed variation in the propensity to adopt evidence-based physiotherapy.

Barriers to implementing a change in specific practice behaviour

One study from the Netherlands was carried out to identify barriers to implementation of a guideline for low back pain (Bekkering et al 2003). One hundred randomly selected physiotherapists were invited to participate and were asked, in a survey, to identify any differences between the guideline recommendations and their current practice. The survey revealed a number of issues, highlighted by discrepancies between guideline recommendations and practice, that might be regarded as barriers to implementation. The most important of these was lack of knowledge or skills of physiotherapists in both diagnostic and treatment processes, particularly where there were

differences between traditional and evidence-based treatment. (For example, passive interventions were traditionally used, but were discouraged by the guidelines.) The second most important difference was an organizational one involving problems with getting the co-operation of the referring physicians (mostly general practitioners). There was also an issue about the expectations of patients. The authors concluded that, because skills and knowledge were the most important barriers, there was a need for continuing postgraduate education to keep knowledge and skills up to date.

In Scotland, a stroke therapy evaluation programme was carried out as a multidisciplinary project. One part of this project was the implementation of evidence-based rehabilitation. Pollock et al (2000) conducted a study to identify barriers to evidence-based stroke rehabilitation among health professionals, of whom 31% were physiotherapists. The study started with focus groups identifying perceived barriers, followed by a postal questionnaire to rate participants' agreement with the identified barriers. The barriers were divided into three areas: ability, opportunity and implementation. The key barriers identified across professionals were lack of time, lack of ability and need for training, and difficulties relating to the implementation of research findings. Physiotherapists felt less put off by statistics than occupational therapists and nurses. Sixty-seven per cent of all respondents agreed that they needed more training in appraisal and interpretation of studies, and only 8% agreed that they had sufficient time to read. Barriers to implementation appeared to be a lack of confidence in the validity of research findings and in the transferability of research findings to an individual's working environment.

What do these studies tell us? There are big variations in the barriers reported, but the main barriers to implementing evidence-based practice relate to time, skills and culture. One barrier that was not identified in the studies reported, but which we believe is relevant, is the lack of high-quality clinical research in some areas. If you go through the steps of formulating a question and searching for evidence without identifying high-quality studies, this must be a barrier to evidence-based practice.

Barriers to implementation of specific behaviour changes are more complex in nature, and specific to the topic under study. Overall, the conclusion seems to be that barriers need to be identified for each project and setting, because different approaches appear to be needed to address them.

Evidence-based implementation

What helps people to change practice?

A range of strategies exists to change the behaviour of health care professionals, with the aim of improving the quality of patient care. Box 9.1 provides examples of interventions that have been evaluated in systematic reviews with a focus on improving practice. The interventions are classified by the Cochrane Collaboration's Effective Practice and Organization

Box 9.1

Examples of interventions to promote professional behaviour change (based on EPOC taxonomy; http://epoc.cochrane.org/)

- **Educational materials** Distribution of published or printed recommendations for clinical care (such as clinical practice guidelines, audio-visual materials, electronic publications)
- **Didactic educational meetings** Lectures with minimal participant interaction
- **Interactive educational meetings** Participation of health care providers in workshops that include discussion or practice
- **Educational outreach visits** A personal visit by a trained person to a health care provider in his or her own setting to give information with the intent of changing practice
- **Reminders (manual or computerized)** Patient or encounter-specific information, provided verbally, on paper or on a computer screen, that is designed or intended to prompt a health professional to recall information
- **Audit and feedback** Any summary of clinical performance of health care over a specified period of time. The summary may also have included recommendations for clinical action
- **Local opinion leaders** Health professionals nominated by their colleagues as being educationally influential are recruited to promote implementation
- **Local consensus process** Inclusion of health professionals in discussions to agree to an approach to managing a clinical problem that they have selected as important
- **Patient-mediated interventions** Specific information sought from or given to patients
- **Multifaceted interventions** A combination of two or more interventions

of Care (EPOC) group (http://epoc.cochrane.org/) and include various forms of continuing education, quality assurance, informatics, and financial, organizational and regulatory interventions that can affect the ability of health care professionals to deliver services more effectively and efficiently. The focus of the EPOC group's work is on reviews of interventions designed to improve professional practice and the delivery of effective health services.

As discussed in the introduction to this chapter, implementation of evidence-based practice can be promoted in different ways or stages. Implementing the steps of evidence-based practice is one option that might lead to changes in specific behaviours.

Implementing the steps of evidence-based practice

Several studies have investigated the effects of teaching critical appraisal (Parkes et al 2001) and of teaching the 'steps' in evidence-based practice (Coomarasamy & Khan 2004, Flores-Mateo & Argimon 2007). These studies indicate that the teaching interventions improve participants' knowledge but have a variable effect on professional behaviour. The available data suggest that teaching of the steps of evidence-based practice is most successful when it takes place in clinical setting, particularly if it focuses on real clinical decisions and actions (Coomarasamy & Khan 2004). One systematic review of qualitative studies that have explored participants' experiences with courses of evidence-based practice supports this, and points out the importance of having clear aims and pre-course reading materials (Bradley et al 2005). Currently, much of the teaching of evidence-based practice involves interactive educational meetings with small group discussions and practice-related questions. There is a need for more research into the best ways to implement the steps effectively. This is closely linked to issues of self-evaluation, which will be discussed in the next chapter.

Implementing a change in specific practice behaviour

The effects of implementation strategies could be assessed by measuring either of two types of outcome. Outcomes can be measured at the level of professional performance, for example by measuring the frequency with which ultrasound is used to treat carpal tunnel syndrome or physiotherapists' compliance with a guideline for the treatment of ankle sprains.

Outcome can also be measured at the level of the patient, for example by measuring changes in pain, disability or time away from work. Studies have evaluated effects of implementation interventions on both types of outcome.

Several interventions have been evaluated, although most of these studies (approximately 90%) are carried out among physicians. The studies have been carried out in both primary care and hospitals, and the focus has often been on improvement in one or more aspects of practice behaviour or compliance with a guideline. As we will demonstrate later in this chapter, it remains unclear how best to implement and sustain evidence-based practice, especially among physiotherapists.

The following section provides an overview of systematic reviews of the effects of interventions aimed at changing professional health care practice. The overview is based on a high-quality evidence-based report (Grimshaw et al 2001), as well as systematic reviews and primary research published subsequently. One systematic review on guideline implementation in physiotherapy is described more in detail. Table 9.1 provides an overview of some relevant reviews on effects of specific interventions to improve practice. Many of the included trials are on implementation of guidelines. You need to bear in mind that the results are based mainly on studies carried out among physicians, but these studies constitute the best available evaluations of implementation strategies.

The title of a systematic review of implementation strategies published in 1995 declared there are 'no magic bullets' when it comes to translating research into practice (Oxman et al 1995). This still seems to be the case. Although no intervention seems to work in all settings, small to moderate improvements can be achieved by many interventions. Several interventions, such as audit and feedback, outreach visits, and educational workshops that involve discussion, reflection and practice, seem to be able to make modest to moderate improvements. Overall multifaceted intervention does not seem to provide better effect than single interventions.

Box 9.2 describes two examples of workplace initiatives designed to facilitate the implementation of evidence-based physiotherapy.

Implementing clinical guidelines

As outlined in Chapter 7, clinical guidelines can be and increasingly are used to improve physiotherapy practice and health care outcomes. Guidelines have the potential to improve quality and achieve better practice by promoting interventions of proven benefit and discouraging ineffective interventions. But do we know whether guidelines are worth the costs associated with their development and on implementation?

Although many countries have developed clinical guidelines in physiotherapy over recent years, very few have evaluated their impact on practice or health care outcome. In a systematic review of the effects of guideline implementation in physiotherapy (van der Wees et al 2008) only three studies were identified up to 2008. The studies evaluated strategies used to implement guidelines in low back pain and whiplash. All studies used multifaceted strategies including educational meetings to implement the guidelines. The studies are described in Table 9.2. The results varied across outcomes but showed some important improvement in outcomes such as 'limiting the number of treatment sessions' for low back pain (risk difference (RD) 0.13, 95% confidence interval (CI) 0.03 to 0.23), and 'using active intervention' (RD 0.13, 95% CI 0.05 to 0.21), 'reassuring the patient' (RD 0.40, 95% CI 0.07 to 0.74) and 'advising the patient to act as usual' in whiplash (RD 0.48, 95% CI 0.15 to 0.80). However, there was no evidence that patient health outcomes were improved or that the cost of care was reduced. The review concluded that multifaceted interventions based on educational meetings to increase implementation of clinical guidelines in physiotherapy may improve some outcomes of professional practice. These findings are comparable with results among other health professions.

Given the limited research on implementation of guidelines in physiotherapy, our impression is that physiotherapy bodies and groups have put a lot of effort and resources into the development process but very few have followed this up with systematic implementation and evaluation processes. In most cases the recommendations of clinical guidelines are passively diffused, or disseminated by post and in national physiotherapy publications. Some guidelines are available only by purchasing them from organizations. There are, however, some examples of more active implementation strategies. In Australia, the implementation of guidelines for low back pain was carried out as a 'road show' and a lot of marketing and advertising was put into the process. In the UK, physiotherapists identified as opinion leaders have been involved in guideline development processes. This is seen both as a strategy for improving the quality and relevance of the guidelines and as a way of

Table 9.1 Systematic reviews on interventions to promote professional behaviour change

Intervention	Reference	Conclusion
Printed educational materials	Farmer et al 2008 (23 included trials)	Printed educational materials when used alone may have a beneficial effect on process outcomes (overall absolute risk difference median of 4.3% on categorical process outcomes, range −8.0% to +9.6%). Despite this wide of range of effects reported, clinical significance of the observed effect sizes is not known. There is insufficient information about how to optimize educational materials. The effectiveness of educational materials compared with other interventions is uncertain
Continuing education meetings and workshops	Forsetlund et al 2009 (81 included trials)	Educational meetings alone or combined with other interventions can improve professional practice (median adjusted risk difference in compliance with desired practice was 6%, interquartile range 2% to 16%)
		There are large variations in the effects found in different studies
		Few studies have compared different types of educational meeting. No firm conclusions can be drawn about what is the most effective form
		The effect appears to be larger with higher attendance at the educational meetings and with mixed interactive and didactic educational meetings
Educational outreach visit (defined as a personal visit by a trained person to a health care provider in his or her own setting)	O'Brien et al 2007 (69 included trials)	Educational outreach visits alone or when combined with other interventions have small to moderate but potentially important effects (median risk difference 6%, interquartile range 3.0% to 10%)
		From this review it was not possible identify key characteristics of educational outreach visits that are important to their success
Computer reminders	Shojania et al 2009 (29 included trials)	Point of care computer reminders generally achieve small to modest improvements in provider behaviour (median 4% improvement, interquartile range 1% to 19%). A minority of interventions showed larger effects, but no specific reminder or contextual features were significantly associated with effect magnitude
Audit and feedback	Jamtvedt et al 2006 (118 included trials)	Audit and feedback alone or combined with other interventions can be effective in improving professional practice. When it is effective, the effects are generally small to moderate (median risk difference 5%, interquartile range 3% to 11%). The relative effectiveness of audit and feedback is likely to be greater when baseline adherence to recommended practice is low and when feedback is delivered more intensively
Local opinion leaders	Doumit et al 2007 (12 included trials)	The use of local opinion leaders can successfully promote evidence-based practice. Overall the median adjusted risk difference was 0.10, representing a 10% absolute decrease in non-compliance in the intervention group. However, the feasibility of its widespread use remains uncertain
Clinical pathways	Rotter et al 2010 (27 included trials)	Clinical pathways are associated with reduced in-hospital complications and improved documentation without negatively impacting on length of stay and hospital costs

Box 9.2

Examples of successful implementation

Example 1

In a community hospital in St Louis, Missouri, USA, the partnership between academic faculty members and a physical therapist at the hospital was used to develop a framework to implement an evidence-based journal club. The partnership blended the expertise of academic faculty members and a physical therapist with knowledge of evidence-based practice who served as the liaison between members of the partnership team and the clinicians at the community hospital. A three-step framework enabled the clinicians to learn about critical appraisal, participate in guided practice of critical appraisal with the liaison, and lead critical appraisal of a paper with the assistance of the liaison as needed (Austin et al 2009).

Example 2

Physiotherapists at the Bankstown-Lidcombe Hospital in Sydney, Australia, hold fortnightly meetings designed to promote evidence-based physiotherapy in their workplace. The meetings have three components:

1. Identification, by the group, of clinical questions that have arisen in the course of recent practice or from reading about emerging areas of practice. Staff, often working in pairs, are allocated the task of conducting a search, identifying key research reports, circulating copies of those reports to the group, and subsequently leading group discussions critically appraising the

research. The group aims to achieve consensus about the implications of the research for clinical practice. Once consensus is reached, discussions are held regarding how the practice will be implemented. Implementation strategies are finalized and tasks are delegated to team members. Reviews regarding adherence to the new practice are held in subsequent weeks.

2. A staff member assesses and treats a patient in the presence of two or three other therapists who use a checklist to record observations of the staff member's skills. After the session the observing therapists provide feedback on the staff member's performance.

3. A group of therapists collectively assesses and treats a patient with particularly difficult problems.

The three components of these meetings ensure both that practice is informed by high-quality clinical research and that staff have the skills necessary to implement evidence in practice. Several years of experience with this process suggests there are two critical features to its success. First, the meetings are timetabled into staff schedules and all staff are expected to attend and contribute. Second, a roster ensures that all staff (junior and senior) contribute to all aspects of the process (searching, leading discussions on critical appraisal, evaluation of clinical performance and discussion of difficult cases).

---

giving the guidelines credibility. However, we have not seen any formal evaluation of these activities.

There are many reasons why we do not see more robust evaluations of the effects on practice after guideline development and dissemination in physiotherapy. Lack of resources is certainly a common factor. Another reason might be a belief that passive dissemination of guidelines and presentation at conferences alone will have an impact on practice and change behaviour if needed. But we do not know whether this approach works among physiotherapists, and we have to admit we have limited knowledge of the effects of guidelines in physiotherapy. Just as specific physiotherapy interventions should be evaluated for their effect, there is a need to evaluate the effects of implementation strategies. Robust design is needed to see whether implementation strategies, or for that matter other quality improvement strategies, have an impact on practice or patients' health.

Grimshaw et al (2004) conducted a systematic review of the effectiveness and costs of different

guideline development, dissemination and implementation strategies in health care from studies published up to 1998. They identified 235 studies that evaluated guideline dissemination and implementation among medically qualified health care professionals. At that time no such study had been carried out in physiotherapy; indeed, 39% of the studies were carried out in primary care. Seventy-three per cent of the comparisons evaluated multifaceted interventions, defined as more than one implementation strategy. Commonly evaluated single interventions were reminders, dissemination of educational materials, and audit and feedback. The evidence base for the guideline recommendations was not clear in 94% of the studies.

Overall the majority of the studies observed improvements in care, but there were large variations both within and across interventions. The improvements were small to moderate, with a median improvement in measures of quality of care of 10% across all studies. One important result, that many will find surprising, is that multifaceted

Table 9.2 Characteristics of implementation trials in physiotherapy

Reference	Design	Intervention	Outcomes
Bekkering et al 2005	Cluster RCT 113 physiotherapists from 68 private clinics treated 500 patients with low back pain Follow-up: 12 months	*Intervention* Two interactive training sessions (2.5 hours each) with interval of 4 weeks, including didactic lecture and role-playing. Dissemination of guidelines, self-evaluation form, forms to facilitate discussion, copy of Quebec back pain disability scale	*Professional practice* Number of sessions Functional treatment goals Active interventions Adequate information All 4 outcomes met
		Control Dissemination of guidelines, self-evaluation form, forms to facilitate discussion, copy of Quebec back pain disability scale	*Patient outcomes* Physical functioning Pain
Rebbeck et al 2006	Cluster RCT 27 physiotherapists from 27 private clinics treated 103 patients with whiplash injury Follow-up: 12 months	*Intervention* One interactive educational session by opinion leaders (8 hours), including interactive sessions, practical sessions and problem-solving. Follow-up of educational outreach (2 hours) after 6 months. Dissemination of guidelines	*Professional practice* Knowledge test Functional outcomes Reassured patient Advised patient to act as usual Prescribe function Prescribe exercise Prescribe medication
		Control Dissemination of guidelines	*Patient outcomes* Disability (Functional Rating Index) Disability (Core Outcome measure) Global Perceived Effect
Stevenson et al 2006	Cluster RCT 30 physiotherapists treated 306 patients with low back pain Follow-up: 6 months	*Intervention* One interactive evidence-based educational session (5 hours), administered by local opinion leaders *Control* One standard in-service training session (5 hours) on clinical management of knee dysfunction	*Professional practice* Advice about work situation Advice return to normal activities Advice to increase activity level Encourage early return to work Encourage activities by themselves Change attitudes/beliefs about pain

RCT, randomized controlled trial.

interventions did not appear more effective than single interventions. Only 29% of the comparisons reported any economic data, and the majority of these reported only the cost of treatment. Very few studies reported costs of guideline development, dissemination or implementation.

The generalizability of the findings from this review to other behaviours, settings or professions is uncertain. Most studies provided no rationale for their choice of intervention and gave only limited descriptions of the interventions and contextual data (Grimshaw et al 2004). The authors of the review wrote that there is a need for a robust theoretical basis for understanding health care provider and organizational behaviour, and that future research is needed to develop a better theoretical base for the evaluation of guideline dissemination and implementation (Grimshaw et al 2004).

Evidence-based physiotherapy in the context of continuous quality improvement

Making evidence-based physiotherapy happen should benefit patients by providing them with better health outcomes. However, in the real world, implementation of evidence-based practice will not always deliver better health outcomes. The degree to which practice is based on evidence is only one dimension of quality improvement. Changes in practice might not be effective if they are implemented in a way that ignores the overall quality of the organizational system. Whether the 'organizational system' is a sole practitioner practice, a 1000-bed hospital, or a community service in a remote setting, there will always be a range of processes or pathways of care for patients. For example, a pathway could extend from the point of entry of a patient into the health care system, to the identification of needs, referral, tests (single or multiple), treatment by a single or team of practitioners, social support, identification of a longer-term plan or strategy for ongoing care or prevention of recurrence ... and so on. The pathway crosses departments and organizations horizontally – it is not hierarchical in nature. The physiotherapist's application of evidence-based physiotherapy needs to be seen in the context of, and must be sensitive to, the whole care pathway.

Good organizations strive continually to improve their processes of care (continuous quality improvement), and physiotherapists should engage in this process. Many of the interventions described in the previous section of this chapter can be used in continuous quality improvement activities.

Physiotherapists 'at the coalface' often know which services function best and what the problems with services are. They are therefore well placed to make improvements. A progressive organization will empower staff to identify the potential for improvement and instigate change. The culture of an organization is all-important. A good organization will have a culture of striving for improvement and places high importance on staff learning. Organizations should also emphasize the importance of involving patients in continuous quality improvement work. Systematic use of findings from surveys of patient experience and patient satisfaction reports should be used to improve quality in physiotherapy practice.

Continual improvement requires leaders who can support and nurture individuals and who believe that individuals want to do better, to learn and to develop. Donald Berwick, a pioneer of continuous quality improvement, once famously said, 'Every process is perfectly designed to achieve exactly the results it delivers,' which suggests that if a process is not working it ought to be changed.[1]

The theme of continuous improvement can also be applied at an individual practitioner level. As discussed at the beginning of this book, part of the responsibility attached to being an autonomous practitioner is a responsibility for keeping up to date and striving for improvement through learning. Physiotherapists can set up their own continuous improvement cycles through the measurement of their practice (audit, outcomes evaluation) and by reflective practice and peer review. We will discuss these more in Chapter 10.

---

[1]When a system is working well, it may be better not to change it (Oxman et al 2005).

References

Agency for Healthcare Research and Quality, 2004. Closing the quality gap: a critical analysis of quality improvement strategies. AHRQ, Rockville.

Austin, M.T., Richter, R.R., Frese, T., 2009. Using a partnership between academic faculty and a physical therapist liaison to develop a framework for an evidence-based journal club: a discussion. Physiother. Res. Int. 14, 213–223.

Bandura, A., 1997. Self-efficacy: towards a unifying theory of behaviour change. Psychol. Rev. 84, 191–215.

Barnard, S., Wiles, R., 2001. Evidence-based physiotherapy. Physiotherapy 87, 115–124.

Bekkering, G.E., Engers, A.J., Wensing, M., et al., 2003. Development of an implementation strategy for physiotherapy guidelines on low back pain. Aust. J. Physiother. 49, 208–214.

Bekkering, G.E., Hendriks, H.J., van Tulder, M.W., et al., 2005. Effect on the process of care of an active strategy to implement clinical guidelines on physiotherapy for low

back pain: a cluster randomised controlled trial. Qual. Saf. Health Care 14, 107–112.

Bradley, P., Nordheim, L., De La Harpe, D., et al., 2005. A systematic review of qualitative literature on educational interventions for Evidence Based Practice. Learning in Health and Social Care 4 (2), 89–109.

Bridges, P.H., Bierema, L.L., Valentine, T., 2007. The propensity to adopt evidence-based practice among physical therapists. BMC Health Serv. Res. 7, 103.

Coomarasamy, A., Khan, K.S., 2004. What is the evidence that postgraduate teaching in evidence based medicine changes anything? A systematic review. BMJ 329, 1017–1021.

Doumit, G., Gattellari, M., Grimshaw, J., et al., 2007. Local opinion leaders: effects on professional practice and health care outcomes. Cochrane Database Syst. Rev. 1, CD000125.

Farmer, A.P., Légaré, F., Turcot, L., et al., 2008. Printed educational materials: effects on professional practice and health care outcomes. Cochrane Database Syst. Rev. 3, CD004398.

Flores-Mateo, G., Argimon, J.M., 2007. Evidence based practice education in postgraduate health care: a systematic review. BMC Health Serv. Res. 7, 119.

Forsetlund, L., Bjørndal, A., Rashidian, A., et al., 2009. Continuing education meetings and workshops: effects on professional practice and health care outcomes. Cochrane Database Syst. Rev. 2, CD003030.

Freeman, A.C., Sweeney, C., 2001. Why general practitioners do not implement evidence: qualitative study. BMJ 323, 1100.

Green, L., Kreuter, M., Deeds, S., 1980. Health education planning: a diagnostic approach. Mayfield, Mountain View, CA.

Grimshaw, J.M., Shirran, L., Thomas, R., et al., 2001. Changing provider behaviour. An overview of systematic reviews of interventions. Med. Care 39 (Suppl 2), II2–II45.

Grimshaw, J.M., Thomas, R., Maclennan, G., et al., 2004. Effectiveness and efficiency of guideline dissemination and implementation strategies. Health Technol. Assess. 8 (6), 1–72.

Humphris, D., Littlejohns, P., Victor, C.J., et al., 2000. Implementing evidence-based practice: factors that influence the use of research evidence by occupational therapists. Br. J. Occup. Ther. 11, 516–522.

Jamtvedt, G., Young, J.M., Kristoffersen, D.T., et al., 2006. Audit and feedback: effects on professional practice and health care outcomes. Cochrane Database Syst. Rev. 2, CD000259.

Kotler, P., 1983. Social marketing of health behaviour. In: Fredriksen, L., Solomon, L., Brehony, K. (Eds.), Marketing health behaviour: principles, techniques and applications. Plenum Press, New York, pp. 23–29.

Lomas, J., 1993. Diffusion, dissemination, and implementation: who should do what? Ann. N. Y. Acad. Sci. 703, 226–235.

Marcus, B.H., Emmons, K.M., Simkin-Silverman, et al., 1998. Motivationally tailored vs standard self-help physical activity interventions at the workplace: a prospective randomized, controlled trial. Am. J. Health Promot. 12 (4), 246–253.

Metcalfe, C., Lewin, R., Wisher, S., et al., 2001. Barriers to implementing the evidence base in four NHS therapies. Physiotherapy 87, 433–441.

O'Brien, M.A., Rogers, S., Jamtvedt, G., et al., 2007. Educational outreach visits: effects on professional practice and health care outcomes. Cochrane Database Syst. Rev. 4, CD000409.

Oxman, A., Flottorp, S., 1998. An overview of strategies to promote implementation of evidence based health care. In: Silagy, C., Haines, A. (Eds.), Evidence based practice in primary care. BMJ Books, London, pp. 91–109.

Oxman, A.D., Thomson, M.A., Davis, D.A., et al., 1995. No magic bullets: a systematic review of 102 trials of interventions to improve professional practice. Can. Med. Assoc. J. 153 (10), 1423–1431.

Oxman, A.D., Sackett, D.L., Chalmers, I., et al., 2005. A surrealistic mega-analysis of redisorganization theories. J. R. Soc. Med. 98, 563–568.

Parkes, J., Hyde, C., Deeks, J.J., et al., 2001. Teaching critical appraisal skills in health care settings. Cochrane Database Syst. Rev. 3, CD001270.

Pollock, A., Legg, L., Langhorne, P., et al., 2000. Barriers to achieving evidence-based stroke rehabilitation. Clin. Rehabil. 14, 611–617.

Prochaska, J.O., Velicer, W.F., 1997. The transtheoretical model of health behavior change. Am. J. Health Promot. 12 (1), 38–48.

Rebbeck, T., Maher, C.G., Refshauge, K.M., 2006. Evaluating two implementation strategies for whiplash guidelines in physiotherapy: a cluster randomised trial. Aust. J. Physiother. 52, 165–174.

Riemsma, P.R., Pattenden, J., Bridle, C., et al., 2003. Systematic review of effectiveness of stage based interventions to promote smoking cessation. BMJ 326, 1175–1177.

Rogers, E., 1995. Diffusion of innovation, fourth ed. Free Press, New York.

Rotter, T., Kinsman, L., James, E., et al., 2010. Clinical pathways: effects on professional practice, patient outcomes, length of stay and hospital costs. Cochrane Database Syst. Rev. 3, CD006632.

Shojania, K.G., Jennings, A., Mayhew, A., et al., 2009. The effects of on-screen, point of care computer reminders on processes and outcomes of care. Cochrane Database Syst. Rev. 3, CD001096.

Stevenson, K., Lewis, M., Hay, E., 2006. Does physiotherapy management of low back pain change as a result of an evidence-based educational programme? J. Eval. Clin. Pract. 12, 365–375.

van der Wees, P.J., Jamtvedt, G., Rebbeck, T., et al., 2008. Multifaceted strategies may increase implementation of physiotherapy clinical guidelines: a systematic review. Aust. J. Physiother. 54, 233–241.

Young, J., Ward, J.E., 2001. Evidence-based medicine in general practice: beliefs and barriers among Australian GPs. J. Eval. Clin. Pract. 7, 201–210.

Am I on the right track?

10

CHAPTER CONTENTS

Overview 161

Assessing patient outcomes:
clinical measurement 161

   How can we interpret measurements
   of outcome? 162

Assessing the process of care: audit 164

   Audit of clinical practice 164
   Clinical audit 164
   Peer review 166
   Reflective practice 166
   Audit of the process by which
   questions are answered 166

Concluding comment 168

References 168

OVERVIEW

In this chapter we consider how physiotherapists can evaluate their practice. Evaluation could involve evaluation of either outcomes or process of practice. Measurement of outcomes potentially provides some insights into the effectiveness of practice. However, clinical measures of outcome need to be interpreted cautiously because they are potentially misleading. We argue that clinical measures of outcome are most useful when there is little strong evidence for the effects of intervention and when outcomes are extreme (either very good or very poor). When the evidence is strong, or when outcomes are less extreme, it is more useful to evaluate processes. Evaluation of the process of clinical practice could involve a formal process audit, peer review of clinical performance, or reflective practice. Finally, we consider the audit of the steps of practising evidence-based physiotherapy, discussed in Chapter 1.

The process of evidence-based physiotherapy begins and ends by questioning one's own practice. Having asked a clinical question, sought out and critically appraised evidence, and implemented evidence-based practice, it is constructive to reflect on whether the process was carried out well and produced the best outcome for the patient. We refer to this as evaluation.

In this chapter we separately consider how to evaluate the *outcomes* of evidence-based practice and to audit the *process*.

Assessing patient outcomes: clinical measurement

Historically, outcome measurement was not a feature of routine clinical practice. Physiotherapists (and, for that matter, most other health professionals) did not systematically collect data on patients' outcomes. Typically, physiotherapists obtained information about the effectiveness of their practice incidentally, from their impressions of clinical outcomes or from patients' comments about their satisfaction (or dissatisfaction) with physiotherapy services.

In more recent times there has been pressure on physiotherapists to become more accountable for their practices. The pressure has come from makers of health care policies, those who allocate and fund health care (government, insurers, managers), and from within the physiotherapy profession. One of the driving forces has been the perception that physiotherapists must justify what they do. It is thought that by providing evidence of good clinical outcomes physiotherapists can demonstrate that what they do is worthwhile.

In the last two decades the physiotherapy profession has taken up the call for more and better clinical measurement. An early landmark was the publication, in 1985, of *Measurement in Physical Therapy* (Rothstein 1985). More recently, there has been a proliferation of textbooks, journal features and websites documenting clinical outcome measures and their measurement properties (Finch et al 2002, Koke et al 1999, Maher et al 2000, Wade 1992; see also the excellent website and on-line database produced by the Chartered Society of Physiotherapy at http://www.csp.org.uk/director/members/practice/clinicalresources/outcomemeasures.cfm and the regular feature entitled *Clinimetrics* in the *Journal of Physiotherapy*). In some countries at least, a large proportion of physiotherapists routinely document clinical outcomes using validated tools. In New South Wales, Australia, the public provider of rehabilitation services for work-related injuries pays an additional fee to practitioners who adequately document measures of clinical outcomes.

The evolution of a culture in which physiotherapists routinely measure clinical outcomes with validated tools may well have produced an increase in the effectiveness of physiotherapy practice, because systematic collection of outcome data focuses both patients and therapists on outcomes. To our knowledge, however, there have been no randomized trials of the effects of routine measures of outcomes on outcomes of care.

Perhaps it is unfortunate that the physiotherapy profession has responded to the perception that physiotherapists must justify what they do by routinely measuring clinical outcomes. The implication is that measures of outcome can provide justification for intervention. Arguably that is not the case.

How can we interpret measurements of outcome?

Outcome measures measure outcomes. They do not measure the effects of intervention. Outcomes of interventions and effects of interventions are very different things.

In Chapter 3 we saw that clinical outcomes are influenced by many factors other than intervention, including the natural course of the condition, statistical regression, placebo effects, polite patient effects, and so on. The implication is that a good outcome does not necessarily indicate that intervention was effective (because a good outcome may have occurred even without intervention). And a poor outcome does not necessarily indicate that intervention was ineffective (because the outcome may have been worse still without intervention). Consequently, we look to randomized trials to find out about the effects of intervention. This implies a belief that clinical outcome measures should not be relied upon to provide dependable information about the effectiveness of interventions. It is illogical, on the one hand, to look to randomized controlled trials for evidence of effects of interventions, while on the other hand to seek justification for the effectiveness of clinical practice with uncontrolled measurement of clinical outcomes.

Taken further, this line of reasoning suggests that, at least in some circumstances, measures of a patient's clinical outcome should have no role in influencing decisions about treatment for that patient. According to this view, randomized trials provide better information about the effects of intervention than measures of clinical outcomes. So decisions about intervention for a particular patient should be based entirely on the findings of randomized trials, without regard to the apparent effects of treatment suggested by measures of clinical outcome on that patient. For example, if a randomized trial suggests that, on average, an intervention produces effects that a patient considers would be worthwhile, the implication is that intervention should continue to be offered even if the patient's outcomes are poor. The reasoning goes that the best we can know of the effects of a treatment (from randomized trials) tells us that this intervention typically produces clinically worthwhile effects. The patient may be one of the unlucky patients who does not benefit from (or is harmed by) this intervention, or it may be that the patient's poor outcomes might have been worse still without the intervention. We cannot discriminate between these scenarios, so we act on the basis of what we think is most likely to be true: on average the intervention is helpful. Consequently we continue to provide the intervention, even though the outcome of intervention is poor.

This view is completely antithetical to the empirical approach to clinical practice exemplified by some authors (notably Maitland et al 2001). In the fully empirical approach, intervention is always followed by assessment. If outcomes improve, the intervention may be continued until the problem is completely resolved. If outcomes do not improve, or worsen, the intervention is modified or discontinued. This approach appears to be reasonable, but it involves making clinical decisions on the basis of information that is very difficult to interpret. The empirical approach, in which clinical decisions are based on careful measurement of outcomes, is not evidence-based physiotherapy. If we base clinical decisions about intervention exclusively on high-quality clinical research, measures of clinical outcome can have little role in clinical decision-making or in justifying clinical practice. Interventions can be recommended without consideration of their outcomes.

Is there any role for clinical outcome measures in clinical decision-making? We think that, when there is evidence of effects of intervention from high-quality clinical trials, a sensible approach to clinical decision-making lies somewhere between the two extremes of the fully empirical approach and a hard-line approach in which clinical decision-making is based only on high-quality clinical research without regard to outcome.[1] As a consequence, extreme clinical observations (very good or very poor outcomes) are likely to be 'real' (bias is unlikely to have qualitatively altered the clinical picture). On the other hand, the qualitative interpretation of typical observations (small improvements in outcome) could plausibly be altered by bias.

> In other words, this approach suggests that clinical decision-making should be influenced by observations of very good and very poor outcomes, but should not be influenced by less extreme observations.

What does this mean in practice? It means, first of all, that there is value in careful measurement of clinical outcomes, because extreme clinical outcomes influence clinical decision-making. It also means that the degree of regard we pay to measures of clinical outcomes depends on how extreme the outcomes are. When outcomes are *very* poor we *should* discontinue the intervention, even if the best clinical trials tell us that the intervention is, on average, effective: a *very* poor outcome is unlikely to be explicable only by

confounding effects such as the natural course of the condition, statistical regression, polite patients and so on – it probably also reflects that this person truly responded poorly to the intervention. On the other hand, less extreme poor outcomes might reasonably be ignored, and an intervention might be persisted with, regardless of moderately poor outcome, if the best clinical trials provide strong evidence that the intervention produces, on average, a clinically worthwhile effect.[2] In all circumstances, clinical decision-making should be informed by patients' preferences and values.

Clinical outcome measures become more important when there is little or no evidence from high-quality randomized trials. In that case, the alternatives are either not to intervene at all, or to intervene in the absence of high-quality evidence and use (potentially misleading) clinical outcome measures to guide decisions about intervention. In contrast, when there is clear evidence of the effects of an intervention from high-quality clinical trials, clinical outcome measures become relatively unimportant and measures of the process of care become more useful.

> When evidence of effects of interventions is strong, we should use process audit to evaluate practice. When there is little or no evidence (i.e. when practice cannot be evidence based) we should use measures of clinical outcomes to evaluate practice.

The preceding discussion assumes that it is not possible rigorously to establish the effects of therapy on a single patient. But, as we saw in Chapter 4, there is one exception: single-case experimental designs (n-of-1 studies) can establish, with a high degree of rigour, the effects of intervention on a single patient. Unfortunately, n-of-1 trials are difficult to conduct as part of routine clinical practice and are, at any rate, suited only to certain conditions (see Chapter 4). A more practical approach is to use less rigorous designs, such as the so-called ABA' design. In ABA' designs, the patient's condition is monitored prior to intervention (period A), during intervention (period B) and following intervention (period A'). The magnitude of the improvement seen in the transition from period A to period B and the magnitude of the decline seen in the transition from period B to

---

[1]The essence of this approach is that it recognizes that person-to-person variability in response to an intervention is likely to be far greater than the bias in inferences about effects of interventions based on measures of clinical outcome. The degree of person-to-person variability can be estimated from randomized trials when it can reasonably be assumed that outcomes of participants in the intervention group are not correlated with the outcomes that the same participants would have obtained if they had not received the intervention (Bell et al 2008).

[2]This theoretical position may be very difficult to maintain in practice. It could be hard to continue a treatment that you expect is effective if clinical observations suggest it is not. And, conversely, it could be hard to resist provision of a treatment when outcomes associated with the treatment are good.

period A′ provide an indication of the effect of intervention on that patient, although this approach should be considered less rigorous than properly designed n-of-1 trials. Smith et al (2004) provide a nice example of how the ABA′ approach can be used in practice, in this case to test the effects of low-Dye taping on plantar fasciitis pain.

Before completing the discussion of the role of clinical measurement, we note that there is another role for measurement of outcomes, other than its limited role in telling us about the effects of intervention. Routine standardized outcome measurements potentially provide us with other useful data. They can be used to generate practice-specific estimates of prognosis. For example, a physiotherapist who routinely assesses the presence or absence of shoulder pain in stroke patients at discharge following an upper limb rehabilitation programme can use those data to generate practice-specific prognoses about the risk of developing shoulder pain by the time of discharge. It is important to recognize that these data have useful prognostic value, but they do not provide good evidence of the effectiveness or otherwise of intervention.

We have argued that clinical outcome measures have two roles. First, they provide limited information about the effects of an intervention on a particular patient; such measures are most useful when there is little or no evidence of the effects of intervention and when extreme outcomes are observed. Second, if standardized outcome data are collected routinely, they potentially provide practice-specific prognostic data. Where physiotherapists measure clinical outcomes for these purposes they ought to use appropriate measurement tools. That is, they should choose tools that are reliable (precise) and valid. We will not consider how to ascertain whether a clinical measurement tool has these properties, as that is the topic of other, more authoritative, texts (Feinstein 1987, Rothstein 1985, Streiner & Norman 2003).

Assessing the process of care: audit

Audit of clinical practice

Clinical audit

Clinical audit has been defined as a 'quality improvement process that seeks to improve patient care and outcomes through systematic review of care against explicit criteria and the implementation of change' (National Institute for Clinical Excellence 2002: 1). Put simply, audit is a method of comparing what is actually happening in clinical practice against agreed standards or guidelines. Audit criteria should be based on high-quality clinical research. As we saw earlier in this chapter, when evidence of the effects of an intervention is strong, audit of process is a more appropriate way to evaluate practice than the use of measures of clinical outcome.

Clinical audit is a cyclical process. The key components of the process are:

- The setting of explicit standards or criteria for practice
- Measurement of actual performance against the pre-determined criteria
- Review of performance, based on the measurements
- Agreement about what practice improvements are needed (if any)
- Action taken to implement agreed improvements
- Measurement of actual performance repeated to confirm improvement (or not)
- Continuation of the cycle.

We present an evidence-based audit cycle in Figure 10.1, which includes all the components discussed above. Additionally, it includes a requirement that the standards or criteria (the foundation of the audit process) have been developed from evidence derived from high-quality clinical research, following the steps described in this book. This means that, if there is adherence with the standards and criteria, practice will be based on an evidence-based process of care.

Audit of practice can be carried out by the individual practitioner (self-audit), but is better undertaken by someone else so that the data are collected systematically, objectively and without bias. Usually, the source of the data is the patient or physiotherapy record. The auditor (or data collector) examines a sample of records to see whether practice, as recorded, has met the evidence-based standards or criteria. The data are then used to review practice, and there is consideration of the extent to which practice adhered to the criteria. If there was a discrepancy between the criteria and then practice, there is consideration of why this occurred. An action plan, or recommendations, can then be drawn up and implemented, after which a further data collection exercise can be carried out to see whether adherence improves.

Figure 10.1 • An evidence-based audit cycle.

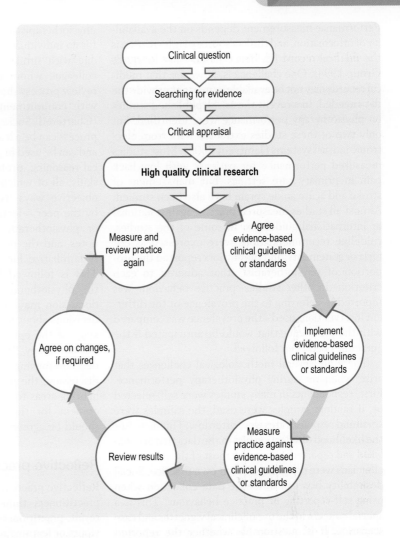

An audit process can be used to describe quality of care by assessing whether the recommendations from high-quality clinical guideline are being adhered to. Here, the guideline recommendations provide the basis for criteria against which to measure clinical practice. Assessing whether practice is evidence based is closely linked to measuring *performance*. Measuring performance refers to the measurement of actual clinical practice and comparing it to desired clinical practice (Akl et al 2007). The aim of performance measurement is to collect the minimum amount of information needed to determine how well health care professionals are performing and whether practice can be improved.

It is often important to measure baseline performance prior to instituting interventions designed to improve performance. This helps to:

- Justify a quality improvement intervention by demonstrating a gap between actual and desired clinical practice.
- Estimate the magnitude of the problem. Low baseline performance indicates there is much room for improvement, whereas high baseline performance indicates there is little room for improvement (ceiling effect).
- Identify practice patterns and the factors that determine them; you can use these factors to tailor intervention.
- Use measurements as part of an intervention involving feedback.
- Assess the impact of the intervention by comparing pre (baseline) and post-intervention performances.

Performance measurement depends on the availability of information, and the key source of information is the medical record (Evidence-Based Care Resource Group 1994). One challenge is, however, that medical records may not be available or may not provide the data needed. In a recent thesis, 11 published studies on physiotherapy performance were identified, but only two of these studies extracted data from electronic journal systems (Jamtvedt 2009). Most studies measured performance for patients with low back pain in primary care settings, but management of stroke and acute ankle sprain have also been studied. Almost all studies measured practice against national or international guidelines. In some of the studies, guideline recommendations were expressed as criteria or statements, and the authors reported the proportion of physiotherapists that adhered to each criterion. In other studies, practice behaviour was reported by referring to the prevalence of the different interventions used – the prevalence was compared with the prevalence that would be anticipated if the guidelines had been followed.

There are several methodological challenges that arise when measuring physiotherapy performance. First, respondents in many studies were self-selected or, if random samples were used, the samples were small and response rates were often low. This increases the likelihood of selection bias in the data that are analysed and reported. Second, in most of the studies the clinicians were reporting on their own practice. Social desirability bias can influence data collection when using self-reporting of practice behaviour. This is a special concern in the use of clinical vignettes and case scenarios. It is questionable whether the reported practice based on clinical vignettes and case scenarios reflects actual practice on real patients.

More commonly, audit of a service is carried out as part of an organization's quality assurance systems. This can provide valuable feedback to individual physiotherapists about their use of evidence in practice. The greatest impact for patients will occur in organizations where there is a culture of continuous improvement and willingness to change. Still, it is necessary to evaluate the impact of quality improvement activities on process and patient outcomes, and there is an ongoing debate on how such evaluations should be conducted (Øvretveit & Gustafson 2003).

Peer review

Another form of audit is peer review, which is assessment of clinical performance undertaken by another physiotherapist (a peer). It provides an opportunity for an individual's practice to be evaluated by someone with similar experience, ideally by a trusted colleague whom the individual has selected. The review process should be approached by both parties with commitment and integrity, as well as trust (Chartered Society of Physiotherapy 2000). The process can be a learning opportunity for both parties and can be used in particular to enhance skills in clinical reasoning, professional judgement and reflective skills, all of which are difficult to evaluate in more objective ways. Normally reviews are carried out by the peer selecting a random set of patient notes or physiotherapy records. The peer reviews the notes, and the physiotherapist being reviewed may re-familiarize himself or herself with the records. This is followed by a discussion that focuses on the physiotherapist's clinical reasoning skills. The discussion may consider assessment and diagnosis, decisions about intervention, and evaluation of each stage of the episode of care (Chartered Society of Physiotherapy 2000). The use of evidence to support decision-making can also be reviewed. Following discussion, the peer has the responsibility for highlighting areas for further training, learning or development for the individual. A timed action plan should be agreed upon.

Reflective practice

Reflective practice is a professional activity in which practitioners think critically about practice. As a result, practitioners may modify their actions, behaviours or learning needs. Reflective practice involves reviewing episodes of practice to describe, analyse and evaluate activity. It enables learning at a subconscious level to be brought to a level where it can be articulated and shared with others. The opportunity to re-think practices becomes a tool for professional learning and contributes to an individual's practice knowledge and clinical expertise (Gamble et al 2001).

Audit of the process by which questions are answered

We hope this book will encourage you to practise evidence-based physiotherapy so that you become not only a reader of research but also a user of high-quality clinical research. As we have seen, evidence-based physiotherapy involves formulating questions, searching for evidence, critical appraisal, implementation and evaluation.

One way of evaluating your performance is to reflect on questions related to each step of the process of evidence-based practice. This part of the chapter will describe the domains in which you might want to evaluate your performance. A summary is found in Box 10.1. Sackett and colleagues (2000) provide further reading on this issue.

To become a user of research you first have to acknowledge your information needs and reflect on your practice. This implies a process that might start with raising awareness and discussing different sources of information, and concludes by framing questions and by finding and applying evidence. Do you think there is a need for high-quality clinical research to inform physiotherapy practice? Do you challenge your colleagues by asking what they base their practice on?

You can also evaluate your performance by asking questions. One way of doing this is by recording the questions you ask and checking whether the questions were answerable and translated into a search for literature. In our experience, when physiotherapists have learned that there are different types of question, asking and searching become much easier. When you become more skilled in formulating questions, you might also start trying to find answers to your colleagues questions and promoting an 'asking environment' in your workplace.

To be able to carry out searches for evidence you need to have access to an information infrastructure. A first step might be to get access to the internet so you can search PEDro, PubMed and, in some countries, the Cochrane Library (see Chapter 4). Refine your search strategies, for example by routinely looking first for systematic reviews. You might need to improve your searching performance by asking a librarian. Librarians are useful people and very important collaborators for evidence-based practice. Perhaps you need to undertake a course to update your literature searching skills, or ask a librarian to repeat a search that you have already done, and compare that with yours.

Next, consider how you read papers. Do you start by assessing the validity of the study (see Chapter 5), or do you only read the conclusion? Reading and discussing a paper together with peers is useful, and can be fun, and you can learn a lot. Do you have a journal club at your workplace? Different checklists are available as useful tools for appraisal. Do you know where to find checklists for different kinds of study? By reading more studies (and this book) you will become more skilled in interpreting measures of effect (see Chapter 6). Do you feel more confident

---

Box 10.1

Evaluating performance of the process of evidence-based physiotherapy

Reflection on practice/raising awareness

- Do I ask myself why I do the things I do at work?
- Do I discuss with colleagues the basis for our clinical decisions?

Asking questions

- Do I ask clinical questions?
- Do I ask well formulated questions?
- Do I classify questions into different types (effect of interventions, prognosis, aetiology, etc.)?
- Do I encourage my colleagues to ask questions?

Searching for evidence

- Do I search for evidence?
- Do I know the best sources for different types of question?
- Do I have ready access to the internet?
- Am I becoming more efficient in my searching?
- Do I start by searching for systematic reviews?

Critical appraisal

- Do I read papers at all?
- Do I use critical appraisal guides or checklists for different designs?
- Have I improved my interpretation of effect estimates (e.g. number needed to treat)?
- Do I promote the reading of research articles at my workplace?

Implementing high-quality clinical research

- Do I use high-quality research to inform or change my practice?
- Do I use this approach to help resolve disagreement with colleagues about the management of a problem?

Self-evaluation

- Have I audited my evidence-based practice-performance?

in reading and applying the results that are presented in research papers?

The most important question of all is perhaps this one: 'Do I use the findings from high-quality research to improve my practice?' If you go through the steps without applying relevant high-quality research to practice then you may have wasted time and resources. If this has happened, consider what barriers prevented you from using research in practice (see Chapter 9). As outlined in Chapter 1, research alone does not make decisions so there can be many legitimate reasons for not practising as the evidence suggests you should. Informed health care decisions are made by integrating research, patient preferences and practice knowledge, so that practice is informed by high-quality clinical research but adapted to a specific setting or individual patient. This can be regarded as the optimal outcome of evidence-based practice.

Concluding comment

Evaluation satisfies more than a technical requirement for quantifying the quality and effects of care. It also provides an opportunity for reflecting on practice. With routine self-reflection, physiotherapists should be better able to combine evidence from high-quality research with patient preferences and practice knowledge, so they should be better practitioners of evidence-based physiotherapy.

References

Akl, E.A., Treweek, S., Foy, R., et al., 2007. NorthStar, a support tool for the design and evaluation of quality improvement interventions in healthcare. Implementation Science: IS 2, 19.

Bell, K.J.L., Irwig, L., Craig, J.C., et al., 2008. Use of randomised trials to decide when to monitor response to new treatment. BMJ 336, 361–365.

Chartered Society of Physiotherapy, 2000. Clinical audit tools. In: Standards of physiotherapy practice pack. CSP, London, pp. 1–56.

Evidence-Based Care Resource Group, 1994. Evidence-based care: 3. Measuring performance: How are we managing this problem? CMAJ 150, 1575–1579.

Feinstein, A.R., 1987. Clinimetrics. Yale University Press, New Haven.

Finch, E., Brooks, D., Stratford, P., et al., 2002. Physical rehabilitation outcome measures: a guide to enhanced clinical decision making, second ed. Lippincott, Williams and Wilkins, Philadelphia.

Gamble, J., Chan, P., Davey, H., 2001. Reflection as a tool for developing professional practice knowledge and expertise. In: Higgs, J., Titchen, A. (Eds.), Practice knowledge and expertise in the health professions. Butterworth-Heinemann, Oxford, pp. 121–127.

Jamtvedt, G., 2009. Physiotherapy in patients with knee osteoarthritis. In: Clinical practice compared to findings from systematic reviews. Thesis. Faculty of Medicine, University of Oslo.

Koke, A.J.A., Heuts, P.H.T.G., Vlaeyen, J.W.S., et al., 1999. Meetinstrumenten chronische pijn. Deel 1 functionele status. Pijn Kennis Centrum S, Maastricht.

Maher, C., Latimer, J., Refshauge, K., 2000. Atlas of clinical tests and measures for low back pain. Australian Physiotherapy Association, Melbourne.

Maitland, G.D., Hengeveld, E., Banks, K., et al., 2001. Maitland's vertebral manipulation. Butterworth-Heinemann, Oxford.

National Institute for Clinical Excellence, 2002. Principles for best practice in clinical audit. Radcliffe Medical Press, Abingdon.

Øvretveit, J., Gustafson, D., 2003. Using research to inform quality programmes. BMJ 326, 759–761.

Rothstein, J.M. (Ed.), 1985. Measurement in physical therapy. Churchill Livingstone, New York.

Sackett, D.L., Straus, S.E., Richardson, W., et al., 2000. Evidence-based medicine: how to practice and teach EBM. Churchill Livingstone, Edinburgh.

Smith, M., Brooker, S., Vicenzino, B., et al., 2004. Use of antipronation taping to assess suitability of orthotic prescription: case report. Aust. J. Physiother. 50, 111–113.

Streiner, D.L., Norman, G.R., 2003. Health measurement scales: a practical guide to their development and use. Oxford University Press, Oxford.

Wade, D.T., 1992. Measurement in neurological rehabilitation. Oxford University Press, Oxford.

Index

NB: Page numbers in *italics* refer to boxes, figures and tables.

A

ABA' designs 163–164
Absolute risk reduction (ARR) 108, *109, 110, 111*
Active dissemination, stage 6 new therapy protocol 146
Aetiology 11
AGREE (Appraisal of Guidelines, Research and Evaluation) Collaboration 138, *138, 139*
see also Critical appraisal
Allocation
  bias 20
  blinding 71–76
  haphazard 66
AMED (Allied and Complementary Medicine Database) 78
American Psychological Association 75
Analysis
  by intention to treat 70, 71
  data 83–84, *84*
  detailed 95–96
  stratified 120–121
  sub-group 95–96
  see also Meta-analysis
Anterior drawer test 130, *131*
Assessment 161–168
  measurement interpretation 162–164
  patient outcomes 167
  process audit 163, 164–168, *167*
Assessors, blinding 71–76
Audit, process 163, 164–168, *167*
Australian Physiotherapy Association (APA) 58

B

Bandura's social cognitive theory 151–152
Baseline risk 113–114
Behaviour, stage models 151–152
  see also Professional behaviour change
Benefit-harm trade-off method 103
Berwick, Donald 159
Best practice 136–137
Bias
  allocation/selection 20
  diagnostic tests 89
  guidelines 137, 140
  measurement 75
  missing data 68–69
  recall 17–18, *18*
Blinding 71–76
  diagnostic tests 88–89, *90*
  double-blinding 75, 76, 80
BMJ BestPractice 40–41, 58
Browsing, electronic databases *59, 60*

C

Campbell Collaboration 30
Case series, effects of intervention 19–21
Case-control studies 33–34, 89
Category foundation 123
Cates' plot *109*
Cause-effect interpretations 17–18
Centre for Evidence-Based Physiotherapy 78

Change 150–153
  barriers to 152–153
  theories of 150–152
CINAHL (Cumulative Index to Nursing and Allied Health Literature) *52,* 55
  clinical guidelines 137
  experiences 55–56, *56, 56*
  prognosis 51–52
  randomized trials 78, 79
Classical model 151
Clinical audit 164–166, *165*
  key components 164
Clinical decision-making 163
  factors influencing 3
  model 2
  process 3–4
Clinical exploration, stage 2 new therapy protocol 146
Clinical guidelines 135–142
  critical appraisal 138–141
  defined 135–136
  developers 138–140, 141
  history/importance 136–137
  implementation 155–158, *158*
  key processes 137
  locating 137–138
  vs systematic reviews *136*
Clinical measurement 161–164
  interpreting 162–164
Clinical observation
  diagnostic tests 32–33
  effects of intervention 16–18, *18*
  experiences 26–27

Clinical observation (*Continued*)
  prognosis 30
  stage 1 new therapy protocol 146
Clinical practice *see* Practice relevance
Clinical questions 9–13
  categorization *10*
  preclinical 11
  process audit 166–168, *167*
  refining 11–13
  relevant 9–11
Clinical reasoning 3–4
Clinical research 5
  diagnostic tests 33–34
  effects of intervention 19–23
  experiences 27–29
  practice gap 5
  prognosis 30–32
  see also High-quality clinical research
Clinical trials, prognosis 31–32
Cluster randomized trials 21–22
Cochrane Back Review Group 80
Cochrane Central Register of Controlled
     Trials (CENTRAL) 48–51
Cochrane Collaboration 5, 80
  diagnostic tests 34–35
  Effective Practice and Organization
     of Care (EPOC) 154, *154*
  effects of intervention 24–25, 30
  Register of Clinical Trials
     (CENTRAL) 78, 79
  systematic reviews 114
Cochrane Database of Systematic
     Reviews (CDSR) 48–51
Cochrane Library 34–35, *57, 58, 167*
  effects of intervention 48–51, *51*
  wild cards 42
Cochrane Qualitative Methods Group 30
Cochrane Review Groups 5
Cohort studies 33, 89
  inception 84, 85–86
  prospective/retrospective 31
Confidence intervals 104–107, *105,
     107, 110, 111, 119,* 121–122,
     126, *127*
Confounding effects of intervention
     16–18
Consecutive cases 84–85, 86
Consolidated Standards of Reporting
     Trials (CONSORT) 69, 121
Contingent valuation 103
Continuous outcomes 100–107, 125
Continuous quality improvement 159
Control groups vs intervention groups
     65–67

Controlled trials
  effects of intervention 19–21
  prognosis 31–32
Critical appraisal 61–92
  approach 97
  clinical guidelines 138–141
  diagnostic tests *81,* 87–89
  effects of intervention 64–81,
     76
  experiences 81–84, *84*
  process 62–64, *63*
  prognosis 84–87, *87*
  see also Practice relevance
Critically Appraised Papers (CAPs)
     59, 60
Crossover trials 21–22
Cross-sectional studies, diagnostic tests
     33–34
Cultural influences 3

D

Data
  analysis 83–84, *84*
  collection 82–83, *84*
Database of Abstracts of Reviews
     of Effects (DARE) 48–51
Databases *see* Electronic databases
Decision support tools 40–41
Decision-making *see* Clinical
     decision-making
Delphi technique 64
Descriptive model 151
Development phase, new therapy
     protocol *145,* 146
Diagnosis
  likelihood ratios 129–132
  questions 12–13
  taxonomies 94–95
  uncertainty 89, *90*
Diagnostic tests, studies
  critical appraisal *81,* 87–89
  electronic databases 51–55
  individual *81,* 88–89
  practice relevance 127–132
  research, types of 32–35
Dichotomous outcomes 99–100,
     107–114, *110,* 125
Dichotomous scale 118
Diffusion of Innovation Theory (Rogers)
     151
Dissemination 154–158
  active 146
Double-blinding 75, *76,* 80

E

EBSCO front-end 56, *56*
Effect modifiers 94
Effects of intervention
  critical appraisal 64–81, *76*
  electronic databases 43–51, *44*
  PICO (mnemonic) 11–12
  practice relevance 99–122
  research 11, 15–26
  size, estimating 101–103, *106*
  smallest worthwhile 102–103,
     106
Electronic databases 39–60
  browsing *59,* 60
  clinical guidelines 137–138
  diagnostic tests 51–55
  effects of intervention 43–51, *44*
  experiences 55–58
  full text 58–59
  prognosis 51–55
  search strategies 39–43
Electrotherapy 96
Embase database *52,* 55
  clinical guidelines 137
  prognosis 51–52
  randomized trials 78, 79
Empirical approach 162–163
Encainide 98
Ethical issues 21, *22*
  data collection 83
EuroQol 97
Evaluation *see* Assessment
*Evidence-Based Healthcare: A Practical
     Guide for Therapists* (Bury &
     Mead) 5
Evidence-Based Medicine (journal)
     60, 121
Evidence-Based Nursing (journal) 60
Evidence-based physiotherapy 1–7
  continuous quality improvement
     159
  defined 1–4
  history 5
  implementation 149–150,
     154–158, *154, 156, 157,
     158*
  importance 4–5
  steps for practising 5–6, 150,
     152–153, 154, 167, *167*
Experiences
  critical appraisal 81–84, *84*
  electronic databases 55–58
  questions 12

research, types of 26–30
studies, practice relevance 122–124
Explanatory approach 73, 76
Extinction, stage 7 new therapies 144

F

Factorial trials 21–22
Findings
diagnostic tests, studies 128–132
effects of intervention, systematic
reviews 115–122
experience, studies 122–124
prognosis, studies 125–127
randomized trials 99–114
Flecainide 98
Follow-up see Loss to follow-up
Forest plots 119, 121
Funders, evidence-based practice,
importance 4–5

G

Grading of Recommendations
Assessment, Development and
Evaluation (GRADE) Working
Group 117, 137, 140–141
Green's precede-proceed model 151
Guidelines see Clinical guidelines
Guidelines International Network
(G-I-N) 138
Guyatt, Gordon 5

H

Hand Movement Scale, 6 point 125
Health Technology Assessment
Database (HTA) 48–51
Heterogeneity 119–120
Hierarchy of evidence 140
High-quality clinical guidelines 138, 141
High-quality clinical research 1–4, 5,
19–23
defined 2
High-quality evidence 117
HINARI website 58

I

Inception cohort studies 84, 85–86
Indications for therapy 95
Individual studies
diagnostic tests 81, 88–89
prognosis 84–87, 87

Information
hierarchy 140
patient 4, 29
see also Clinical questions; Electronic
databases
Innovation-decision process 151
Institutional models 152
Internet see Electronic databases
Interpretive research 124
Intervention
appropriate application 96–97
groups vs control groups 65–67,
94–96
sham 71–76
see also Effects of intervention
Intuition 131

J

Journal of the American Medical
Association (JAMA) Users'
Guide 64
Journal of Physiotherapy 60, 145,
162

K

Knowledge see Practice knowledge

L

Laboratory studies, stage 1 new therapy
protocol 146
Lachman's test 130, 132
Learning theory 152
Levels of evidence 116–117, 116, 121,
140–141
Likelihood ratios 128–132
nomogram 130–131, 130
Longitudinal studies 30–31
Loss to follow-up
effects of intervention 67–71, 69
prognosis 86–87
Low-quality clinical guidelines 138
Low-quality evidence 117
very 117

M

Maastricht scale 80
McKenzie's theory of low back pain
94–95
Manual Therapy (journal) 145
Marketing approaches 152

Measurement bias 75
see also Clinical measurement
Measurement in Physical Therapy
(Rothstein) 162
Mechanisms, theories 18–19
Medical innovation see New therapies
MEDLINE database 52
clinical guidelines 137
prognosis 51–52, 53
randomized trials 78, 79
Meta-analysis 117–120, 121–122
vs systematic reviews 25, 25
Meta-regression 120
Moderate-quality evidence 117
Motivational theories 151–152
Multivariate predictive models 127

N

Narrative reviews 24
National Electronic Library for Health
58
National Guidelines Clearing House 138
National Institute for Health and
Clinical Excellence 141
National Library of Medicine 55
Natural recovery 16
Naturalistic inquiry see Qualitative
methods
New therapies 143–148
case study 145
life cycle stages 143–145
objections 146–147
protocol 145–146, 145
N-of-1 randomized trials 22–23
Non-adherence (non-compliance) 70
Number needed to treat (NNT)
108–112, 109, 111

O

Observation see Clinical observation
Odds ratio 118
Organizational theory 152
Ottawa Model of Healthcare Research
151
Ottawa Model of Research Use 151
Outcomes
continuous 100–107, 125
dichotomous 99–100, 107–114, 110,
125
self-reports 16–17
usefulness 97–99
Outpatient Service Trialists 114

P

Passive diffusion 149
Patient outcomes
  assessment 167
  measurement interpretation 162–164
Patient-physiotherapist relationship 28
Patients
  evidence-based practice,
    importance 4
  information 4, 29
  preferences, defined 2
  treatment demand 152
  see also Intervention groups
Pattern recognition 123
PEDro database 55, 167
  advanced search 46–48, *56*
  clinical guidelines 137–138
  detailed search 45, *46*
  effects of intervention 44–48, *48*
  randomized trials *44*, 63, *63*, 78, 79
  scale 64, 80
  simple search 44–46, *45*
  systematic reviews *44*, 62
  wild cards 42
Peer review 166
Performance, measuring 165–166, *167*
Physiotherapists, evidence-based
    practice, importance 4
PICO (mnemonic) 11–12
Pilot studies, stage 3 new therapy
    protocol 146
Pivot shift test 130
Placebo effect 17, 71–76
Planned change models 151
Post-test probabilities 131
Practical considerations 21, *22*
Practice knowledge 16
  defined 3
Practice relevance 93–134
  diagnostic test, studies 127–132
  evidence-based approach,
    implementation 149–150,
    154–158, *154, 156,*
    157, 158
  experience, studies 122–124
  new therapies 143–148
  prognosis, studies 124–127
  randomized trials 93–114
  specific behaviour 150, 152, 153,
    154–155
  systematic reviews, effects of
    intervention 114–122
Pragmatic approach 73, *76*

Precede-proceed model (Green) 151
Predictive models, multivariate 127
Preferences, patient 2
Probabilities
  pre-test 131, 132
  post-test 131
Process audit 163, 164–168, *167*
Professional adoption, stage 2 new
    therapies 144
Professional behaviour change 154–155,
    154
  barriers 153
  systematic reviews *156*
Professional craft knowledge 16
Professional denunciation, stage 6 new
    therapies 144
Professional interests, evidence-based
    practice, importance 4
Prognosis
  critical appraisal 84–87, *87*
  electronic databases 51–55
  individual studies 84–87, *87*
  questions 12
  research, types of 30–32
  studies, practice relevance
    124–127
  systematic reviews 87
  variables 126–127
Promising Report, stage 1 new therapies
    144
Protocol
  new therapies 145–146, *145*
  violation 70
PsycINFO database *52*, 55
  prognosis 51–52
  randomized trials 78, 79
Public acceptance, stage 3 new therapies
    144
PubMed database 55, 167
  clinical queries home page 53
  experiences 56–58, *57, 57*
  prognosis 51–52
  randomized trials 78, *78*
  wild cards 42

Q

Qualitative methods 27–29
  experiences 81–82, 83–84
  findings 122–123
  guidelines 140
  implementation barriers 152–153
  validity 122
  value 123–124

Quality
  assurance systems 166
  of evidence 140–141
  improvement, continuous 159
  intervention 121–122
  of life 97, 98
  management, total 152
Quantitative methods 27, 28, 122
Questions *see* Clinical questions; Critical
    appraisal
Quotations 123

R

Randomized clinical trials
  cluster 21–22
  diagnostic tests 34
  effects of intervention 21–22,
    65–76
  ethical/practical considerations
    21, *22*
  forest plots *119*
  N-of-1 22–23
  PEDro *44*, 63, *63*
  practice relevance 93–114, *114*
  prognosis 31–32
  quality 80–81, *81*
  stage 4 new therapy protocol 146
  stage 5 new therapies 144–145
  systematic reviews 77–81, *78, 79*
Rational system models 152
Reasoning, clinical 3–4
Recall bias 17–18, *18*
Recommendations
  critical appraisal 138–141
  development 140–141
  strength of 140–141
Reference standards 88, *90*
Refinement and Dissemination phase,
    new therapy protocol *145*,
    146
Refinement studies, stage 5 new therapy
    protocol 146
Reflective practice 166, *167*
Regional factors 3
Relative risk 118
  reduction (RRR) 108, 113
Reliability, quantitative methods 122
Research *see* Clinical research
Resources, availability 3
Risk
  absolute risk reduction (ARR) 108,
    109, 110, 111
  baseline 113–114

relative risk reduction (RRR) 108,
  113
Rogers' Diffusion of Innovation
  Theory 151

S

Sampling
  diagnostic tests 89, *90*
  representative 84–85
  strategy 82, *84*
Screening tests, research, types of 34
Search strategies
  combining terms 42–43, *43*
  electronic databases 39–43, *79*
  selecting terms 41–42
Selection bias 20
Self-reports, of outcomes 16–17
Sensitivity, diagnostic tests 128
Settings, test 128
Sham intervention 71–76
Short Form 36 (SF-36) 97, 98
Skills, test 128
Snowball sampling 82
Social cognitive theory (Bandura)
  151–152
Social marketing model 151
Social psychological theories 151–152
Social Sciences Citation Index 55
Specificity, diagnostic tests 128
Stage models of behaviour 151–152

Stakeholders 138–140
Standard Practice, stage 4 new therapies
  144
Statistical regression 16, *17*
Stratified analysis 120–121
Stress urinary incontinence 145
Strong evidence, defined 117
Sub-group analysis 95–96
Subjectivity 131
Survival curves 125–126, *126*
Systematic reviews
  vs clinical guidelines *136*
  diagnostic tests 34–35
  effects of intervention 23–25,
    114–122
  experiences 29–30
  high-quality 5
  vs meta-analyses 25, *25*
  PEDro *44*, 62
  professional behaviour change *156*
  prognosis 32, 87
  prospective 25
  randomized trials 77–81, *78*, *79*
  stage 4 new therapy protocol 146
  validity 77–80, *78*

T

Testing phase, new therapy protocol
  145, 146
Theoretical framework 123

Theory, development 28
Therapy
  indications for 95
  new *see* New therapies
  see also Effects of intervention
Thrombolytic therapy 5
'Top-down' approach 149–150
Total quality management 152
Tree plots 104, *106*

U

Ultrasound 18–19
Uncertainty
  diagnostic 89, *90*
  estimating 102–103, *110*
  living with 104–107, *107*
UpToDate 40–41

V

Validity, qualitative methods 122
Very low-quality evidence 117
Vote counting 115–116, 121

W

Wild cards 42
World wide web 40–41
  see also Electronic databases